Applied Kinesiology

Applied Kinesiology

The Scientific Study of Human Performance

Clayne R. Jensen

PROFESSOR AND ASSISTANT DEAN
COLLEGE OF PHYSICAL EDUCATION
BRIGHAM YOUNG UNIVERSITY

Gordon W. Schultz

ASSOCIATE PROFESSOR OF HEALTH EDUCATION
CENTRAL MICHIGAN UNIVERSITY

McGraw-Hill Book Company

New York   St. Louis   San Francisco   London   Sydney   Toronto
Mexico   Panama

Applied Kinesiology

Library of Congress Catalog Card Number 72-76145

32462

2 3 4 5 6 7 8 9 0   MAMM   7 6 5 4 3 2 1 0

This book is sincerely dedicated to those great athletes who have achieved excellence in performance and to the teachers and coaches who have devoted their lives to helping others achieve.

Preface

Through the ages man's struggle to achieve excellence in motor performance has been vigorous and constant. Seemingly, he has always wanted to jump higher, run faster, and demonstrate greater strength and skill. He has delighted in putting himself in contest with opponents to determine who is the superior performer. Man is by nature highly competitive and in search of excellence in performance.

Bit by bit a scientific field of knowledge relative to motor performance has been established, and the field has been divided into phases. One of the most common and useful phases of this important field is kinesiology, a subject which is now standard in the professional preparation of physical educators, athletic coaches, and physical therapists. While becoming established as a separate subject, kinesiology was associated with several divisions of the college curriculum. It has found its home in physical education and related areas, and it is now offered as a course in almost all colleges and universities in the United States.

Physical education, the area of the curriculum in which human performance receives the greatest emphasis, deals with the specific components of performance and methods of improving performance. Through this phase of education, men and women become involved with the improvement of running, jumping, throwing, and other *basic skills*. They also learn *specific skills* which demand great accuracy and precision. Physical educators are especially concerned that human performance be graceful, efficient, and effective.

Because kinesiology has become so strongly identified with this area of education, this text emphasizes the physical education approach, rather than kinesiology as it relates to occupational skills. The content of the text is especially selected and arranged to help people perform more skillfully and effectively and to give teachers, coaches, and therapists additional insight into teaching others how to perform. The book is specifically designed to serve as a college text for undergraduate students.

We believe this book follows the most logical approach to the study of kinesiology at the undergraduate level. It contains the most current and useful information available on the subject. To make the book highly readable, many useful illustrations are included, and to make it more meaningful, numerous practical examples are given. In the latter part of the book practical application is made to the basic performance patterns.

The authors express sincere appreciation to Drs. Blauer Bangerter, Julia Carver, Boyd Call, and the numerous other colleagues who have given sound advice on the book's content. Also, appreciation is expressed to our students who have worked with us in developing the text.

Clayne R. Jensen
Gordon W. Schultz

Contents

1

Introduction

Kinesiology is a term unfamiliar to most people. It is derived from the Greek *kinesis*, meaning "motion," and *logos*, meaning "word" or "knowledge." Kinesiology, then, was originally defined as the study of motion. The subject contains an organized and systematized body of knowledge, and, therefore, it is referred to as a science. Because it deals with motions involved in human performance, it is precisely defined as "the study of the science of human motion."

Kinesiology today is related to, and draws from, four commonly known fields of knowledge: anatomy, physiology, physics, and geometry. From these fields it takes only facts which relate directly to human performance. Therefore, it may be said that kinesiology is based specifically on biomechanics, musculoskeletal anatomy, and neuromuscular physiology.

The human body, which is very complex, is subject to both mechanical and biological laws and principles. How effectively and efficiently it performs is dependent upon both its mechanical and biological functions. Kinesiology emphasizes the mechanical aspects, but by necessity it also includes biological functions as they relate directly to performance. Therefore, some of the subsequent chapters deal in a special way with biological functioning, while other chapters deal with mechanics of body structure and movement.

Many performances involve more than movements of the body and its parts. They involve the manipulation of implements such as balls, bats, rackets, poles, clubs. The use we make of these implements and how we handle them influence performance. Therefore, kinesiology must also deal with factors affecting the use of implements, such as force, friction, elasticity, projections, and angles. In summary, then, kinesiology includes a study of human movement and of implements and objects used in performance. We study kinesiology to learn how to analyze

1

performance better and how to apply underlying principles to improve performance.

The foundation on which kinesiology is based is almost as old as recorded history. Aristotle, one of the greatest of ancient Greeks, is often termed the father of kinesiology, for he was the first person on record to study, teach, and write about mechanical principles relating to performance. He is credited as the one whose work on mechanics started the chain of thought that has led us to our present approach to mechanical analysis. Living more than 300 years before Christ, Aristotle demonstrated remarkable understanding of the center of gravity in man, laws of gravity and motion, and principles of leverage.

Another great Greek, Archimedes, developed the hydrostatic principles governing floating bodies in water. By means of a pulley arrangement, he launched a ship that many men were unable to move. To further emphasize the usefulness of mechanical advantage, he stated, "Give me a place to stand on and I can move the earth."

Claudius Galen (A.D. 131–201), a Roman physician for the gladiators, is considered the first athletic team physician. He had opportunity to observe and study parts of the human body laid open in mortal combat, and he developed a substantial knowledge of the human anatomy and physiology which underlie kinesiological study. Through the epics of time many other scientists have added bits of knowledge which help to form the subject we now call kinesiology.

Even though kinesiology is based on highly standardized fields of knowledge, it has remained dynamic in nature. The human in performance, one of our most complex and interesting phenomena, has attracted some of our best thinkers. These people have discovered additional knowledge of better methods of teaching, how to apply basic laws and principles to performance, and how to use new devices, such as high-speed photography, television replay, the electrogoniometer, and the electromyograph, to analyze performance more effectively. This flow of new knowledge has helped to develop kinesiology into a highly practical, useful subject. Additional development of the subject continues, stimulated by the ever-present desire of man to improve his performance.

Part 1

Muscular actions—the key to human movement

Because of man's structure he is able to accomplish a variety of performances that other forms of life cannot accomplish. But some other species can perform practically every kind of movement better than man. Man tends to be highly versatile, but not highly specialized in motor performance. Man can walk, run, hop, climb, jump, swing, throw objects, and manipulate implements. This great versatility is primarily due to the complexity and refinement of his muscular, skeletal, and nervous systems. The muscular system is the focal point in movement, while the nervous system works through the muscles by providing impules to control their contractions, and the skeletal system provides the levers against which the muscles apply force to cause bodily movement.

If we want to be able to move with greater force, we *strengthen* the muscles involved. If we want to continue movement for a longer time, we *increase the durability* of the muscles. When we desire faster movements, we attempt to *speed the rate of muscle contractions*. If we desire to perform a movement more efficiently and smoothly, we *increase the coordination* of the muscles involved. And if we desire to alter body proportions, we may *increase or decrease the size* of muscles.

The muscular system is uniquely structured to perform its specific functions well. Each muscle is shaped and sized according to its position in the body and the functions it is to serve. Each muscle attaches at exact locations on the skeletal system and is able to contract with a certain amount of speed and force to cause its assigned movements.

The eight chapters in Part 1 of the text are specifically designed to help the reader understand how the muscular system is put together, how it contributes to performance, and how its functions can be improved. Chapter 2 describes important facts about muscle tissue and how it functions. Chapter 3 explains the inter-

3

related actions of the muscular and skeletal systems in causing movement. Chapter 4 illustrates the great versatility of muscles—how they may be used in a variety of ways during performance. Chapters 5 to 7 give explanations and illustrations of the locations and the specific actions of individual muscles and muscle groups. Chapter 8 tells how to improve the effectiveness of muscle contractions in performance, and Chapter 9 is an example of how to perform a muscle analysis of a specific skill.

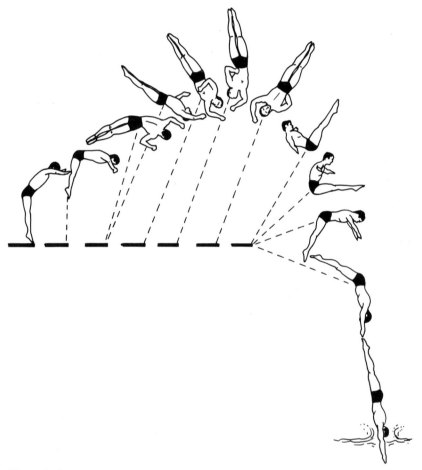

Figure 1–1.
Diver executing a forward 1½ somersault with two twists in the free position. (*After Billingsley, Hobie: "Diving Illustrated," The Ronald Press Company, New York, 1965.*)

To illustrate the complexity and the marvel of muscular actions in the human body, the following illustration is given of a forward 1½ somersault with two twists. During this dive, which is completed in about one second, well over 100 muscles contract as agonists to cause the desired movements. Many additional muscles contract to play the role of stabilizers and neutralizers. All totaled, practically every motor muscle in the body contributes in some way to this very quick and complex performance. Many of the muscles act in two or more different roles during the performance. For example, at one moment a muscle may be a prime mover, the next moment it may become antagonistic to the next desired movement, and a moment later it may play the role of stabilizer or neutralizer. All this may occur within a fraction of a second. Many other performances call for coordinations equally complex as those in this illustration.

A study of the chapters in this part will increase the reader's knowledge of exactly what is involved in a performance in terms of body movements and muscular actions. This increased knowledge will better prepare him to detect and correct errors. It will make him more able to increase coordination (skill) and strengthen specific muscles to cause improved performance.

2

The human muscular system

*M*uscle tissue, which constitutes 40 to 50 percent of the adult human body, is one of the most interesting tissues of creation. Its special characteristics are *excitability* (irritability), *contractability, extensibility,* and *elasticity.* Excitability means that it is able to receive and respond to a stimulus. Under normal conditions the stimulus is supplied by the nervous system. Contractability means that the muscle changes shape as a result of stimuli, usually becoming shorter and thicker. Extensibility means that the muscle can be stretched (extended) beyond its normal length. And, elasticity means that it readily returns to its normal length when the stretching force is eliminated.

All movements in the human body involve muscular contractions. These movements include motor actions, contractions of the heart and vessels, actions in the intestines, and many other specific movements of and within the body. The common acts of walking, picking up food, and breathing all depend directly upon muscular contractions, while such vigorous and complex performances as throwing the discus, pole vaulting, and field running in football depend on a large number of muscles and complex neuromuscular coordinations.

Three different kinds of muscle tissues are responsible for body movements. They are known as *skeletal, cardiac,* and *smooth* muscles. The different kinds of muscles have some characteristics in common, but they differ in several ways. For instance, the contractile process is the same in each, but the speed of contraction, duration of contraction, and purposes which they serve differ greatly. Each kind of muscle is especially adapted to the job it is to perform. In fact, each specific muscle of the body is especially suited in both structure and function to its particular task.

Even though cardiac and smooth muscles are essential to life, they are relatively unimportant in the study of human movement to which the actions of skeletal muscles are of prime importance because they attach to the skeletal system and cause it to move. Therefore, this chapter includes only brief points of information about cardiac and smooth muscles, but it expounds on the structure and function of skeletal muscle.

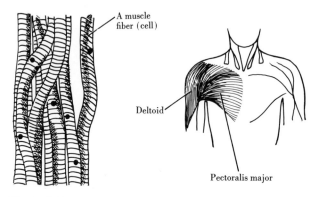

Figure 2–1.
Skeletal muscle tissue. Right diagram shows deltoid and pectoralis major muscles. Left diagram shows magnified muscle tissue. Note cross-striations of the skeletal muscle fibers. Because they are so long, only part of their length shows on a microscope slide. (*After Anthony, Catherine Parker: "Structure and Function of the Body," The C. V. Mosby Company, St. Louis, 1960.*)

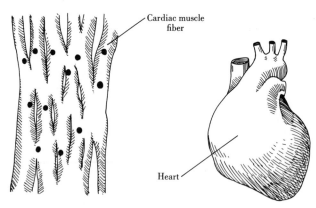

Figure 2–2.
Cardiac muscle tissue. Right diagram shows the heart, the only organ composed of cardiac muscle tissue. Left diagram shows tissue magnified by a microscope. Note how its fibers branch into each other. (*After Anthony*)

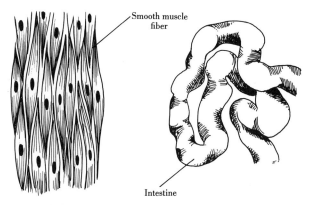

Smooth muscle
fiber

Intestine

Figure 2–3.
Visceral (smooth) muscle tissue. Right diagram shows part
of the intestine, one of the many internal organs composed
partly of smooth muscle. Left diagram shows smooth muscle
tissue magnified by a microscope. Its fibers are "smooth";
that is, they do not have cross-striations and are shorter than
skeletal muscle fibers. (*After Anthony*)

Skeletal muscle

There are more than 430 named skeletal muscles in the human body, almost all
of which appear in pairs on the right and left sides. However, most vigorous movements, as in physical education performances, are caused by less than 80 pairs of
muscles. Skeletal muscles are voluntarily controlled by nervous impulses transmitted from the central nervous system. As a result of their contractions made in
correct sequence with sufficient force, we are able to walk, run, swim, throw
objects, breathe, and perform numerous other movements.

Some muscles, such as those involved in breathing, are both voluntary and
involuntary; that is, breathing can be controlled at will to a certain extent, but
ordinarily it continues without conscious attention of the individual.

Structure of skeletal muscle

Muscles vary greatly in size, ranging in length from less than 1 inch to more
than 24 inches in adults. Also, muscles vary greatly in shape. Some are long and
slender, while others are short, chubby, round, flat, or fan-shaped. Most muscles
are *uniceps*, meaning they taper into only one tendon at each end (one-headed).
For example, the rectus femoris is a unicep muscle. A muscle is called a *biceps*
(two-headed) muscle when it is divided at one end, to form two tapering ends.

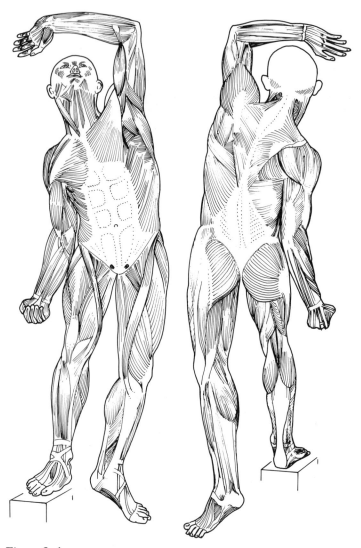

Figure 2–4.
Superficial skeletal muscles, anterior and posterior views.

The muscle in the front of the arm between the shoulder and elbow (biceps brachii) is an example of a biceps muscle. A *triceps* (three-headed) muscle is one that divides into three tapering sections at one end, such as the muscle at the back of the upper arm.

Each muscle is composed of a great number of fibers (cells). Fibers are the basic units of muscle structure. The fibers of skeletal muscles are very slender (10 to 100 microns in diameter) and vary greatly in length. Some fibers run the full length of the muscle, whereas others may run only part way through the muscle. Each fiber is enclosed by a membrane called the *sacrolemma*, a word which means skin. Immediately underneath the sacrolemma is a plasma membrane which has the capacity to transmit nerve impulses throughout the fiber. The fibers are connected by tissue which is penetrated by nerve fibers, through which nerve impulses enter the muscle fibers, and by blood vessels which carry oxygen and nutrients to the muscle fibers.

In skeletal muscles two types of fibers are present, red and white. Generally, rapid movements are performed by muscles in which white cells predominate, while slower, more sustained movements are performed by muscles in which red cells predominate.

Each fiber has cross strips (striations) at right angles to its long axis. The striations, which are visible under a powerful microscope, give the muscle the name *striated* or *striped* muscle (Figure 2–1). A single muscle fiber contains 1,000 or more long, thin parts called *myofibrils* arranged in bundles longitudinally within the fiber. The myofibrils are composed mainly of two proteins: myosin, which is especially abundant, and actin. The striations in the muscle fibers arise from variations in the density of these proteins at different places along the myofibrils. Apparently these proteins are the actual contractile elements of the muscle (**43**).

Figure 2–5a illustrates a skeletal muscle made up of many thousands of fibers, a small section of which is magnified in Figure 2–5b. The small branching structures attached to the fibers are *end plates* of a motor nerve fiber branch which conducts signals for the muscle fibers to contract. The lines circling the fibers are striations. A small section of a single fiber is enlarged in Figure 2–5c, giving a better view of the striations and illustrating the myofibrils of which the fiber is composed. In Figure 2–5d a small, greatly enlarged section of a myofibril is shown, and the striation pattern of light and dark bands is illustrated in much greater detail. Figure 2–5e illustrates a single striation and identifies its different parts, the Z lines, I bands, A band, and H zone. Figure 2–5f illustrates how the arrangement of myosin and actin filaments causes the light and dark zones in the myofibril, thereby giving the muscle fiber a striated appearance. It is rather well established that the thicker filaments are myosin molecules, while the thinner filaments are primarily actin molecules. Notice that the dark A band of the striation is caused by overlapping of myosin and actin (both filaments). The medium-colored H zone consists only of the thicker filaments (myosin), while the lighter I zone is composed of the thinner filaments (actin). Figure 2–8c shows an electromicrographic view of a skeletal muscle in which all the different parts of a striation pattern are apparent (**43**).

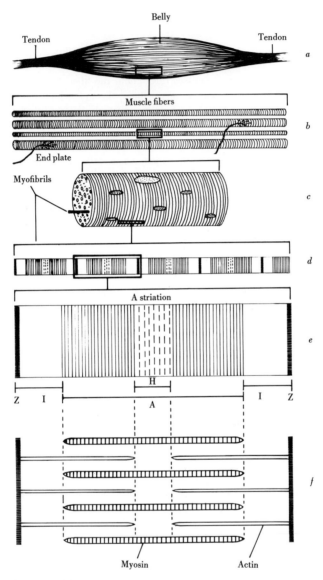

Figure 2–5.
The details of the structure of skeletal muscle. (*After Huxley, H. E.: The Contraction of Muscle, Sci. Am., vol. 199, p. 67, 1958.*)

Muscle attachments

When the muscle receives a stimulus, the belly portion contracts, exerting pull on the tendons. The tendons, in turn, pull on the bones to which they are attached, and if the pull is great enough, the bones move in the desired direction. The two attachments of a muscle are the *origin* and the *insertion*. The origin is usually at the *proximal* end of the muscle, meaning that in muscles lying vertically the origin is usually the upper attachment, and in muscles lying horizontally the origin is usually the attachment nearest the midline of the body. The origin is attached to the more stable portion of the skeleton, and the body of the muscle (belly) usually lies closer to the origin. The insertion is at the *distal* attachment, where the skeletal system is more freely movable, and the distal tendon is usually the longer of the tendons. The tendons actually grow onto the bones at locations especially shaped to accommodate the attachments.

When the muscle contracts, it does not pull mostly on the distal attachment, but rather it pulls toward the middle, exerting equal force on attachments at both ends, in an attempt to pull them toward each other. Which bone moves as a result of the force depends on the relative stability of the bones at that particular time. To a large extent, stability of a bone at a given time is determined by contractions of muscles acting as stabilizers.

Muscle contraction

All forms of animals move by contracting their muscles; therefore, muscle contraction is one of the key processes of life. A muscle has the capacity only to contract or not to contract (relax). It is said to contract when its fibers respond to a stimulus. Muscles can contract in more than one way, as demonstrated later in this chapter, and they may contract with varying degrees of force. Following is an explanation of how muscles contract.

The fibers of a skeletal muscle are organized into motor units, each consisting of approximately 150 muscle fibers (this number varies greatly in different muscles). A motor unit is all the muscle fibers served by a single motor nerve fiber. A motor nerve fiber originates at the central nervous system and enters the skeletal muscle which it serves. Near its end, the nerve fiber separates into many branches, and each branch attaches to a muscle fiber. When the nerve fiber transmits impulses, the impulses pass through the branches of the fiber and go to all the muscle cells served by that fiber. All the active muscle fibers (those capable of responding to the stimulus) within the motor unit then respond in unison. It is important to note that muscle fibers in a motor unit are not grouped together but are dispersed throughout the muscle. Therefore, if a single motor unit were stimulated, it would appear that the total muscle contracted very mildly. If additional motor units were stimulated, the muscle would contract with greater force.

Those muscles which control very fine movements and which contract rapidly usually have only a few muscle fibers in each motor unit, meaning that the ratio

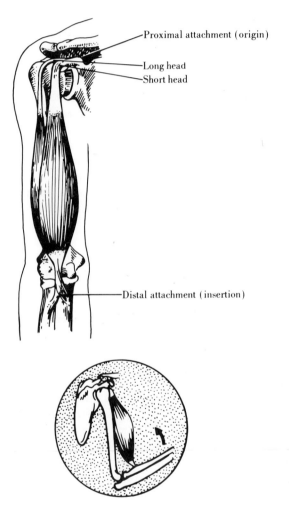

Figure 2–6.
Attachments of the biceps brachii muscle, and the action it causes when it contracts.

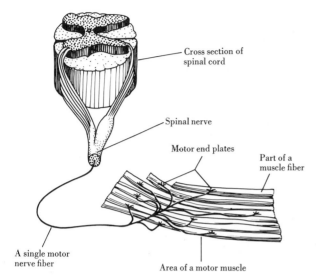

Cross section of
spinal cord

Spinal nerve

Motor end plates

Part of a
muscle fiber

A single motor
nerve fiber

Area of a motor muscle

Figure 2–7.
Motor unit. A typical motor unit includes many more
muscle fibers than appear here.

of nerve fibers to muscle fibers is very high. For instance, muscles which control
eye movements have no more than 10 to 25 muscle fibers in each motor unit, while
slower-contracting muscles which cause less refined movements, such as the soleus
muscle, may have more than 500 muscle fibers in a motor unit.

When the central nervous system provides a stimulus to a particular motor nerve
fiber, the fiber either responds or fails to respond, depending on whether the
stimulus is strong enough to exceed the threshold of the fiber. If the threshold is
exceeded, impulses are transmitted through the fiber to all the muscle fibers
which it serves (motor unit).

When the impulses reach the nerve ending (neuromyal junction), calcium ions
flow in rapidly, creating an electric potential called the *end plate potential*. This
excites the entire muscle fiber and causes it to contract. The contraction actually
results from interaction between the layers of myosin and actin filaments, which
causes the actin filaments to be pulled inward among the myosin filaments, thus
shortening the muscle (Figure 2–8). The exact details of the cause of this interaction between myosin and actin remain unknown.

Once the calcium ions have been released into the interior of the muscle fiber,
the contraction will continue until they are removed. Fortunately, within the
muscle fiber is a substance called *relaxing factor* which has a natural affinity for

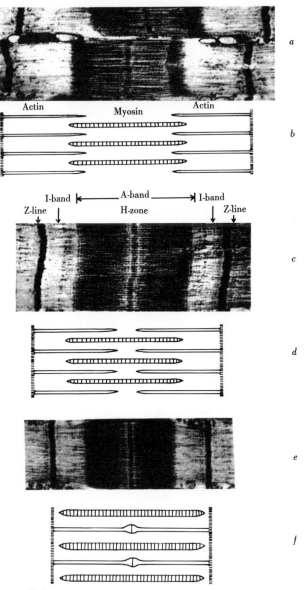

Figure 2–8.
Electron micrographic views of myofibrils of skeletal muscle. In (*a*) the muscle is stretched. In (*c*) it is in normal extended position. (*e*) represents partial contraction. (*b*), (*d*), and (*f*) illustrate the relative positions of myosin and actin filaments when the muscle moves from stretch to normal extended length, then to partial contraction. (*After Huxley*)

calcium ions and combines with them within a few hundredths of a second; this action neutralizes the calcium and causes the muscle fiber to relax.

In short, the nerve impulses cause a pulsation of calcium ions inside the muscle fibers. The calcium concentration goes up very rapidly, causing the fibers to contract, and then it falls to zero within a few hundredths of a second. This total process, including the initiation of the stimulus, transmission of the impulses, contraction of the muscle fibers, and relaxation of the fibers, may occur within a small fraction of a second.

The all-or-none law.   The all-or-none law applies to contraction of skeletal muscle fibers in exactly the same way it applies to transmission of impulses over a nerve fiber. That is, once the fiber has become excited (received an impulse), an action potential spreads along its membrane, and the entire fiber responds. A muscle fiber cannot be partially excited; either it does not become excited at all, or it becomes excited in its entirety. The all-or-none law does not imply that the strength of contraction is the same each time the fiber contracts. Sometimes, the contractile elements of the fiber are weaker than at other times. Because of fatigue, lack of nutrients, or other causes, the entire fiber responds with different amounts of force at different times. In essence, then, the all-or-none law means that when a muscle fiber is excited, the entire fiber contracts to the full extent of its *immediate ability to contract*.

Force of contraction.   In different performances it is important that a particular muscle be able to contract with different degrees of force. This is controlled by two variables. The first variable is the *number of motor units* contracting at once. When a weak contraction is desired, only a few units contract; when a maximum contraction is desired, an attempt is made to contract simultaneously as many motor units as possible. All gradients of muscle contractions between minimal and maximal can be attained by varying the number of contracting motor units, as illustrated in Figure 2–9, which shows the force of various numbers of motor units contracting simultaneously.

The second variable influencing force of contraction is the *summation wave*. Summation waves occur when a wave of successive impulses is sent to the muscle fibers, causing the fibers to contract many times in rapid succession. If the impulses are close enough, each new contraction will occur before the previous one is over. Therefore, each succeeding contraction adds to the force of the previous one. Figure 2–10 illustrates the buildup of the contractile force as the rate of impulses per second increases. In the case of large skeletal muscles, when the rate of impulses reaches about 35 per second, the muscle tetanizes, meaning that the responses to individual impulses are no longer detectable, and the contraction becomes smooth and continuous. Maximum contractile force occurs at about 50 impulses per second in large skeletal muscles. However, in smaller muscles which cause highly precise and rapid movements, such as those of the eye, maximum contraction comes at 400 to 600 impulses per second.

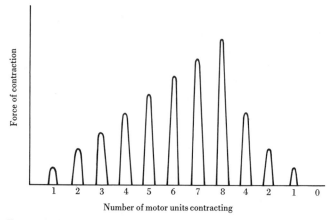

Figure 2–9.
Multiple motor unit summation illustrating the progressive in-
crease in contractile force caused by increasing numbers of mo-
tor units contracting simultaneously. (*After Guyton, Arthur C.:
"Function of the Human Body," 2d ed., W. B. Saunders Co.,
Philadelphia, 1965.*)

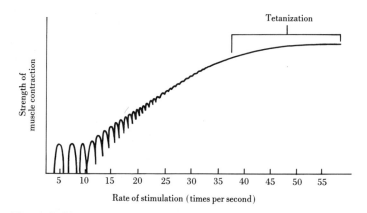

Figure 2–10.
Wave summation, showing progressive summation of successive contractions as the rate of stimulation is increased. Tetanization occurs
when the rate of stimulation reaches approximately 35 per second,
and maximum force of contraction occurs at approximately 50 per
second for large skeletal muscles. (*After Guyton*)

Types of muscle contractions

The term *contraction* means that a muscle responds to a stimulus. When a
muscle responds, tension, which may cause shortening, develops. Following are
different ways a muscle can contract.

Concentric contraction.   When a stimulated muscle develops tension sufficient to move a body segment, the muscle shortens and the body segment moves.
The muscle is then said to have contracted concentrically (see Figure 2–6). For
example, in a pull-up, the biceps brachii (and other muscles) contract, causing
the elbow to bend, thus drawing the shoulder close to the hand. In vigorous motor
movements, such as in athletics, most of the apparent contractions are concentric,
but many of the less apparent constructions are either eccentric or static in nature.
Eccentric contraction.   A muscle contracts eccentrically when it responds to
a stimulus and applies tension which is overcome by the external resistance, thus
causing the muscle to lengthen instead of shorten. Eccentric contraction is demonstrated by moving slowly from a standing to a squatting position. To allow this
movement, the leg extensor muscles must lengthen while their contractions tend to
oppose lengthening. In other words, these muscles apply tension which is less
than the force of gravity pulling the body downward. However, the tension is
sufficient to control the speed at which the body lowers. Eccentric contraction is
also demonstrated in the actions of the biceps when the body is lowered from a
pull-up position, and in the actions of the triceps in lowering the body from the
push-up position.

In all eccentric contractions, the movement is directly opposite the action ordinarily assigned to the muscle. In lowering from the pull-up, the movement is elbow
extension, but the active muscles are the elbow flexors. Eccentric contractions are
common in wrestling and football, where force applied by the opponent often
causes muscles to lengthen while in contraction, and in gymnastics, where the
body, in arm-supported positions, is often lowered slowly. When the body lands, or
when a heavy object is received, the muscles contract eccentrically to absorb the
shock of the force. It should be noted that the lengthening of a muscle in a relaxed
condition (no tension) due to contraction of opposite muscles is not considered
eccentric contraction.

Isotonic (dynamic or phasic) contraction.   Both concentric and eccentric
contractions are isotonic in nature, meaning the body segment moves as the muscle
shortens or lengthens. All motor movements involve isotonic contractions.

Isometric (static or tonic) contraction.   A muscle contracts isometrically
when it attempts to shorten (applies tension) but does not overcome the resistance; therefore, shortening of the muscle and movement of the body segment fail
to occur. Isometric contraction occurs when a person pushes or pulls against an
immovable object, or when the muscular tension equals the opposing force. Such
contractions are used frequently in stabilizing the body or portions of the body.

Important qualities of skeletal muscles

If skeletal muscles are to perform their functions effectively, they must possess
certain qualities in sufficient amounts. Most important are the abilities to (1) con-

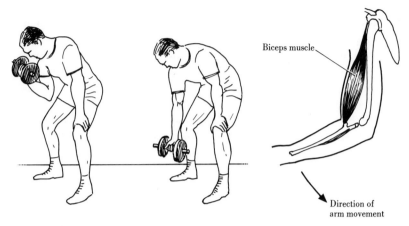

Figure 2–11.
Muscles contracting eccentrically as weight is lowered. The elbow extends, but the elbow flexor muscles contract (eccentrically) to control the rate of extension.

tract forcefully, (2) contract rapidly, (3) endure repeated contractions, and (4) remain in good tone.

Contractile force.   Every muscle, unless totally paralyzed, has ability to contract with some force (tension). This ability varies greatly among the different muscles of the body and in the same muscles of different individuals. This quality changes considerably in a particular muscle at different times, depending on the state of conditioning. The force with which a muscle can contract is related to and influenced by the following:

Size (cross-sectional measurement) of the muscle. The ability of a muscle to contract forcefully varies approximately in proportion to its cross-sectional measurement. That is, if a muscle develops until its cross-sectional area doubles, its strength will approximately double. Increased muscle size results primarily from increased size of individual fibers, but the number of fibers remains constant. An increase in muscle size results from either (1) normal growth during the formative years, or (2) consistent and systematic overloading of the muscle (contracting it against greater resistance than it is accustomed).

Proportion of active fibers. Only a portion of the fibers in a muscle is capable of contraction, and this portion increases as the condition of the muscle improves. As a result of training, inactive (dormant) fibers are reactivated. As they are reactivated, they increase in size, as do the active fibers, and thus contribute to the increased size of the total muscle. If the percentage of active fibers in a muscle can be increased by about 10 percent, then obviously the contractile force of the muscle will increase.

Strength of stimulus. To contract with maximum force, a muscle must receive a stimulus to all available motor units simultaneously, and the stimulus must produce a summation wave of impulses sufficient to effect maximum contraction of the muscle fibers.

Speed of contraction. Certain muscles are able to contract with much greater speed than other muscles because they are designed to perform functions requiring fast contractions. Similarly, muscles in different individuals vary in their ability to contract rapidly. Speed of contraction against resistance can be increased slightly by training techniques which emphasize fast contractions. Such training increases the efficiency of the total contractile process. Maximum power (as required in putting the shot) results from the best combination of speed of contraction and application of force.

Endurance of muscles. Every muscle is able to contract repeatedly against a given resistance; in other words, it has a certain ability to resist fatigue. Endurance of a muscle is influenced primarily by (1) contractile force (strength) of the muscle, (2) efficiency of the circulorespiratory functioning (most important is internal respiration), and (3) ability of the nervous system to continue to provide sufficiently strong stimuli. To illustrate:

1. If muscles of varying strengths were called upon to contract against an equal resistance, the weaker muscles would have to contract near maximum, while the stronger muscles could repeat the action considerably more times than the weaker muscles before being overcome by fatigue.

2. Circulorespiratory functioning directly influences a muscle's ability to endure because the muscle fibers depend on the circulorespiratory system to keep them supplied with oxygen and nutrients and to clear them of waste products which contribute to fatigue. If circulorespiratory functioning is insufficient, muscle fatigue occurs.

3. Muscle fibers contract only when they receive a stimulus. When partial failure occurs in the transmission of impulses to muscle fibers, those fibers fail to contract, resulting in a weaker total muscle contraction. In such a case, the point of fatigue is in the nervous system, but the result is a weaker muscle contraction, and it appears as though muscle fatigue has occurred.

Muscle tone. Tone is the quality which gives firmness and proper shape to muscles. Skeletal muscles have a certain amount of tone, depending on their state of conditioning. Well-conditioned muscles possess good tone, while poorly conditioned muscles are poorly toned.

Cardiac (heart) muscle

Cardiac muscle (Figure 2–2) forms the walls and partitions of the heart. Like all other muscle tissue, it is composed of thousands of fibers (cells). The most striking characteristics of its fibers are (1) they are involuntary, meaning we cannot voluntarily prevent them from contracting or cause them to contract; (2) they are striated, similar to skeletal muscle (see Figure 2–1); and (3) the fibers are arranged in syncytia, meaning they appear to be interconnected with each other. Recent discoveries have shown that the fibers are actually separate in structure but function as syncytia.

The heart is composed of two syncytia, one forming the wall and septum of the atria and the other forming the wall and septum of the ventricles. When one of the syncytia receives an impulse, all the fibers in that syncytium become stimulated. In other words, the whole syncytium contracts as a single unit, meaning that the all-or-none law of muscle contraction applies to the syncytium as a whole.

Physiologically, cardiac muscle differs from skeletal muscle in two ways: (1) Skeletal muscle normally contracts only when stimulated by nerve impulses, whereas cardiac muscle contracts consistently and rhythmically without receiving impulses from the nervous system. The cardiac contraction is caused by a stimulus which originates within the cardiac muscle. Among adults this occurs about once every $\frac{8}{10}$ second (72 times per minute) under conditions of rest or very moderate activity and is hastened with increased exercise or emotional excitement. (2) Another striking difference between cardiac and skeletal muscles is the rate of depolarization (time required for relaxation) following contraction. Cardiac muscle remains depolarized for about $\frac{3}{10}$ second, while the depolarization period of skeletal muscle is about $\frac{1}{500}$ second. This simply means that cardiac muscle remains contracted for about $\frac{3}{10}$ second each time it contracts under normal conditions; apparently this prolonged contraction is necessary for the heart to force blood from its chambers.

Smooth (visceral) muscle

Smooth muscle is located in the walls of the internal (visceral) organs other than the heart, such as the blood vessels, intestines, alimentary tract, and stomach. Like cardiac muscle, it contracts involuntarily. It is under the control of the involuntary portion of the nervous system, known as the autonomic system. Smooth muscle is characterized by smooth-appearing (nonstriated) muscle cells which are slender and tapered toward both ends (Figure 2–3). The cells are much smaller ($\frac{1}{100}$ to $\frac{1}{500}$ inch in length) than those found in most skeletal muscles. Even though smooth muscle is found in almost every internal organ, its specific characteristics and functions vary from one organ to another; for example: (1) smooth muscle around the pupil of the eye is a different type than that in the walls of the stomach and performs quite a different function; (2) contraction of smooth muscle which lines the hollow organs causes the organs to empty, as in the case of the intestinal tract, where waves of contractions push the inner content onward; (3) if additional contraction occurs in the smooth muscle of the blood vessels, circulation is impeded and blood pressure rises.

Compared with skeletal muscle, smooth muscle possesses (1) greater extensibility, (2) greater sensitivity to temperature and chemical stimuli, (3) greater ability for sustained contraction, and (4) more sluggishness in its movements.

Recommended supplementary reading

deVRIES, HERBERT A.: "Physiology of Exercise for Physical Education and Athletics," chaps. 1 and 2, William C. Brown Co., Dubuque, Iowa, 1966.

GUYTON, ARTHUR C.: "Function of the Human Body," 2d ed., chap. 21, W. B. Saunders Company, Philadelphia, 1965.

HUXLEY, H. E.: The Contraction of Muscle, reprinted from *Sci. Am.*, November, 1958.

RASCH, PHILLIP J., and ROGER K. BURKE: "Kinesiology and Applied Anatomy," 3d ed., chaps. 3 and 4, Lea and Febiger, Philadelphia, 1967.

3

Musculoskeletal action

*I*t would be impossible for skeletal muscles to perform their functions without the assistance of the skeletal system, for this system provides levers to which the muscles apply force and provides joints (fulcrums) around which movements occur. Amazing versatility is displayed in the human skeleton. It is a complex network composed of several types of bones, joints, and connective tissues, designed to serve several purposes. The skeletal system is another marvel of the human structure, and students of kinesiology must visualize its role clearly to understand human performance.

The skeletal system is composed of 206 named bones and more than 200 joints (articulations) between bones. Most of the bones and joints appear in pairs, with one on the right side and one on the left side of the body. When the skeleton is classified into major divisions, the number of bones in each division is cranium 8, face 14, ear 6, hyoid 1, spine 26, sternum and ribs 25, upper extremities 64, and lower extremities 62.

Functions of the skeleton

The skeletal system serves five important functions: (1) to give form and structure to the body, (2) to protect internal organs, (3) to produce blood cells, (4) to store calcium and phosphorus, and (5) to serve as levers and joints in body movements. Visualize what the body would be like without this system. It would have no definite shape and could not stand upright; vital organs would be almost totally unprotected, and motor movements would be impossible.

Of the skeletal system's five important functions, the last one mentioned, *to serve as levers and joints in movement,* is of greatest concern in the study of perfor-

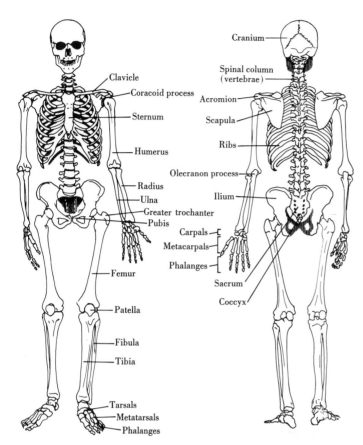

Figure 3–1.
Front and back views of the human skeletal system.

mance. Almost every bone attaches to another bone to form a joint, and in motor movements the joint serves as an axis (fulcrum) and the bones serve as levers. All skeletal muscles attach to bones or to connective tissue, which in turn attaches to bones; therefore, when muscles contract (apply force), the lever (bone) moves around the fulcrum (joint), provided the muscular force is great enough to overcome the resistance applied to the lever.

Bones of the body

No two bones on the same side of the body are shaped alike; each bone is uniquely shaped to best perform its special functions. The femur (thigh bone),

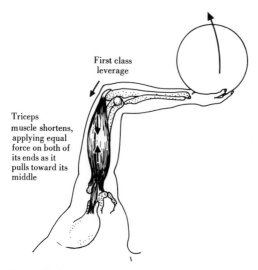

First class
leverage

Triceps
muscle shortens,
applying equal
force on both of
its ends as it
pulls toward its
middle

Figure 3–2.
The movement of a body lever as a result of
muscular force.

for example, is especially designed to withstand the great stress produced by the
body in vigorous performances and to serve as a lever against which the strong
muscles about the thigh exert tremendous force. Also, the femur is precisely
designed on the upper end to form part of the hip (ball-and-socket) joint and on
the lower end to form part of the knee joint. It has bumps and plateaus especially
designed for the attachment of specific tendons, ligaments, and fleshy tissue. If
the femur, or any other bone, deviated only slightly from its present form, it would
not effectively serve its purposes. There are many different sizes and shapes of
bones, and they are classified as *long, short, flat,* and *irregular.* Several of each
type can be readily identified in Figure 3–1.

Long bones

Long bones consist of slender shafts composed of compact tissue with hollowed
interiors. They are usually thicker toward both ends where tendons and fascia
sheets attach, and thinner toward the middle. The two ends of a long bone are
especially shaped to form portions of the joints which they help to compose. The
proximal end is usually the head, and the distal end is the foot of the bone.
Typically, both ends display protrusions called *tuberosities* which are located to
serve as attachments for ligaments and tendons. The two extreme ends are uniquely
designed to articulate with other bones to form joints. The shaft of the bone is

hollowed and filled with marrow, and the hollow is surrounded by compact bone. The thickness of the compact bone layer varies to accommodate the amount of stress applied to the bone at any particular point. The bones seem to be designed to conserve weight (tubular and hollow) and still withstand heavy stress. Long bones are found in the arms and legs. Examples are the femur, radius, and humerus bones (Figure 3–1). Long bones are designed for sweeping-type movements of great speed and long range, and their muscle attachments are usually located to enhance speed of movement.

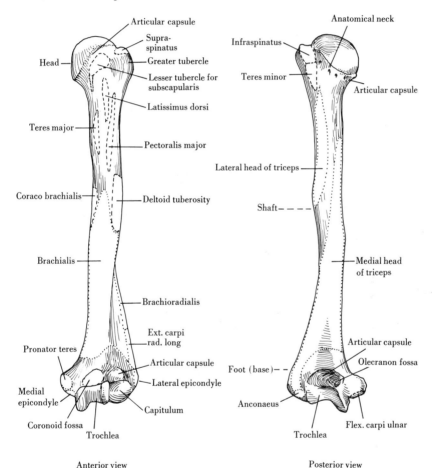

Anterior view   Posterior view

Figure 3–3.
Parts of a long bone (the left humerus) with positions of muscle attachments indicated. (*After Goss, C. M.: "Gray's Anatomy," 27th ed., Lea and Febiger, Philadelphia, 1959.*)

Short bones

Short bones are the carpals (16), the tarsals (14), and the patellae (2). These bones are composed of spongy-type tissue with a thin, hard surface. Their shapes tend toward roundness as opposed to flat, irregular, or shaftlike structures. Even though they contribute significantly to movement, their role in movement is much less dramatic than that of long bones.

Flat bones

Flat bones are those with broad and smooth surfaces, such as the bones of the cranium. They are composed of two thin layers of hard surface tissue, with variable amounts of spongy tissue enclosed between the layers. Except for the scapulae and pelvis, flat bones serve little purpose in movement. They exist primarily in the skull and face, and their main function is to protect vital organs.

Irregular bones

All bones that do not fit into one of the above three categories are classified as irregular. Examples of irregular bones are vertebrae, ear bones, and bones of the face. Vertebrae form the spinal column, and they are among the most used bones in body movements. Practically every vigorous motor movement involves the spinal column.

Joint actions

A *joint*, which is one of the most specialized and perfectly formed structures in the body, is a point in the skeletal system where two or more bones meet (articulate). The bones are usually attached to each other by connective tissue. Practically all bones have articulating surfaces which form joints, so that various body movements may be accomplished. Joints vary considerably in the amount of movement they allow and are classified generally as *immovable, slightly movable*, and *freely movable*. Examples of each type are illustrated in Figure 3–1.

Immovable joints

An immovable joint is an articulation of two bones that have fused together. Such joints are not capable of movement, and for all practical purposes, they could as well not exist. Examples of immovable joints are those found in the cranium and face.

Slightly movable joints

These joints are not firmly fixed as are immovable joints, but the structure of bones and connective tissues in and around the joints restricts the range of motion to only a few degrees. Examples of slightly movable joints are those located in the spine. Every two vertebrae are separated by a disk which is compressible, allowing the vertebrae to be moved a very limited amount in any direction. However, the combined movements of all the joints in the spine result in extensive spinal action. Slightly movable joints are also found between the sacrum and ilia and at several places in the rib cage.

Freely movable joints

These joints have a relatively large range of movement and are of prime importance in motor performances. They are located in the upper and lower extremities. Examples of freely movable joints are the shoulder, elbow, wrist, hip, and knee joints.

Types of joint movements

Some joints permit only two movements, extension and flexion, whereas others permit several additional movements. A few joints, such as the shoulder and hip joints, allow a large number of different kinds of movements. Following are descriptions of all the movements that occur in body joints. The movements that can be performed at each joint are given in Chapters 5 to 7.

Flexion (bending). Movement of a segment of the body which causes a decrease in the angle at the joint, such as bending the arm at the elbow or the leg at the knee.

Lateral flexion. The trunk and neck can bend (flex) forward or sideways. Bending sideways is lateral flexion (left or right).

Horizontal flexion. Flexion with the segment in a horizontal position. The arm moves through horizontal flexion in throwing the discus.

Extension (straightening). Movement in the opposite direction from flexion which causes an increase in the angle at the joint, such as straightening at the elbow or at the knee.

Horizontal extension. Extension with the body segment in a horizontal position. In putting the shot the opposite arm moves through horizontal extension.

Hyperextension. Extension of a body segment to a position beyond its normal extended position, such as arching the back or extending the leg at the hip beyond its normal vertical position.

Abduction. Movement in the lateral plane away from the midline of the body, such as raising a leg or an arm sideward.

Adduction. Movement in the lateral plane toward the midline of the body, as moving the arm from a downward horizontal to vertical position alongside the body.

Circumduction. Circular or conelike movement of a body segment, such as swinging the arm in a circular movement at the shoulder joint. This type of movement is also possible in the wrist, trunk, hip, and ankle joints.

Rotation. Movement of a segment around its own longitudinal axis. A body segment may be rotated inward (medially) or outward (laterally). The scapulae may be rotated upward or downward, and the spine may rotate to the right or left.

Pronation. Rotation of the hand and forearm, resulting in a "palm-down" position.

Supination. Rotation of the hand and forearm, resulting in a "palm-up" position.

Inversion. Rotation of the foot, turning the sole inward.

Eversion. Rotation of the foot, turning the sole outward.

Dorsiflexion. Movement of the top of the foot toward the tibia; cocking the foot at the ankle.

Plantar flexion (extension). Movement of the top of the foot away from the tibia, as in raising onto the toes or pressing downward on the gas pedal. This movement is also referred to as ankle extension.

Adduction and abduction at the wrist are based upon the anatomical position (hands at sides with palms forward) and are confusing because movements are rarely made from that position. More convenient terms are *radial flexion* (bending toward the thumb side—actually abduction) and *ulnar flexion* (bending toward the little finger—actually adduction).

Joint structure

The structure of each joint is best for the functions of that joint. The structure determines the actions and range of motion of which the joint is capable. The structure of an immovable joint amounts to two bones fused together with a thin layer of fibrous tissue between them, such as the joints in the cranium.

Slightly movable joints are of two types: ligamentous and cartilaginous. A ligamentous type is two bones bound together by ligaments, in such way that only a meager amount of movement results, and no disk is present within the joint. An example is the mid-radioulnar joint near the wrist. A cartilaginous joint is two bones bound together by ligaments and separated by a cartilage-type disk, such as the joints of the spinal column. In this type of joint, movement results from compression of the disk.

Freely movable joints are especially structured to allow for great sweeping and rapid motor movements. In these joints the articulating surfaces are covered with a layer of cartilage known as articular cartilage (Figure 3–4a) which prevents direct wearing on the bones and helps to absorb shocks. The bones are bound together by ligaments, and a ligamentous sleeve (capsular ligament) completely encloses the joint and attaches firmly all the way around both bones of the joint (Figure 3–4c). The interior of this sleeve-type ligament is lined with a membrane

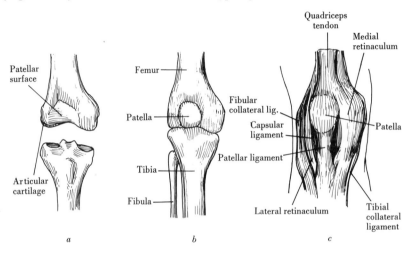

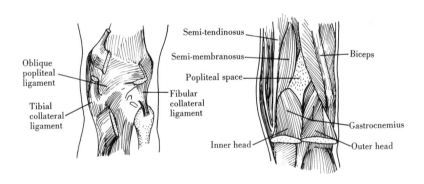

Figure 3–4.
Structure of a freely movable joint (the knee joint). (*a*) The joint spread apart, showing the articulating surfaces. (*b*) Bone structure of joint. (*c*) Front view showing ligaments. (*d*) Back view showing ligaments. (*e*) Back view of muscles and tendons which cross over the joint and add support to it.

which secretes fluid into the interior of the joint to keep it lubricated. In most freely movable joints several additional ligaments assist the capsular ligament in binding the two bones together (Figures 3–4c and 3–4d).

Muscles or their tendons extend across most movable joints (Figure 3–4e) and assist the ligaments by holding the joints closed and preventing them from dislocating. Added muscular strength and tone will strengthen joints, because stronger muscles hold the joints more tightly intact. Muscles (and tendons) are responsible for withstanding much of the force of gravity, which tends to separate or dislocate the joints.

Freely movable joints are of six different structural types, each especially designed to accommodate the movements of the particular segment of the body. See Figure 3–1.

Gliding joints

Gliding joints permit only gliding movements, as the joints between the carpal bones of the wrist or between the tarsal bones of the ankle. The gliding surfaces of these bones are nearly flat, or one may be slightly concave and the other slightly convex. During movement the surfaces simply slide across each other.

Hinge joints

These joints are similar to a door swinging on its hinges. Examples of this type are the elbow and the first and second joints of the phalanges. Hinge joints allow movement in only one plane; in other words, they allow only flexion and extension.

Condyloid joints

This type of joint is characterized by an oval-shaped head (condyle) of bone fitted into a shallow cavity, such as the joints between the metacarpals and phalanges (except the thumb). Movements permitted in these joints are extension, flexion, abduction, adduction, and circumduction. The movements are through two planes. Condyloid joints are similar to ball-and-socket joints, except they are shallower, and the muscle arrangements around them do not usually allow rotation.

Saddle joints

These joints function very much like condyloid joints, but their structure is different. From one angle the articular surfaces appear convex, and from the opposite angle they appear concave. This type of joint consists of two saddlelike structures fitted into each other. The movements in saddle joints are the same as in condyloid joints. The carpal-metacarpal joint of the thumb is an example of the saddle type.

Pivot joints

Pivot joints allow only one type of movement—rotation around the longitudinal axes of the bones involved. The articulating surfaces in this type of joint consist of a ring-shaped bony structure rotating around a pivotlike process. An example of a pivot joint is the proximal articulation of the radius and ulna immediately below the elbow.

Ball-and-socket joints

Characterized by a ball-shaped bone inserted into a concave socket, these joints afford a greater variety of movements and a larger range of movement than any other type of joint. They permit angular movement in all directions in addition to rotary movements. Examples of ball-and-socket joints are the shoulder and hip joints.

Range of motion

Range of motion is the amount of movement through a particular plane that can occur in a joint. It is expressed in degrees. Range of motion in any joint is dependent upon three factors: (1) bone structure of the joint itself; (2) amount of bulk (muscle and other tissue) near the joint, which may restrict movement; and (3) elasticity of the muscles, tendons, and ligaments around the joint. The following examples illustrate how each factor may restrict range of motion.

Example A: The range of motion in the elbow joint is restricted by the bony structure which allows the arm to extend no farther than the straight position. It can bend, then straighten, but because of the joint structure, it cannot bend in the opposite direction. Due to its bone structure, the thoracic spine can do little more than rotate, and most spinal rotation is from that portion of the spine. In contrast, the lumbar spine provides considerable flexion, extension, hyperextension, and lateral flexion, though hardly any rotation. Meanwhile, the cervical spine (neck) is capable of all these movements. *Example B:* As the biceps of the arm increases in size, extreme flexion at the elbow is restricted. If the biceps becomes excessively large, then range of motion at the elbow may be reduced considerably. *Example C:* A person may be unable to bend over and touch his toes with his hands while his knees are straight, because the muscles and connective tissues of the lower back and upper legs are not elastic (flexible) enough to allow this much movement. In such a case, inadequate elasticity of muscles and connective tissues restricts range of motion.

Inadequate range of motion in certain joints may restrict one's ability to perform. Often range of motion can be increased by regular exercises which stretch muscles and connective tissues in opposition to the particular movement. Inflexibility acts as a resistance or a "brake" to both speed and strength of movement. Continual overcoming of such resistance hastens fatigue and thus reduces endurance. Also, inflexibility of muscles may contribute to injury of those muscles when they are forced to stretch beyond the customary amount. However, it is important to recognize that increased flexibility reduces joint stability, and this may contribute to joint injuries in such sports as football, soccer, and wrestling. In some instances, stability of the joint is more important than additional range of motion.

Recommended supplementary reading

EVANS, F. GAYNOR: "Stress and Strain in Bones," Charles C Thomas, Publisher, Springfield, Ill., 1957.

RASCH, PHILLIP J., and ROGER K. BURKE: "Kinesiology and Applied Anatomy," 3d ed., chap. 2, Lea and Febiger, Philadelphia, 1967.

WELLS, KATHERINE F.: "Kinesiology," 4th ed., chap. 4, W. B. Saunders Company, Philadelphia, 1966.

Student projects

A. Identify the different bones of the body (excluding the head) and indicate the type (long, short, flat, or irregular) of each bone. Treat the following bones as groups rather than list them individually: phalanges, metacarpals, carpals, ribs, vertebrae, tarsals, and metatarsals.

B. Identify the various joints of the body (excluding the head), indicate the type of joint (ball-and-socket, hinge, etc.), and name the movements of which each joint is capable. Group certain joints as the bones were grouped in A above.

4

Specific muscle uses

A muscle can only contract or relax, and under normal conditions contraction results only from a series of nerve impulses. A muscle may contract fully or partially, with maximum force or less. A muscle may contract isometrically or isotonically, singly (in rare instances) or as a member of a group. Because muscles can contract in these different ways, they have the ability to act in different roles and to change quickly from one role to another.

Roles of muscles

At any given time a particular skeletal muscle may play the role of *agonist, antagonist, stabilizer, neutralizer,* or *synergist.* It may change from one role to another instantly, and during a motor performance, a particular muscle may function in all the different roles at different times. The role of a muscle is determined by its particular function at a given time during performance.

Agonist (mover) muscles

A muscle is a mover (agonistic to the movement) when its concentric contraction contributes to the desired movement of a segment of the body. For instance, in flexion at the elbow, the biceps brachii is a mover, as are seven other muscles in this particular case. Some muscles are movers for more than one action in a particular joint, and some cause movements in more than one joint. For instance, the biceps brachii may cause elbow flexion, shoulder flexion, or lower arm supination, depending on the simultaneous actions of other muscles. If the biceps contracted singly, all three of its movements would occur simultaneously. If only one or two of the movements are desired, then the other movements may be omitted by the coordinated contractions of other muscles. When this is done, the other muscles are said to neutralize part of the functions of the biceps.

Mover muscles are classified as *prime movers* and *assistant movers*. The former is a muscle whose primary function is to cause the particular movement, and one which makes a strong contribution to that movement. The latter is a muscle which has the ability to assist in the movement but is of only secondary importance to the movement. An example is the triceps brachii, a prime mover in elbow extension but only an assistant mover in shoulder extension. In shoulder extension, the latissimus dorsi and teres major muscles are the prime movers, and when the load is heavy, the triceps muscle (and others) is called upon for assistance. There is usually more than one prime mover in a particular joint action, and there are often several assistant movers.

Antagonist muscles

A muscle is antagonistic to a movement when it must relax to allow the movement to occur. Antagonist muscles cause actions opposite those caused by the agonist muscles. The triceps brachii is antagonistic to flexion at the elbow; therefore, the triceps must relax in order to allow flexion to occur. In elbow extension the triceps becomes an agonist and the biceps an antagonist; in other words, the biceps and triceps are antagonistic to each other. Generally, extensors and flexors are antagonistic to each other, as are abductors and adductors and medial rotators and lateral rotators.

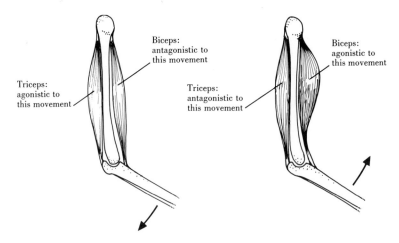

Figure 4—1.
Biceps and triceps muscles exchanging roles as the arm movement changes from extension to flexion.

Stabilizer (fixator) muscles

In order for a segment of the body to move, the body part on which the segment moves must be stable. For instance, when the arm moves at the shoulder joint, the shoulder girdle must be held firm by the contraction of specific muscles in that region. Without being stabilized, the shoulder girdle would move and thus reduce the force which the muscles of the shoulder joint could exert on the arm. The same could be said about movement of the leg around the hip joint (pelvic region must be stable) or about movement at numerous other joints. When acting as a stabilizer, a muscle usually contracts statically (isometrically) because its role is to hold the body segment motionless, or nearly motionless. Therefore, the muscle shortens very little, if any, during its contraction, and it causes very little, if any, movement. A clear example is the action of the abdominal muscles during floor push-ups. If these muscles did not contract statically, the back would bow, causing the trunk to sway so the exercise could not be performed effectively.

Neutralizer muscles

A muscle plays the role of neutralizer when it equalizes or nullifies one or more actions of another muscle. To neutralize each other, two muscles must cause opposite movements. For example, the pectoralis major and the latissimus dorsi muscles are both movers in adduction of the humerus; in addition, the pectoralis major flexes the humerus while the latissimus dorsi extends it. When the two muscles neutralize each other's functions of flexion and extension, the result is adduction. Another example occurs in the sit-up exercise where the right and left external oblique muscles combine to contribute to trunk flexion, neutralizing each other's functions in trunk lateral flexion and trunk rotation. Besides causing forward trunk flexion, the right external oblique muscle, if contracted singly, would laterally flex the trunk to the right and rotate it to the left. The left external oblique muscle would laterally flex the trunk to the left and rotate it to the right. In other words, the two muscles perform one common movement, trunk forward flexion, and two opposite movements, trunk lateral flexion left and right and trunk rotation left and right. To cooperate in forward trunk flexion, the two muscles neutralize each other's roles as lateral trunk flexors and rotators.

Occasionally, a portion of a muscle must neutralize another portion of the same muscle. An example is the contraction of the deltoid muscle to abduct the humerus. The anterior portion of the deltoid also causes horizontal flexion, while the posterior portion also causes horizontal extension. The horizontal extension and flexion movements are neutralized when pure abduction is performed. The anterior deltoid rotates the humerus inwardly, and the posterior deltoid rotates it outwardly. These rotations are also neutralized in pure abduction of the humerus.

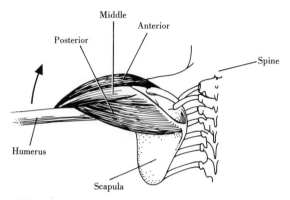

Figure 4–2.
The three portions of the deltoid muscle contract to cause shoulder abduction. Middle portion causes pure abduction, while the anterior and posterior portions neutralize the other functions of each other.

Coordinated actions of muscles

Motor muscles nearly always act in groups rather than individually; whenever a major motor movement occurs, many muscles contract and numerous coordinations take place. Those muscles which are agonistic to the movement contract concentrically and must be coordinated with each other in order to produce maximum total contractile force. Those muscles antagonistic to the movement must relax and must be coordinated with the agonist muscles, or they provide resistance to the movement. Numerous other muscles must contract to stabilize parts of the body on which the active segments move, and these muscles must be coordinated with the agonists and antagonists. Also, many other contractions are required to neutralize undesired actions of some muscles.

Visualize the tremendous number of muscular actions involved in various roles during the common, but very complex overarm pitch. Also, visualize the complex coordinations involved in the pole vault, discus throw, swimming the crawl stroke, or field running in football. It is absolutely amazing that so many muscles can be so precisely coordinated into so many different functions within a brief moment. The extent to which the necessary contractions can be effectively coordinated with each other is the prime element of what is known as *skill*. Hence, when we practice to improve skill, we attempt to perfect the coordinated contractions of the many different muscles involved.

Mechanics of muscle use

Usually the proximal end of a muscle is attached to the more stable body portion, and this causes most of the body movement to occur in the segment to which the distal end of the muscle attaches. However, it is erroneous to assume that a muscle pulls toward its proximal attachment. The pull is from both ends toward the muscle's belly (middle) along the length of its fibers. The conception that all force from a muscle is directed toward the distal attachment is misleading and untrue. For example, in Figure 4–3, the teres major is pulling equally at its two ends, but the humerus, which is the least stable of the two segments, performs most of the movement.

The amount of movement that occurs in any body segment as a result of muscle contraction is determined by the relative stability of the segment. For example, when the deltoid contracts, the arm usually moves on the shoulder girdle because the shoulder girdle is the more stable of the two segments, and other muscles contract to reduce its movement further. If the shoulder girdle were less stable than the arm, then it would move on the arm because the amount of tension applied to both segments by the deltoid is equal. Following are reasons why some segments are less movable (more stable) than others.

1. *Segment structure.* If a muscle attaches on both the scapula and the humerus (see teres major, Figure 4–3), the pull on the humeral attachment can cause free movement of the humerus at the shoulder joint (ball-and-socket joint). The pull on the scapula can only produce a movement of the scapula over the rib cage, and the scapula is not highly movable and is easily stabilized. Its movement is greatly restricted by the structure of that region of the body. Therefore, when the muscle applies equal force to the scapula and the humerus, the humerus moves the greater amount because it is freer to move.

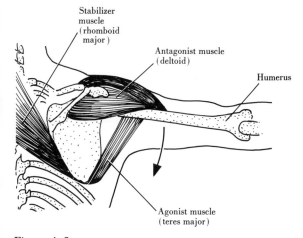

Figure 4–3.
Teamwork of three muscles in arm adduction: teres major as agonist, deltoid (middle) as antagonist, rhomboid major as stabilizer of the scapula.

2. *Stabilizing actions of muscles.* The extent to which muscles are used to stabilize a segment influences its movability. For example, the rhomboid muscle often works in connection with the teres major to stabilize the scapula. The action of the rhomboid is in direct opposition to the movement caused by the teres major on the scapula, and the two forces cancel each other, causing stability of the scapula. As a result of this, all the force of pull by the teres major can now be directed to its attachment on the humerus making this action more effective than would be possible if both segments moved with the freedom allowed by the structure of the shoulder joint.

Assume you were involved simultaneously in two tugs-of-war with two ropes, each pulling in opposite directions. You would be attempting to defeat both opponents at one time, thus dividing the force you could apply; you would then be playing a role similar to that of a muscle working alone. Now, suppose you eliminated one opponent, substituting a telephone pole for him (this would represent the stabilizing action of the rhomboid). You could now direct all of your force to overcome the remaining opponent. Under this condition you would be more successful even though you have no more force available than you had when working against two opponents.

In some instances a muscle will reverse its customary function. This means the proximal attachment becomes the movable part. For example, think of the hip flexors raising the legs in a forward and upward direction as in running. But, when we perform a sit-up, the same hip flexors pull the same way except the legs are stabilized, causing the trunk to be the movable part. If both the trunk and legs are equally free to move, the result is an exercise called the V-sit, in which both the legs and upper body leave the floor simultaneously and move toward each other.

Another essential consideration is that most muscles are single units, meaning they are not capable of contracting in portions. In other words, when they contract, they contract throughout. However, a few muscles are subdivided into parts, and any part can contract separately to cause an action which the whole muscle cannot cause. Examples of such muscles are the trapezius (Figure 5–15), which is divided into parts I, II, III, IV, and the deltoid (Figure 5–13), which has three parts, anterior, middle, and posterior. The anterior deltoid causes arm horizontal flexion while the posterior portion causes the opposite movement (horizontal extension), and the middle portion abducts the arm. If all three portions were contracted simultaneously, the arm would only abduct.

A single muscle, because of its position of attachment, may contribute to more than one movement. It is established that all a muscle can do is contract and relax; therefore, it is apparent that when a muscle contracts, it tends to cause all the movements of which it is capable. The only way any of the movements can be prevented is for another muscle to contract simultaneously and neutralize the undesired actions. For example, the serratus anterior muscle (Figure 5–16) causes abduction and upward rotation of the scapula. It is not possible for that muscle to contract to cause only abduction or only upward rotation. Therefore, when only abduction is desired, another muscle must be called upon to nullify the upward rotation action. In this case, the most logical choice is the pectoralis minor (Figure 5–16), whose function is also dual—to abduct and downward rotate the scapula. The two muscles neutralize each other's rotational actions, and they complement each other as prime movers in the one desired action, abduction of the scapula.

Types of muscle actions

A muscle contraction varies in speed, force, and duration to cause different kinds of movements, which vary in relative importance in different performances.

Maximum force movements

In maximum force movements the agonist (mover) muscles apply near-maximum force and contract at near-maximum speed, resulting in fast and forceful movement. An example is putting a shot where the resistance provided by the antagonist muscles is held to a minimum, although resistance always exists to some degree. One's ability to reduce resistance to a particular movement is one key factor in the speed of that movement. Maximum force movements may be of two types, *continuous force* and *ballistic*.

Continuous force

Continuous force movements occur when near-maximum muscle tension is applied throughout the range of the movement, as in executing a heavy weight lift or performing a pull-up. In such movements the muscles contract at nearly the same intensity all through the movement. Sometimes this type of movement demands near-maximum contraction over a relatively long time.

Ballistic movements

A ballistic movement occurs when the body or a segment is put into rapid motion by fast, but very brief, contractions of the mover muscles. After the initial tension has been applied, the remainder of the movement results from momentum of the moving parts. Examples of ballistic movements are swinging a golf club, tennis racket, or baseball bat. These are all explosive movements in which the implement is put into motion by vigorous, very brief contractions. After movement has quickly reached the desired velocity, it continues as a result of built-up momentum. When muscle contraction stops, the velocity of movement gradually reduces because of (1) internal resistance in the joints, (2) resistance of antagonist muscles, and (3) external resistance. To stop the movement at the desired time, the antagonist muscles must apply resistance through eccentric contractions.

Sometimes ballistic movements occur in repetition, such as movements of the arms during running and movements in the wrist when dribbling a ball. This calls for quick reversal of ballistic movements.

Slow tension movements

When speed and force are not of prime importance, and great steadiness and accuracy are needed, slow tension movements are used. Examples are threading a needle, slow and graceful movements in modern dance and ballet, and slow, steady, and precise gymnastic movements. In these kinds of movements the forces applied by the opposite muscle groups are almost equal to each other. If the opposite forces were equal, the body part would be stabilized and steady. As the force of one muscle group overcomes that of the opposite group, slow and steady movement occurs. The fact that all opposing muscle groups apply almost equal tension causes the body part to be highly stable and subject to quick adjustment in direction and rate of movement. One's ability to keep the forces of opposing muscles equal is the limiting factor in steadiness.

Multijoint muscle actions

As the name implies, a *multijoint* muscle is one that extends across more than one joint and contributes to movement in each joint that it crosses. Examples of such muscles are the biceps brachii, which flexes the elbow and shoulder, and the triceps brachii, which extends both the elbow and the shoulder. The hamstring group, located in the back of the thigh, flexes the knee and extends the hip, while the rectus femorus extends the knee and flexes the hip. Several muscles of the lower arm, which contribute to movement of the fingers, act upon several joints. The same is true of the muscles of the lower leg, which contribute to toe movements. Of course, numerous muscles of the back contribute to movement in a series of joints in the spinal column, but this is not a comparable situation because joints of the spine do not usually act separately. Spinal joints work in groups to cause a single movement.

An interesting characteristic of many multijoint muscles is that they do not allow complete range of motion in all joints at one time. For example, the wrist cannot be fully flexed at the same time that the fingers are fully flexed. This is partly because multijoint flexors cannot contract far enough to cause complete flexion in all of the joints simultaneously and partly because the multijoint extensors are unable to stretch far enough to allow complete flexion. To demonstrate

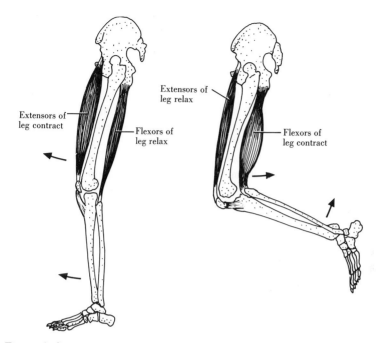

Extensors of
leg relax

Extensors of
leg contract

Flexors of
leg relax

Flexors of
leg contract

Figure 4–4.
Side view of two joint muscles with opposing action. Rectus femoris
(front of leg) extends the knee and flexes the hip; the hamstring group
(back of leg) flex the knee and extend the hip.

this characteristic, flex the wrist as far as possible while the hand is gripped
tightly, then release the grip and notice that the wrist is able to flex an additional
amount. Because the hamstring muscles cross over both the hip and knee joints,
the hip cannot be fully flexed at the same time the knee is fully extended, except
in a few individuals who have devoted much time to increasing flexibility (some
dancers and acrobats).

When a multijoint muscle contracts, it tends to perform its assigned movements
in all the joints on which it acts. For instance, if the rectus femoris contracts, it
flexes the hip and extends the knee. If only one of the actions is desired, then the
other action must be nullified (neutralized) by contractions of other muscles.
Through coordination with other muscles, a multijoint muscle can contribute to
any portion of the total movements that it is capable of causing.

Postural muscles

There are two types of posture: dynamic and static. Both kinds depend primarily
upon muscular contractions, and the muscles involved most are referred to as the

postural (or antigravity) muscles. The muscles most obviously involved in posture are the extensors of the legs, back and neck. These muscles must contract for the body to maintain any kind of erect position. The abdominal muscles contract to prevent sag of the visceral organs. Numerous other muscles are less important but also involved in posture, including the trunk and neck flexors and lateral flexors, leg abductors and adductors, and pronators and supinators of the foot. If all of the antigravity muscles were to relax, the body would collapse.

We know that a muscle contracts only when it receives a stimulus; therefore, postural muscles must receive constant stimulation to carry on their functions., Although much remains to be learned about the exact process by which these muscles are stimulated, it is currently believed that the stimulus comes from two main sources: (1) stretch reflexes, which are initiated from within the skeletal muscles, and (2) the five "righting reflexes," which consist of:

     a. Optical righting reflexes
     b. Body righting reflexes acting upon the body
     c. Body righting reflexes acting on the head
     d. Neck righting reflexes
     e. Labyrinthine righting reflexes

Whenever a body segment deviates from the desired postural position, the appropriate reflex mechanisms initiate a stimulus which causes muscle contractions necessary to correct the deviation. The classic illustration is the swaying action of a person attempting to hold a perfectly erect position. The body repeatedly moves in various directions away from perfect balance. When a certain amount of movement occurs in a given direction, the appropriate reflex mechanism is activated, and the imbalance in position is quickly corrected. This process is continuous during the standing position.

Recommended supplementary reading

RASCH, PHILLIP J., and ROGER K. BURKE: "Kinesiology and Applied Anatomy," 3d ed., pp. 44–48, 50–51, Lea and Febiger, Philadelphia, 1967.

WELLS, KATHERINE F.: "Kinesiology," 4th ed., chap. 5, W. B. Saunders Company, Philadelphia, 1966.

5

Muscular actions of the upper extremities

he upper extremities include the hands, arms, and shoulder girdles. In terms of movement these are the most versatile of the large portions of the body; they are used in the greatest variety of ways. Feature, for example, the numerous movements that occur in the upper extremities during an overhead badminton shot, a baseball pitch, or a batting action. Few performances result from the upper extremities alone. In almost all cases, their movements must be closely coordinated with and assisted by movements in the neck, trunk, and lower extremities. More than 40 pairs of skeletal muscles contribute to movement in the upper extremities, and practically all of those muscles contribute to more than one movement.

Muscular actions in the hand

Man's hand has played a significant role in his daily activities. Its ability to manipulate in a variety of ways is yet unequaled by machines. Of all the specific segments of the body, the hand is the most versatile.

The great mobility of the hand is owed to its many joints and elaborate muscular system. There are 14 joints in the hand alone and several additional joints in the wrist, which contribute directly to the usefulness of the hand. Ten muscles are located in the hand and nine additional muscles, which manipulate the fingers and thumb, are located in the forearm. These nineteen muscles work together in different combinations so that a muscle, through interaction with other muscles, may contribute to more than one movement. Several of the muscles are multijoint muscles.

All joints in the hand are capable of flexion and extension, and the third joint (the one closest to the wrist) of each finger and the second joint of the thumbs are

45

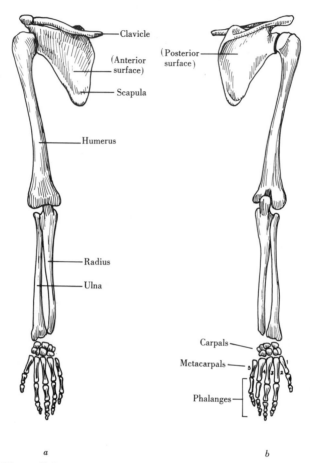

Figure 5–1.
Anterior (*a*) and posterior (*b*) views of the bone structure
of the upper extremity.

also capable of abduction, adduction, and circumduction. The hand movement of
greatest significance to performance is flexion, which results in the gripping action.

Handgrip

In sports performances, the grip is a highly significant movement, used extensively in catching, throwing, and swinging objects and in supporting the body
with the hands. In addition, the grip is very important in tennis, golf, ball games
involving batting, catching, and throwing, the javelin and discus throw, badminton, gymnastics, combatives, and many other athletic performances. Gripping

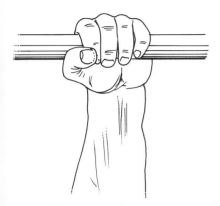

Figure 5–2.
The gripping action of the hand is
very strong and is important in many
performances.

action is important to practically all activities in which an implement is manip-
ulated with the hands.

The muscles causing the grip are listed and illustrated below. Also given is a
description of each muscle and the body movements which it causes. There are
several muscles in the hand which are not mentioned in this text, because they
contribute to hand movements not considered herein.

MUSCLE	DESCRIPTION AND ACTIONS
*Flexor digitorum profundus (Figure 5–5)	Attaches proximally on the anterior and medial surfaces of the ulna, approximately halfway up the forearm. It extends down the arm, and its tendons extend across the wrist and hand and attach at the bases of the distal phalanges of the four fingers. It flexes the distal phalanges, contributes to flexion of the other finger joints, and flexes the wrist.
*Flexor pollicis longus (Figure 5–6)	Attaches proximally at the anterior surface (middle one-third) of the radius, extends down the anterior of the arm, and attaches to the distal phalanx of the thumb. It crosses three joints and causes flexion of the thumb (both joints) and wrist.
*Flexor digitorum sublimis (Figure 5–5)	The proximal attachment is on the medial epicondyle of the humerus, the coronoid process of the ulna, and the upper portion of the radius. It extends down the anterior side of the forearm and attaches to the second phalanges of the four

MUSCLE	DESCRIPTION AND ACTIONS
	fingers. It crosses over four joints, causes flexion of the middle and proximal phalanges, and assists in flexing the wrist and elbow.
*Lumbricalis (Figure 5–3)	Proximal attachment is on the tendons of the flexor profundus muscle, located in the palm of the hand. It extends downward and attaches to the tendons of the extensor communis, which attaches to the back of the distal phalanges of the fingers. It causes flexion of the first phalanges and extension of the distal phalanges of the fingers. Also, it aids in finger abduction.
*Flexor pollicis brevis (Figure 5–3)	Proximal attachment is on the trapezium, trapezoid, and capitate bones of the wrist. It extends down the front of the thumb and attaches on the proximal phalanx of the thumb. It flexes and adducts the thumb.
Adductor pollicis (Figure 5–3)	Proximal attachment is on the second and third metacarpal bones on the palm side near the wrist. It extends down the front of the thumb and attaches to the first phalanx of the thumb on the inner surface. It crosses the two joints of the thumb, and it adducts and flexes the thumb.
Abductor digiti quinti (Figure 5–3)	Attaches proximally to the ulna side of the heel of the hand and extends downward to its distal attachment at the first phalanx of the little finger. It flexes the little finger.
Abductor pollicis brevis (Figure 5–3)	Attaches proximally to the navicular and trapezium bones of the wrist and the transverse carpal ligament. It extends downward and attaches distally to the base of the first phalanx of the thumb. It abducts and flexes the thumb.

* Throughout this chapter, this device indicates prime mover muscle.

Muscular actions in the wrist

The wrist is composed of a cluster of eight small bones with numerous joints at their points of articulation. There are six muscles of the forearm which cause movement in the wrist only. Nine additional muscles, which move the thumb and fingers, also contribute to wrist movements. The wrist, which is highly useful in athletic performance, is capable of flexion, extension, abduction (radial flexion), adduction (ulnar flexion), and circumduction.

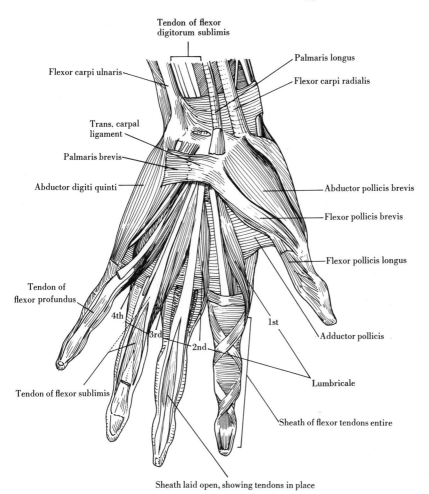

Figure 5–3.
Muscles of the palm of the left hand. (*After Goss*)

Wrist flexion

Flexion is a very strong movement and one used extensively in throwing, swinging, lifting, pushing, and pulling actions. Wrist flexion is very important in throwing objects such as a baseball or softball; striking as in badminton, squash, handball, and the tennis serve; supporting and thrusting the body as in gymnastic movements and pole vaulting; and putting actions as in the shot put. Following is information about the muscles which cause the wrist to flex.

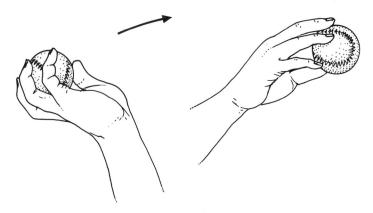

Figure 5–4.
Wrist flexion, one of the most important contributing movements in throwing.

MUSCLE	DESCRIPTION AND ACTIONS
*Flexor carpi ulnaris (Figure 5–6)	Proximal attachment of the two heads are at the medial epicondyle of the humerus and the olecranon process of the ulna. It extends down the medial side of the arm and attaches to the fifth metacarpal and the pisiform bone of the wrist. It crosses two joints, and it flexes and adducts the wrist and flexes the elbow.
*Flexor carpi radialis (Figure 5–6)	Attaches proximally on the medial epicondyle of the humerus, extends down the anterior of forearm, and attaches distally at the base of the second metacarpal bone. It crosses two joints, and it flexes and abducts the wrist and flexes the elbow.
Palmaris longus (Figure 5–6)	Attaches proximally on the medial epicondyle of the humerus, extends down the anterior of the forearm, and attaches to the carpal ligament in the palm of the hand. It crosses over two joints and contributes to flexion of the wrist and flexion of the elbow.
Flexor digitorum profundus (Figure 5–5)	See Handgrip, page 47.
Flexor digitorum sublimis (Figure 5–6)	See Handgrip, page 47.

MUSCLE	DESCRIPTION AND ACTIONS
Flexor pollicis longus (Figure 5–5)	See Handgrip, page 47.

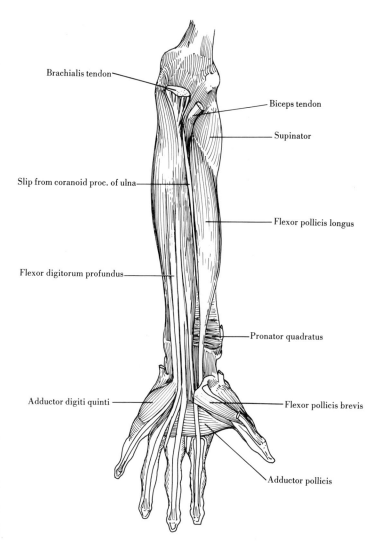

Figure 5–5.
Deep muscles of the front of the forearm. (*After Goss*)

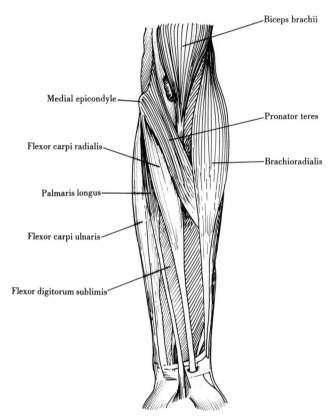

Figure 5–6.
Superficial muscles in the front of the forearm. (*After Goss*)

Wrist extension

Wrist extension is a relatively weak, but necessary movement in sports activities. When wrist extension occurs beyond the straight (180°) position, the movement is called *hyperextension*. The wrist extensor muscles are of prime importance in such performances as badminton and squash backhand shots, golf swings, and batting actions. In the tennis backhand drive and other similar performances, the wrist extensors contract to stabilize the wrist in the desired position. If the wrist is to be held in a fixed position, the extensor muscles must be strong enough to equalize a strong contraction by the opposing muscles (flexors). Following are the muscles which cause wrist extension.

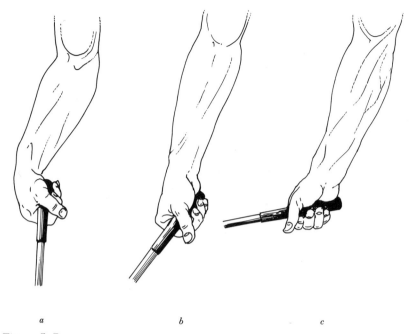

a   b   c

Figure 5–7.
Wrist extension, important in such performances as the badminton or squash backhand shot.

MUSCLE	DESCRIPTION AND ACTIONS
*Extensor carpi radialis brevis (Figure 5–9)	Proximal attachment is on the lateral epicondyl of the humerus. It lies down the posterior of the forearm and attaches on the posterior surface of the third metacarpal bone. It crosses over two joints, and it extends and abducts the wrist and extends the elbow.
*Extensor carpi radialis longus (Figure 5–9)	Attaches proximally on the lateral epicondyle of the humerus, lies down the posterior of the forearm, and attaches onto the second metacarpal of the index finger. It crosses two joints, and it extends and abducts the wrist and extends the elbow.
*Extensor carpi ulnaris (Figure 5–9)	Proximal attachment is on the lateral epicondyle of the humerus and the posterior of the ulna at the elbow joint. It lies down the back of the forearm and attaches to the fifth metacarpal. It crosses two joints, and it extends and adducts the wrist and extends the elbow.

MUSCLE	DESCRIPTION AND ACTIONS
Extensor digiti quinti (Figure 5–9)	Proximal attachment is on the tendon of the previous muscle, approximately 3 inches above the wrist, along the posterior of the forearm. It extends downward and attaches to the fifth metacarpal bone. It extends the wrist.
Extensor digitorum communis (Figure 5–9)	Attaches proximally on the lateral epicondyle of the humerus, lies down the posterior of the forearm, and attaches on to the distal phalanges of the fingers. It crosses over five joints, and it extends the fingers, the wrist, and the elbow.
Extensor indicis (Figure 5–8)	Attaches proximally on the lower posterior surface of the ulna, extends downward, and attaches distally on the second and third phalanges of the index finger. It extends the index finger and the wrist.
Extensor pollicis longus (Figure 5–8)	Proximal attachment is on the lower one-third of the ulna on the posterior surface. It extends down the back of the arm and attaches onto the base of the distal phalanx of the thumb. It crosses three joints, and it extends the thumb and the wrist.

Wrist abduction (radial flexion)

Wrist abduction is a movement of the hand toward the thumb side. It is a relatively weak, seldom-used movement. However, it is important in such skills as the back swing in golf and batting, and the cocking of the wrist for throwing the football and javelin. Also, it is a very important movement in throwing the discus. Five muscles contribute to wrist abduction.

MUSCLE	DESCRIPTION AND ACTIONS
*Flexor carpi radialis (Figure 5–6)	See Wrist Flexion, page 50.
*Extensor carpi radialis brevis (Figure 5–9)	See Wrist Extension, page 53.

MUSCLE	DESCRIPTION AND ACTIONS
Extensor carpi radialis longus (Figure 5–9)	See Wrist Extension, page 53.

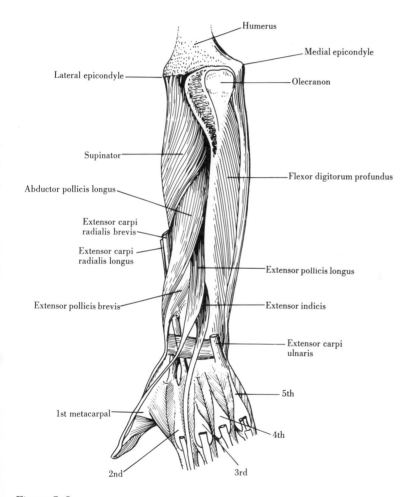

Figure 5–8.
Deep muscles of the posterior surface of the forearm (*After Goss*)

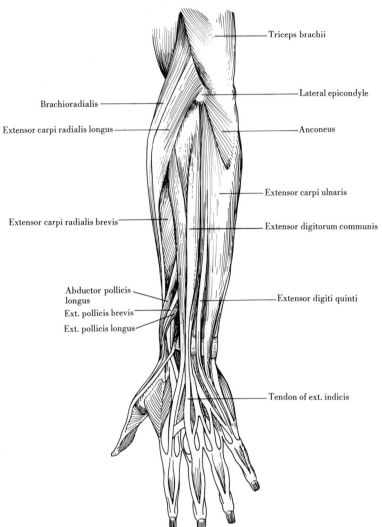

Triceps brachii

Lateral epicondyle

Brachioradialis

Extensor carpi radialis longus

Anconeus

Extensor carpi ulnaris

Extensor carpi radialis brevis

Extensor digitorum communis

Abductor pollicis
longus

Ext. pollicis brevis

Ext. pollicis longus

Extensor digiti quinti

Tendon of ext. indicis

Figure 5–9.
Superficial muscles of the posterior surface of the forearm. (*After Goss*)

MUSCLE	DESCRIPTION AND ACTIONS
Abductor pollicis longus (Figure 5–8)	Proximal attachment is on the inside of the radius and the outside of the ulna about halfway up the forearm. It lies diagonally down the front of the forearm and attaches on the radial side of the first metacarpal of the thumb. It abducts the thumb and wrist.

MUSCLE   DESCRIPTION AND ACTIONS

Extensor   Proximal attachment is on the posterior surface of the radius
pollicis   approximately 1½ inches above the wrist. It extends down
brevis   the back of the arm and attaches to the first phalanx of the
(Figure 5–8)   thumb. It extends and abducts the thumb and abducts the
                        wrist.

Wrist adduction (ulnar flexion)

Adduction of the wrist moves the hand toward the side of the small finger. It is
a short-range movement with a fair amount of application in athletics. It is used
in the lead hand in the golf swing and in batting actions and is important in the
football pass, javelin throw, and some shots in badminton, squash, volleyball, and
some hand-supported gymnastic movements. It is also used to give spin to a baseball causing it to curve. Two muscles are responsible for wrist adduction.

*Flexor   See Wrist Flexion, page 50.
carpi ulnaris
(Figure 5–6)

*Extensor   See Wrist Extension, page 53.
carpi ulnaris
(Figure 5–9)

Wrist circumduction

Circumduction is movement in a circular, cone-shaped pattern. It is simply a
sequential combination of flexion, abduction, extension, and adduction. Circumduction is caused by the muscles which contribute to the four movements which
compose it. Even though it is not a frequently used movement in sports activities,
it is used a limited amount in such performances as the sidearm throw and certain
handball shots.

Muscular actions of the lower arm

A segment rotates when it moves in a circular direction around its own longitudinal axis. Because of the ability of the radius bone to turn around the ulna,
the lower arm may be rotated either medially or laterally. These rotary movements
are frequently used. Supination is the same as lateral rotation of the lower arm,

resulting in the supine position of the hand (palm up). Pronation is the same as medial rotation, resulting in a prone position of the hand (palm down).

Lower arm lateral rotation (supination)

This movement is important in such performances as the underhand pitch, the front crawl stroke and breaststroke in swimming, the tennis backhand drive, and in throwing a curve ball. The supinator and biceps brachii muscles cause the movement.

Supinator (Figure 5–8)	Attaches proximally on the lateral epicondyle of the humerus and the radial ligament of the elbow. It extends downward to the posterior and lateral surfaces of the upper radius. It supinates the lower arm.
Biceps brachii (Figure 5–12)	This is a two-headed muscle. The proximal attachment of the long head is on the top of the scapula at the glenoid process. The short head attaches at the coracoid process of the scapula. The muscle extends down the anterior of the upper arm and attaches to the olecranon process of the ulna, just below the elbow. It crosses two joints, and it flexes the elbow and supinates (rotates laterally) the lower arm. The short head also assists in shoulder flexion and medial rotation, while the long head assists in shoulder abduction.

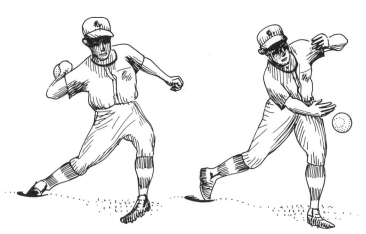

Figure 5–10.
Lateral rotation of the arm, used to good advantage in the underarm pitch.

Lower arm medial rotation (pronation)

This movement is used extensively in handling balls, such as dribbling a basketball, certain arm-supported gymnastic movements, and wrestling. It is a stronger movement than lateral rotation, and it is caused by four muscles.

*Pronator quadratus (Figure 5–5)	Attaches proximally to the lower fourth of the anterior of the ulna and extends downward to its distal attachment on the lower fourth of the radius. It pronates (medially rotates) the forearm.
*Pronator teres (Figure 5–6)	Attaches proximally to the medial epicondyle of the humerus and the coronoid process of the ulna, extends down the lateral side of the arm, and attaches onto the upper third of the radius. It pronates the lower arm and flexes the elbow.
Anconeus (Figure 5–9)	Proximal attachment is on the lateral epicondyle of the humerus. It extends diagonally around the arm to the posterior surface of the ulna and attaches at the olecranon process of the ulna. It pronates the forearm and extends the elbow.
Flexor carpi radialis (Figure 5–6)	See Wrist Flexion, page 50.

Muscular actions in the elbow

The elbow joint is formed by the articulation of the ulna and radius with the humerus. Because this joint is a hinge type, it is capable only of two kinds of movements—flexion and extension. Eight muscles contribute to flexion, and six contribute to extension. Of these fourteen muscles, nine are multijoint, some of which extend across the elbow and shoulder joints, while others cover the joints of the elbow and wrist.

Elbow flexion

Elbow flexion is one of the most powerful movements of the upper extremities and is used in a great variety of performances. Utilized frequently in pulling and lifting actions, elbow flexion is also a strong contributor to chinning, climbing, pole vaulting, several gymnastic movements, wrestling, football tackling, and curl lifts. In addition, it is the movement that must precede elbow extension, another frequently used movement. Eight muscles cause the elbow to flex.

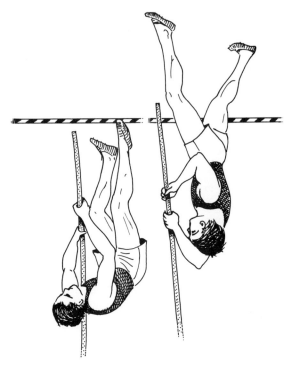

Figure 5–11.
Elbow flexion, an important contributor in pole vaulting.

Biceps brachii (Figure 5–12)	See Lower Arm Lateral Rotation, page 58.
Brachialis (Figure 5–12)	Attaches proximally to the lower half of the humerus, extends down the front of the arm, and attaches at the coronoid process of the ulna. It flexes the elbow.
Brachio-radialis (Figure 5–6)	Proximal attachment is on the lateral surface of the lower third of the humerus. It extends downward and inserts at the base of the styloid process of the radius. It flexes the elbow.
Pronator teres (Figure 5–6)	See Lower Arm Medial Rotation, page 59.

Palmaris longus (Figure 5–6)	See Wrist Flexion, page 50.
Flexor carpi ulnaris (Figure 5–6)	See Wrist Flexion, page 50.
Flexor carpi radialis (Figure 5–6)	See Wrist Flexion, page 50.
Flexor digitorum sublimis (Figure 5–6)	See Handgrip, page 47.

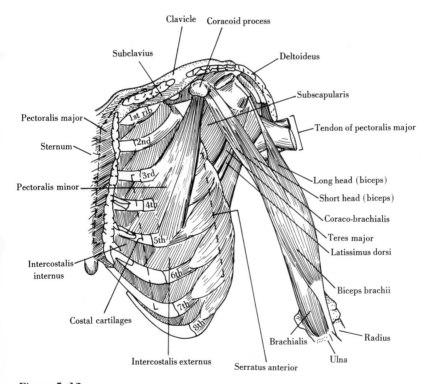

Figure 5–12.
Deep muscles of the upper arm and chest. (*After Goss*)

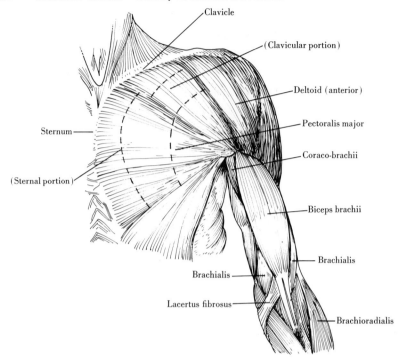

Figure 5–13.
Superficial muscles of the upper arm and chest. (*After Goss*)

Elbow extension

Elbow extension is considerably weaker than elbow flexion, but it is no less significant in performance. Extension is a prime movement in such activities as the overarm throw (Figure 19–3), shot put (Figure 19–6), tennis serve (Figure 12–9), basketball push shots, push-ups, numerous gymnastic movements, and some badminton, squash, and handball shots. Six muscles cause elbow extension.

*Triceps brachii (Figure 5–14)	This is a three-headed muscle. Proximal attachments are (1) long head, on the scapula behind and below the shoulder joints, (2) lateral head, upper posterior of the humerus, (3) medial head, lower and middle posterior of the humerus. Its distal attachment is on the olecranon process of the ulna. It extends the arm and assists in shoulder extension and adduction.
Extensor carpi ulnaris (Figure 5–9)	See Wrist Extension, page 53.

Extensor
digitorum
communis
(Figure 5–9)

See Wrist Extension, page 54.

Extensor
carpi
radialis
brevis
(Figure 5–9)

See Wrist Extension, page 53.

Extensor
carpi
radialis
longus
(Figure 5–9)

See Wrist Extension, page 53.

Anconeus
(Figure 5–9)

See Lower Arm Medial Rotation, page 59.

Muscular actions in the shoulder

The shoulder joint is formed by articulation of the humerus and scapula. It is one of the most versatile and frequently used joints in the body. A ball-and-socket joint, it allows seven different movements—flexion, extension, abduction, adduction, medial and lateral rotation, and circumduction. Twelve muscles, most of which are very powerful, cause movements in this joint. Each of the muscles contributes to more than one movement.

Shoulder flexion

Flexion at the shoulder is caused by four muscles, one of which (biceps) extends across both the elbow and shoulder joints. Shoulder flexion is very important in the common activities of walking and running and is a strong contributor to the underhand throw (see Figure 19–1), pushing, striking, bowling, jumping, hurdling, some strokes in tennis, badminton, squash, and handball, and certain frequently used dance movements. Shoulder flexion may occur with the upper arm in the vertical position, as in the underarm pitch, in the horizontal position, as in the discus throw, and in an intermediate position, as in the sidearm throw (baseball). When flexion occurs in the horizontal plane, it is referred to as horizontal flexion. Muscles which cause shoulder flexion are listed below.

*Deltoid
(anterior)
(Figure
5–13)

The deltoid muscle consists of three parts—anterior, middle, and posterior. The muscle attaches proximally on the anterior surface of the lateral third of the clavicle, the top of the acromion, and the outside edge of the spine of the scapula. It extends downward across the front, top, and back of the shoulder joint and attaches on the lateral side of the middle portion of the humerus. The anterior fibers cause shoulder flexion, abduction, and medial rotation. The middle fibers cause shoulder abduction. The posterior fibers cause shoulder extension, abduction, and lateral rotation.

*Pectoralis
major
(Figure
5–13)

The pectoralis major consists of two parts—the clavicular (upper) portion and the sternal (lower) portion. Its proximal attachment is on the anterior of the clavicle, the whole length of the sternum, and the cartilages of the first six ribs. The muscle lies horizontally, and the distal end attaches to the anterior of the humerus, about one-third of the way between the shoulder and elbow. The clavicular portion causes flexion, horizontal flexion, adduction, and medial rotation at the shoulder. The sternal portion causes shoulder adduction, horizontal flexion, medial rotation, shoulder extension when the arm is in a flexed position, and flexion when the arm is hyperextended. The total muscle is a strong contributor to horizontal flexion at the shoulder.

Biceps
brachii
(short head)
(Figure
5–12)

See Lower Arm Lateral Rotation, page 58.

Coraco-
brachialis
(Figure
5–12)

Attaches proximally onto the coracoid process of the scapula, extends diagonally downward, and attaches distally to the inner surface of the humerus about one-third of the way down the humerus. It contributes to flexion at the shoulder, especially when the arm is in the horizontal position, and adduction.

Shoulder extension

Seven different muscles cause extension at the shoulder. One of these, the triceps, is a two-joint muscle. Shoulder extension is another very powerful movement and is important in such activities as chinning, climbing, pole vaulting, running, walking, rises in gymnastics, and opposite arm movements in the discus throw and shot put. Like flexion, shoulder extension may occur with the upper arm in a vertical, horizontal, or intermediate position. Shoulder extension beyond the anatomical position may occur and cause the arm to move to the rear of the body, a movement known as hyperextension. Muscles causing shoulder extension are the following:

*Latissimus dorsi (Figure 5–15)	Proximal attachment is on the spinous processes of the six lower thoracic and all of the lumbar vertebrae, the sacrum, the crest of the ilium, and the three lowest ribs. It extends diagonally up the back and attaches onto the upper anterior surface of the humerus. It extends, adducts, and medially rotates the arm at the shoulder.
*Teres major (Figure 5–14)	Proximal attachment is on the posterior surface of the lower scapula. It extends diagonally upward and attaches onto the anterior surface of the humerus. It causes extension, adduction, and medial rotation at the shoulder. Its actions are the same as the latissimus dorsi.
*Pectoralis major (sternal portion) (Figure 5–13)	See Shoulder Flexion, page 64.
*Deltoid (posterior) (Figure 5–15)	See Shoulder Flexion, page 64.
Triceps brachii (long head) (Figure 5–14)	See Elbow Extension, page 62.
Infraspinatus (Figure 5–14)	Proximal attachment is on the infraspinous fossa of the scapula (posterior surface and lower portion). It extends diagonally upward and attaches onto the posterior surface of the humerus near the shoulder joint. It rotates the arm laterally and extends it in the horizontal position.
Teres minor (Figure 5–14)	Proximal attachment is on the lower posterior border of the scapula. It extends diagonally upward and attaches onto the posterior surface of the humerus near the shoulder joint. Its actions are the same as the infraspinatus muscle.

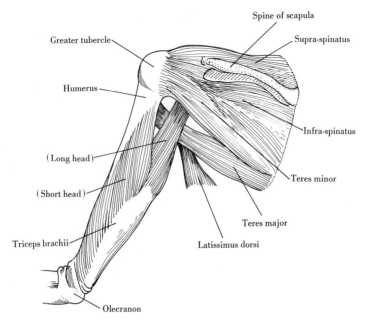

Figure 5–14.
Triceps and deep muscles of the scapula. (*After Goss*)

Shoulder abduction

This is probably the weakest movement of the shoulder joint. It is caused by the supraspinatus, biceps, and deltoid muscles. The pectoralis major (clavicular) also contributes to abduction above the horizontal position only. Although it is not considered a significant contributor in sports performances, this movement is used in elbow thrusting actions in football, soccer, and other body contact games, in basketball hookshots and passes, and in modern dancing and ballet. Also, it is used with shoulder flexion in jumping actions and for maintaining balance as in the football punt, skiing, skating, and beamwalking.

*Deltoid
(Figures
5–13 and
5–15)

See Shoulder Flexion, page 64.

*Supra-spinatus
(Figure
5–14)

Attaches proximally to the supraspinous fossa of the scapula (upper posterior portion), lies horizontally, and attaches onto the greater tubercle (top) of the humerus. It abducts the arm at the shoulder.

Biceps
brachii
(long head)
(Figure
5–12)

See Lower Arm Lateral Rotation, page 58.

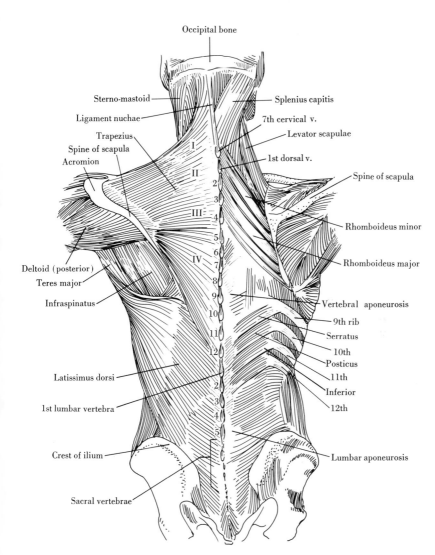

Occipital bone

Sterno-mastoid

Ligament nuchae

Trapezius

Spine of scapula

Acromion

Splenius capitis

7th cervical v.

Levator scapulae

1st dorsal v.

Spine of scapula

Rhomboideus minor

Rhomboideus major

Deltoid (posterior)

Teres major

Infraspinatus

Vertebral aponeurosis

9th rib

Serratus

10th

Posticus

11th

Inferior

12th

Latissimus dorsi

1st lumbar vertebra

Crest of ilium

Sacral vertebrae

Lumbar aponeurosis

Figure 5–15.
Superficial muscles of the back and posterior of the shoulder. (*After Goss*)

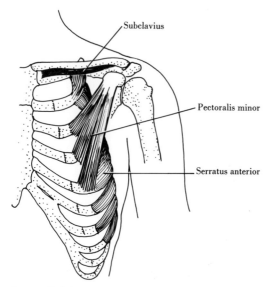

Figure 5–16.
Serratus anterior, subclavius, and pectoralis minor
muscles.

Shoulder adduction

Shoulder adduction is another strong movement. It is used often in arm-supported gymnastic movements, the swimming breaststroke, to some extent in the crawl stroke, and in numerous dance movements. Six muscles contribute to this movement.

*Latissimus dorsi (Figure 5–15)	See Shoulder Extension, page 65.
*Pectoralis major (Figure 5–13)	See Shoulder Flexion, page 64.
*Teres major (Figure 5–14)	See Shoulder Extension, page 65.

Triceps brachii (Figure 5–14)	See Elbow Extension, page 62.
Subscapularis (Figure 5–12)	Proximal attachment is on the anterior (front) side of the scapula, known as the subscapular fossa. It lies horizontally and attaches onto the lesser tubercle (top portion) of the humerus on the anterior surface. It medially rotates and adducts the arm at the shoulder.
Coracobrachialis (Figure 5–12)	See Shoulder Flexion, page 64.

Medial rotation at the shoulder

This movement is very significant. Frequently used in performance, it is vital in the forehand tennis stroke, sidearm and overarm throws, certain badminton, squash, and handball shots, rope climb, and the swimming crawl stroke, butterfly stroke, and breaststroke. Six muscles contribute to the movement. (Note: Care must be taken to be sure humeral rotation is not confused with forearm rotation.)

*Subscapularis (Figure 5–12)	See Shoulder Adduction, page 69.
*Teres major (Figure 5–14)	See Shoulder Extension, page 65.

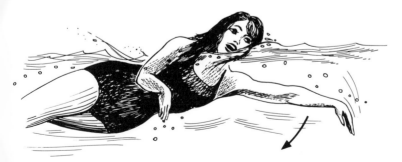

Figure 5–17.
Shoulder adduction, a very strong movement in the sidestroke.

*Pectoralis
major
(Figure
5–13)

See Shoulder Flexion, page 64.

*Latissimus
dorsi
(Figure
5–15)

See Shoulder Extension, page 65.

*Deltoid
(anterior)
(Figure
5–13)

See Shoulder Flexion, page 64.

Biceps
brachii
(short head)
(Figure
5–12)

See Lower Arm Lateral Rotation, page 58.

Lateral rotation at the shoulder

Some of the sports performances in which the upper arm is rotated laterally are the backhand tennis drive, the underhand pitch, preparation for throwing, and the golf swing (forward arm in the downswing, backward arm in the backswing). The movement is caused by the coordinated actions of three muscles.

*Infra-
spinatus
(Figures
5–14 and
5–15)

See Shoulder Extension, page 65.

*Teres minor
(Figure
5–14)

See Shoulder Extension, page 65.

Deltoid
(posterior)
(Figure
5–15)

See Shoulder Flexion, page 64.

Shoulder circumduction

Circumduction at the shoulder, a weak movement not frequently used, results from the sequential combination of shoulder flexion, abduction, extension, and adduction.

Muscular actions in the shoulder girdle

The bone structure of the shoulder girdle consists of the scapula and clavicle. The shoulder girdle is capable of only a small amount of movement in any direction, but some of the movements have great significance in performance. The six movements performed by the shoulder girdle are elevation, depression, protraction, retraction, and rotation downward and upward. Ten muscles work together in different combinations to cause these movements.

It is interesting to note the tremendous cooperation between the movements of the shoulder girdle and the upper arm. Whenever the humerus moves, the clavicle and scapula seem to follow so that the glenoid cavity tends to point in the direction of the axis of the humerus. If the humerus is abducted, the scapula rotates upward. If the humerus is moved out front, as in flexion, the scapula abducts and tries to "turn the corner," following the curvature of the rib cage. Any movement of the humerus toward the rear, as in hyperextension, results in scapular retraction. It is important to note that the humerus does not drag the shoulder girdle along, but rather those muscles which move the shoulder girdle work cooperatively with the muscles causing the corresponding movement in the upper arm.

Shoulder girdle elevation

Elevation of the shoulder girdle is important in lifting, vertical jumping where the arms and shoulders are thrust upward, and in over-the-head reaching. Some specific performances in which the movement is significant are the tennis serve, handstand, shot put, pole vault (pushing action), basketball push shots and rebounding, volleyball spike and overhead push shots, and the high jump and broad jump. Two muscles cause the shoulder girdle to elevate.

*Levator scapulae (Figure 5–15)	Proximal attachment is on the transvere processes (side) of the four upper cervical vertebrae. It extends diagonally downward and attaches onto the upper and medial portion of the scapula. It elevates the shoulder girdle. It may also laterally flex the neck.
*Trapezius (I and II) (Figure 5–15)	This large fan-shaped muscle consists of four parts: I, II, III, and IV. The proximal attachment of the total muscle is on the base of the skull, ligaments of the neck, and the spinous processes down to and including the twelfth thoracic

vertebra. It attaches onto the outer portion of the clavicle, the acromion process, and the upper surface of the scapular spine. Part I elevates the girdle; part II elevates, upward rotates, and retracts the girdle. Part III retracts, and part IV causes upward rotation, depression, and retraction.

Shoulder girdle depression

Depression is the opposite movement from elevation. It is a very strong movement caused by three different muscles. Specific performances in which it is a strong contributor are the pole vault (pulling action), chinning, climbing, swimming (pulling action), and numerous gymnastic activities such as the dip, iron cross (see Figure 20–5), giant swing, and parallel bar movements. Three muscles cause this movement.

*Pectoralis minor (Figure 5–16)

This muscle is underneath and entirely covered by the pectoralis major. Its proximal attachment is on the upper and outer surfaces of the third, fourth, and fifth ribs near their cartilages. It extends diagonally upward and attaches onto the coracoid process of the scapula (anterior surface). It depresses and protracts the shoulder girdle and rotates the scapula downward.

*Subclavius (Figure 5–16)

Proximal attachment is on the anterior of the first rib and its cartilage. It extends upward and attaches along the middle underside of the clavicle. It depresses the shoulder girdle.

*Trapezius IV (Figure 5–15)

See Shoulder Girdle Elevation, page 71.

Shoulder girdle protraction (abduction)

Protraction occurs when the scapulae move outward from the spine, resulting in broadening of the shoulders. It is caused by the pectoralis minor and serratus anterior muscles. Protraction is important in performances such as baseball batting, the ball throw, discus throw, tennis forehand drive, and any performance in which reaching sideward is involved.

*Pectoralis
minor
(Figure
5-16)

See Shoulder Girdle Depression, page 72.

*Serratus
anterior
(Figure
5-16)

Proximal attachment is on the upper-outer surfaces of the first eight ribs. The fibers extend upward and backward and attach to the medial border of the anterior surface of the scapula. It protracts the shoulder girdle and rotates it upward.

Shoulder girdle retraction (adduction)

Retraction is opposite from protraction, meaning the scapulae move toward the spine. This movement is short, but strong, and it is important in pull-ups, dips, climbing, and some gymnastic performances, such as the iron cross. Three muscles contribute to the movement.

*Rhomboi-
deus major
(Figure
5-15)

Proximal attachment is on the spinous processes of the upper thoracic vertebrae. It extends diagonally downward and attaches to the lower half of the medial border of the scapula. It retracts and downward rotates the shoulder girdle.

*Rhomboi-
deus minor
(Figure
5-15)

This muscle lies immediately above and parallel to the rhomboid major. Its proximal attachment is on the spinous processes of the last cervical and first thoracic vertebrae. The distal attachment is on the middle portion of the medial edge of the scapula. It retracts and downward rotates the girdle.

*Trapezius
(II and III)
(Figure
5-15)

See Shoulder Girdle Elevation, page 71.

Shoulder girdle rotation upward

Upward rotation of the shoulder girdle occurs when the scapulae rotate around their own centers, with the lower point moving away from the spine while the upper point moves toward the spine. For example, upward rotation occurs when the arm is raised overhead. This movement is often accompanied by shoulder girdle elevation and abduction. It is caused by two muscles.

*Serratus   See Muscle Girdle Protraction, page 73.
anterior
(Figure
5–16)

*Trapezius   See Shoulder Girdle Elevation, page 71.
(II and IV)
(Figure
5–15)

Shoulder girdle rotation downward

Actually, when the anatomical position is assumed, the shoulder girdle is rotated downward almost to its maximum; however, it may be purposely rotated slightly beyond that position. From the upward rotated position, the shoulder girdle may be rotated downward to the anatomical position. Three muscles cause this movement.

*Pectoralis   See Shoulder Girdle Depression, page 72.
minor
(Figure
5–16)

*Rhomboi-   See Shoulder Girdle Retraction, page 73.
deus major
(Figure
5–15)

*Rhomboi-   See Shoulder Girdle Retraction, page 73.
deus minor
(Figure
5–15)

Recommended supplementary reading

RASCH, PHILLIP J., and ROGER K. BURKE: "Kinesiology and Applied Anatomy," 3d ed., chaps. 9–12, Lea and Febiger, Philadelphia, 1967.

THOMPSON, CLEM W.: "Kranz Manual of Kinesiology," 5th ed., chaps. 2–5, The C. V. Mosby Company, St. Louis, 1965.

WELLS, KATHERINE F.: "Kinesiology," 4th ed., chaps. 14–16, W. B. Saunders Company, Philadelphia, 1966.

A. After carefully studying the muscular actions of the upper extremities, indicate, on the following muscle action table, which muscles cause each movement. Mark PM to indicate prime mover and AM to indicate assistant mover.

B. On the skeletal charts at the end of this chapter (Figures 5–18 and 5–19), place drawings of the muscles of the upper extremities which have been discussed in this chapter. Trace additional charts if needed.

Muscle Action Table: **Upper Extremities**

	GRIP	Wrist FLEXION	Wrist EXTENSION	Wrist ABDUCTION	Wrist ADDUCTION	Lower Arm MEDIAL ROTATION	Lower Arm LATERAL ROTATION	Elbow FLEXION	Elbow EXTENSION
Flexor pollicis longus									
Adductor pollicis									
Abductor digiti quinti									
Abductor pollicis longus									
Lumbricalis									
Flexor digitorum profundus									
Flexor pollicis longus									
Flexor digitorum sublimis									
Flexor carpi ulnaris									
Flexor carpi radialis									
Palmaris longus									
Extensor carpi radialis brevis									
Extensor carpi radialis longus									
Extensor carpi ulnaris									
Extensor digiti quinti									
Extensor digitorum communis									
Extensor indicis									
Extensor pollicis longus									
Extensor pollicis brevis									
Supinator									
Pronator quadratus									
Anconeus									
Pronator teres									
Brachialis									
Brachioradialis									
Biceps									
Triceps									

	Shoulder						Shoulder Girdle					
	FLEXION	EXTENSION	ABDUCTION	ADDUCTION	MEDIAL ROTATION	LATERAL ROTATION	ELEVATION	DEPRESSION	PROTRACTION	RETRACTION	UPWARD ROTATION	DOWNWARD ROTATION
Biceps												
Coracobrachialis												
Deltoid (anterior)												
Deltoid (middle)												
Deltoid (posterior)												
Pectoralis major (clavicular)												
Pectoralis major (sternal)												
Latissimus dorsi												
Infraspinatus												
Teres major												
Teres minor												
Triceps (long head)												
Supraspinatus												
Subscapularis												
Levator scapulae												
Trapezius I												
Trapezius II												
Trapezius III												
Trapezius IV												
Subclavius												
Serratus anterior												
Rhomboideus major												
Rhomboideus minor												
Pectoralis minor												

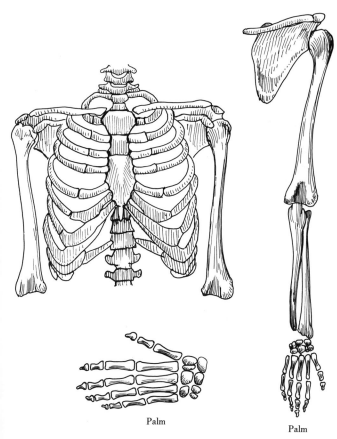

Palm

Palm

Figure 5–18.
Skeleton of the upper extremities (anterior).

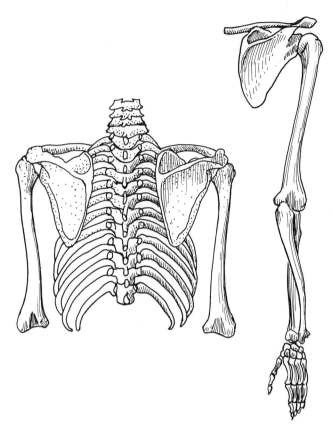

Figure 5–19.
Skeleton of the upper extremities (posterior).

6

Muscular actions of the trunk and neck

*T*he trunk includes about one-half the total body weight. The neck and extremities attach to the trunk, which is the stable unit on which they move. The bone structure of the trunk includes: (1) all the spinal column extending downward from the base of the neck (excluding only the cervical vertebrae), (2) bones of the rib cage, and (3) bones of the pelvic region. The bone structure of the neck consists of the cervical vertebrae and hyoid bone. In other words, except for the upper extremities, the trunk and neck include all the bone structure between the base of the skull and the hip joints. In addition to causing a variety of movements, the muscles of the trunk often play the role of stabilizers, and many of them are among the postural (antigravity) muscles which must remain in partial contraction to hold the body erect.

This chapter covers only the large muscles of the neck and trunk, and those which contribute most to the particular movements discussed. Many smaller muscles in the spinal column and rib cage are not discussed because they are less significant in analysis of vigorous body movements. The smaller muscles of the spine are illustrated in Figure 6–5.

Muscular actions of the trunk

Excluding respiratory action and movement of the abdomen, all trunk actions involve movement in the spine. The structure of spinal vertebrae and the sponge-like disks that separate them make possible a small amount of movement in any direction between each pair of vertebrae. When the movement between all vertebrae is combined, the result is extensive movement of the trunk. The trunk is capable of seven different movements: flexion, extension, lateral flexion to the right and left, rotation to the right and left, and circumduction.

The muscular system of the spine is very complex. It includes many small muscles which connect the individual vertebrae together and add support and stability to the spinal column. There are a few larger spinal muscles which are very significant in vigorous trunk movements. Added to these, the abdominal muscles and muscles of the pelvic region complete the muscular system of the trunk.

Trunk flexion (forward bend)

This movement occurs mostly in the lumbar (lower) region of the spine and is used in almost all athletic performances. It is a prime contributor in trampoline and diving maneuvers which involve the tuck and pike positions, several gymnastic movements, the pole vault, javelin throw, butterfly swimming stroke, over-

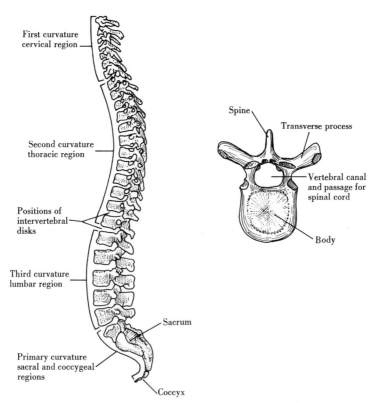

Figure 6–1.
Side view of the spinal column, and cross section of a vertebra.

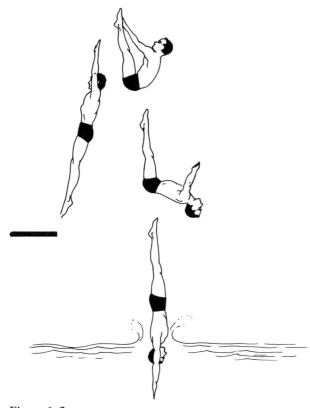

Figure 6–2.
Trunk flexion, essential in a back dive, pike position, and
many other performances.

arm ball throw, and hurdling. Trunk flexion is caused by contraction of the
muscles of the abdominal wall, plus the psoas major.

MUSCLE	DESCRIPTION AND ACTIONS
Rectus abdominis (Figure 6–3)	The two rectus abdominis muscles lie vertically up the front of the abdomen. Proximal attachment of each muscle is on the pubis bone and the ligaments covering the front of the pubis. The distal attachment is on the cartilages of the fifth, sixth, and seventh ribs. The muscle compresses the abdomen and flexes the trunk. When only one of the muscles is contracted, it contributes to trunk lateral flexion.

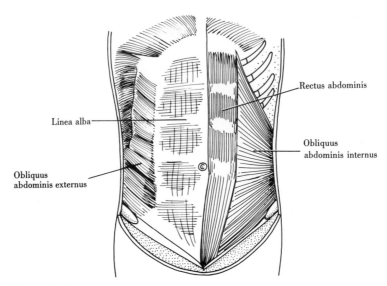

Linea alba

Rectus abdominis

Obliquus
abdominis internus

Obliquus
abdominis externus

Figure 6–3.
Muscles of the abdominal wall. On the left side, the obliquus abdominis externus and the anterior wall of the sheath of the rectus abdominis have been removed.

MUSCLE	DESCRIPTION AND ACTIONS
*Obliquus abdominis externus (Figure 6–3)	This muscle lies diagonally across the front and side of the abdomen. Proximal attachment is on the eight lowest ribs. It extends diagonally downward and attaches onto the upper crest of the ilium, the pubis, and the linea alba. It compresses the abdomen and causes trunk flexion, lateral flexion to the same side, and rotation to the opposite side.
*Obliquus abdominis internus (Figure 6–3)	This muscle lies underneath the external oblique muscle, and the fibers of the two muscles run at right angles to each other. Proximal attachment is on the crest of the ilium. It extends diagonally upward and forward and attaches to the six lowest ribs and the linea alba. It compresses the abdomen and causes trunk flexion, lateral flexion, and rotation to the same side.
Psoas major (Figure 6–4)	See Hip Flexion, page 95.

* Throughout this chapter, this device indicates prime mover muscle.

Trunk extension (straightening)

Like trunk flexion, this movement occurs mostly in the lumbar region of the spine. It is the most powerful movement of the trunk and is very significant in athletics. Used in almost every type of performance, trunk extension is of prime importance in several dance movements, the shot put, butterfly stroke, discus throw, lifting, wrestling, hurdling (final phase), and football blocking and tackling. In addition to the three muscles discussed below, several of the deep, small spinal muscles, especially the rotator muscles, contribute to extension. They are illustrated in Figure 6–6.

MUSCLE	DESCRIPTION AND ACTIONS
*Semi- spinalis (thoracic) (Figure 6–5)	The muscle lies diagonally up the spine. The proximal attachment is on the transverse processes of the sixth to tenth thoracic vertebrae. It attaches distally to the spinous processes of the upper thoracic and lower cervical vertebrae. When the two muscles act together, they extend the trunk. Separately, they laterally flex the trunk and rotate it to the opposite side.

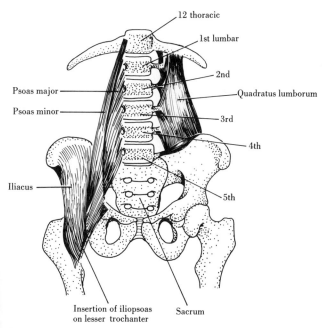

Psoas major
Psoas minor
Iliacus

12 thoracic
1st lumbar
2nd
Quadratus lumborum
3rd
4th
5th

Insertion of iliopsoas
on lesser trochanter
Sacrum

Figure 6–4.
Muscles inside the pelvic region.

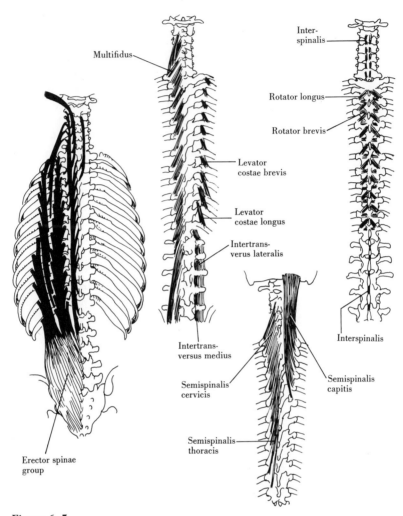

Figure 6–5.
Back muscles which act on the spinal column. They contribute to trunk and neck extension, rotation, and lateral flexion.

MUSCLE	DESCRIPTION AND ACTIONS
Erector spinae (Figure 6–5)	This massive back muscle consists of three branches: the iliocostalis (lateral portion), longissimus (middle portion), and spinalis (medial portion). The muscle attaches proximally on the posterior surface of the sacrum, crest of the ilium, and spines of the lumbar and thoracic vertebrae. It

MUSCLE | DESCRIPTION AND ACTIONS

extends up the back and attaches to the back portion of the ribs at several places, to the posterior of the thoracic and cervical vertebrae, and to the base of the skull. It extends, rotates, and laterally flexes the trunk and neck.

Multifidus
(Figure 6–5)

This muscle lies down the side of the spine. The proximal attachment is on the posterior of the sacrum, the top of the iliac, and the transverse processes of the lumbar and thoracic vertebrae. The muscle extends diagonally upward and attaches to the spinous processes of the spine. Acting together, the two muscles extend the trunk and neck; singly, they cause trunk and neck rotation to the opposite side and lateral flexion.

Trunk lateral flexion (sideward bend)

The trunk may be flexed to either the right or the left by simultaneously contracting the trunk flexor and extensor muscles on the side where lateral flexion is desired. Trunk lateral flexion is especially important in shot-putting, throwing, sideward lifts, and numerous gymnastic and dance movements. Practically all the trunk flexor and extensor muscles contribute to lateral flexion.

MUSCLE | DESCRIPTION AND ACTIONS

Rectus abdominis
(Figure 6–3)

See Trunk Flexion, page 81.

Obliquus abdominis externus
(Figure 6–3)

See Trunk Flexion, page 82.

Obliquus abdominis internus
(Figure 6–3)

See Trunk Flexion, page 82.

Erector spinae
(Figure 6–5)

See Trunk Extension, page 84.

MUSCLE	DESCRIPTION AND ACTIONS
*Semi-spinalis (thoracic) (Figure 6–5)	See Trunk Extension, page 83.
*Multifidus (Figure 6–5)	See Trunk Extension, page 85.
*Quadratus lumborum (Figure 6–4)	This muscle lies up the side of the trunk between the ilium and the bottom of the rib cage. The proximal attachment is on the crest of the ilium and transverse processes of the four lowest lumbar vertebrae. It extends upward and backward toward the spine and attaches to the upper two lumbar vertebrae and the last rib. It causes lateral trunk flexion.

Trunk rotation

In addition to the deep rotator muscles of the spine, there are five larger muscles which cause trunk rotation. Of prime importance in the twisting actions in diving, trampoline, and dance, trunk rotation is also used very extensively in throwing, batting, golf, tennis and badminton strokes, handball shots, the shot put (Figure 19–6), discus throw, swimming, and other physical education performances.

*Obliquus abdominis externus (Figure 6–3)	It rotates the trunk to the opposite side. See Trunk Flexion, page 82.
*Obliquus abdominis internus (Figure 6–3)	It rotates the trunk to the same side. See Trunk Flexion, page 82.
*Erector spinae (Figure 6–5)	It rotates the trunk to the same side. See Trunk Extension, page 84.
*Semi-spinalis (thoracic) (Figure 6–5)	It rotates the trunk to the opposite side. See Trunk Extension, page 83.
*Multifidus (Figure 6–5)	It rotates the trunk to the opposite side. See Trunk Extension, page 85.

Trunk circumduction

Circumduction of the trunk is not a frequently used movement. It results from a sequential combination of flexion, lateral flexion, extension, and hyperextension.

Muscular actions in the neck

The bone structure of the neck consists of the upper seven (cervical) vertebrae of the spinal column. In addition to the smaller muscles of the spine, there are seven larger and more powerful muscles which cause movement in the neck. The neck is capable of extension (backward head tilt), flexion (forward head tilt), lateral flexion (sideward head tilt) to the right and left, rotation to the right and left, and circumduction.

Neck flexion

The neck is flexed by the coordinated actions of the three scalenus muscles and the sternocleidomastoid. Neck flexion, which is a much weaker movement than extension, is important in hurdling (Figure 9–1), diving and trampoline stunts where the pike and tuck positions are used, swimming, several dance movements, and "setting" the neck for contact in football.

Sterno-cleido-mastoid (Figure 6–6)	Attaches proximally on the upper portion of the sternum and on the medial and upper side of the clavicle; extends upward and attaches to the outer lower portion of the occipital bone. It contributes to neck flexion, lateral flexion, and rotation to the opposite side.
Scalenus (anterior, medius, and posterior) (Figure 6–6)	The proximal attachment is on the transverse processes of the middle four cervical vertebrae. It extends diagonally downward, and the anterior and medius muscles attach to the superior surface of the first rib. The posterior muscle attaches to the second rib. The muscles flex the neck laterally and assist in forward flexion.

Neck extension

Extension is the most powerful neck movement. It is caused by five large muscles, plus some of the smaller muscles which connect the vertebrae. Extensor muscles are used frequently in such performances as modern dance and ballet, wrestling, high-jumping, some swimming strokes, especially the breaststroke and butterfly stroke, crouched and three- and four-point football positions, and tumbling and gymnastic movements, especially those involving head support positions.

Erector spinae (Figure 6–5)	See Trunk Extension, page 84.
Semispinalis (capitis) (Figure 6–5)	Attaches proximally onto the articular and transverse processes of the lower four cervical and the upper six thoracic vertebrae. It extends diagonally upward and attaches to the base of the skull at the occipital bone. It contributes to extension, lateral flexion, and rotation of the neck.
Semispinalis (cervicis) (Figure 6–5)	The proximal attachment is on the spinous processes of the lower cervical and upper thoracic vertebrae. It extends upward and attaches to the spinous processes of the upper cervical vertebrae. It contributes to extension, lateral flexion, and rotation of the neck to the opposite side.
Splenius (capitis and cervicis) (Figure 6–6)	The proximal attachment is on the spinous processes of the seventh cervical and first three thoracic vertebrae. It extends upward and outward and attaches to the base of the skull on the occipital and temporal bones. It contributes to neck extension, lateral flexion, and rotation to the same side.
Multifidus (Figure 6–5)	See Trunk Extension, page 85.

Lateral flexion of the neck

Lateral flexion is caused by the following seven large muscles, plus smaller muscles which help connect the vertebrae together. Muscles on the right side cause lateral flexion to the right, while those on the left cause lateral flexion to the left. This movement is used frequently in such activities as modern dance and ballet, twisting and turning movements in diving and gymnastics, wrestling, putting the shot, and hard thrusting sideward and turning movements as in football blocking and tackling.

Splenius (capitis and cervicis) (Figure 6–6)	See Neck Extension, page 88.

*Sterno-
cleido-
mastoid
(Figure 6–6)

See Neck Flexion, page 87.

*Scalenus
(anterior,
medius, and
posterior)
(Figure 6–6)

See Neck Flexion, page 87.

*Semi-
spinalis
(cervicis and
capitis)
(Figure 6–5)

See Neck Extension, page 88.

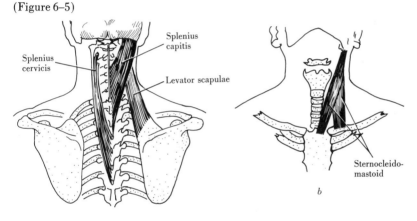

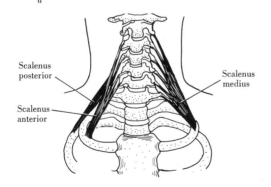

Figure 6–6.
Major muscles of the neck.

*Erector
spinae
(Figure 6–5)
    See Trunk Extension, page 84.

*Multifidus
(upper
portion)
(Figure 6–5)
    See Trunk Extension, page 85.

*Levator
scapulae
(Figure 5–15)
    See Shoulder Girdle Elevation, page 71.

Neck rotation

Four muscles on each side of the body contribute to neck rotation. Three of the muscles are opposite side rotators, meaning that when the left muscle contracts, the neck rotates to the right. Neck rotation is very important in total body twisting and turning movements, swimming (crawl stroke), all throwing activities, and modern dance and ballet. This movement is used to some extent in almost all performances.

*Sterno-
cleido-
mastoid
(Figure 6–6)
    It rotates the neck to the opposite side. See Neck Flexion, page 87.

*Semi-
spinalis
(cervicis and
capitis)
(Figure 6–5)
    It rotates the neck to the opposite side. See Neck Extension, page 88.

*Multifidus
(upper
portion)
(Figure 6–5)
    It rotates the neck to the opposite side. See Trunk Extension, page 85.

*Splenius
(cervicis and
capitis)
(Figure 6–6)
    It rotates the neck to the same side. See Neck Extension, page 88.

Neck circumduction

This movement is not frequently used. As is the case of other body segments capable of this movement, circumduction in the neck results from a combination of other movements; it is the sequential combination of flexion, lateral flexion, and hyperextension.

Recommended supplementary reading

RASCH, PHILIP J., and ROGER K. BURKE: "Kinesiology and Applied Anatomy," 3d ed., chaps. 13–14, Lea and Febiger, Philadelphia, 1967.
THOMPSON, CLEM W.: "Kranz Manual of Kinesiology," 5th ed., chap. 9, The C. V. Mosby Company, St. Louis, 1965.
WELLS, KATHERINE R.: ("Kinesiology," 4th ed., chaps. 12 and 13, W. B. Saunders Commedius, and posterior)

Student projects

A. After carefully studying the muscular actions of the neck and trunk, indicate on the following muscle action table which muscles cause each movement. Mark PM to indicate prime mover and AM to indicate assistant mover.

B. On the skeletal charts at the end of this chapter place drawings of the muscles of the trunk and neck discussed in this chapter. Trace additional charts if needed.

Muscle Action Table: Trunk and Neck

	Trunk				Neck			
	FLEXION	EXTENSION	LATERAL FLEXION	ROTATION	FLEXION	EXTENSION	LATERAL FLEXION	ROTATION
Rectus abdominis								
Obliquus externus								
Obliquus internus								
Psoas								
Semispinalis (thoracis)								
Semispinalis (capitis)								
Semispinalis (cervicis)								
Sacrospinalis								
Multifidus								
Quadratus lumborum								
Splenius (cervicis)								
Splenius (capitis)								
Sternocleidomastoid								
Scalenus (anterior, medius, and posterior)								

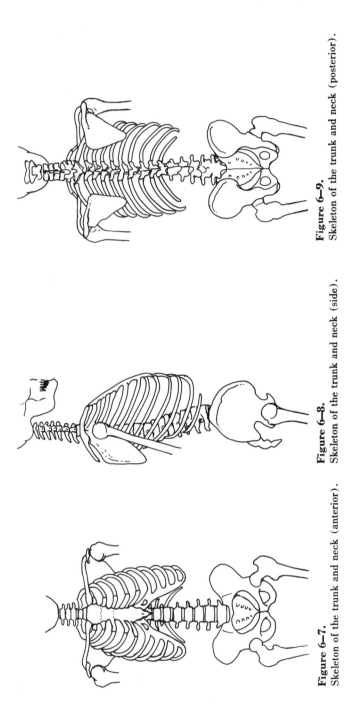

Figure 6–9.
Skeleton of the trunk and neck (posterior).

Figure 6–8.
Skeleton of the trunk and neck (side).

Figure 6–7.
Skeleton of the trunk and neck (anterior).

7

Muscular actions of the lower extremities

*T*his chapter includes the different movements that occur in the joints of
the lower extremities, along with information about the muscles causing
the movements. As in the two previous chapters, an illustration of each
muscle is given.

The lower extremities include the feet and legs. It is the portion of the body
which is used most extensively in locomotion, and in body support in an upright
position. Because of these functions the lower extremities are very important in
practically all performances.

Muscular actions in the hip

The joint at the hip is a ball-and-socket type, and is formed by the articulation
between the femur and pelvis. It is capable of flexion, extension, abduction,
adduction, rotation medially and laterally, and circumduction. It should be noted
that the upper leg may be flexed and extended in either the vertical or horizontal
position, or any position between the vertical and horizontal. Also, the leg may be
hyperextended a small amount, meaning that extension may continue beyond the
vertical (anatomical) position. The twenty muscles surrounding the hip are some
of the largest and most powerful muscles in the body. They contract in different
combinations to cause the seven hip movements. Six of the twenty muscles cross
the knee joint, and contribute to movements in that joint.

Hip flexion

This is one of the strongest movements of the body, and it is caused by the
contraction of nine muscles. Four of the muscles contribute all the way through

93

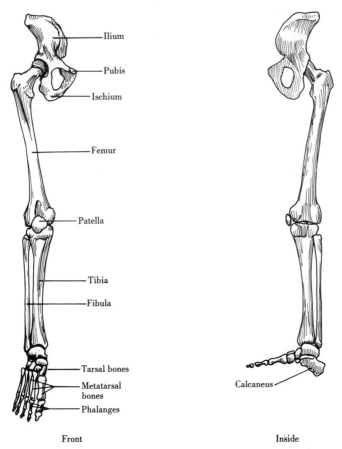

Front   Inside

Figure 7–1.
Front and side views of the skeletal structure of the lower extremity.

the range of motion, while another four (adductor brevis, adductor longus, gracilis, and pectineus) contribute only during the early phase of flexion. Three of the muscles (rectus femoris, gracilis, and sartorius) are two-joint muscles and contribute to actions at both the hip and knee. This movement is used in almost all locomotion including the very common activities of walking and running. In this way hip flexion becomes a part of almost every performance. Among other activities in which hip flexion is of prime importance are swimming, hurdling, high-jumping (swinging leg), pole vaulting, kicking actions as in football, soccer, and speedball, dancing, diving, trampolining, gymnastics, and sit-ups.

MUSCLE	DESCRIPTION AND ACTIONS
*Rectus femoris (Figure 7–3)	This large and powerful muscle lies vertically down the front of the thigh. It attaches proximally by two tendons, one from the front and lower portion of the iliac spine, and the other just slightly higher on the iliac. Its distal attachment is on the upper patella. It flexes the hip and extends the knee.
*Pectineus (Figure 7–3)	The proximal attachment is on the lower surface of the pubis bone. It extends diagonally downward and attaches to the posterior surface about halfway down the femur. It adducts, flexes, and rotates the thigh laterally.
*Psoas major (Figure 7–3)	This strong muscle runs vertically through the inside of the pelvic region. The proximal attachment is on the bodies and transverse process of the last thoracic vertebra and all of the lumbar vertebrae. It extends downward and attaches to the inside of the head of the femur. It flexes and rotates the thigh laterally and assists in trunk flexion.
*Iliacus (Figure 7–3)	Attaches proximally on the interior surface of the iliac crest. It extends downward and joins the distal tendon of the psoas which attaches to the back of the upper portion of the femur

* Throughout this chapter, this device indicates prime mover muscle.

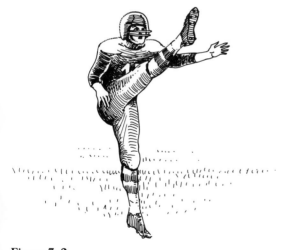

Figure 7–2.
Hip flexion, a prime contributor in the football punt.

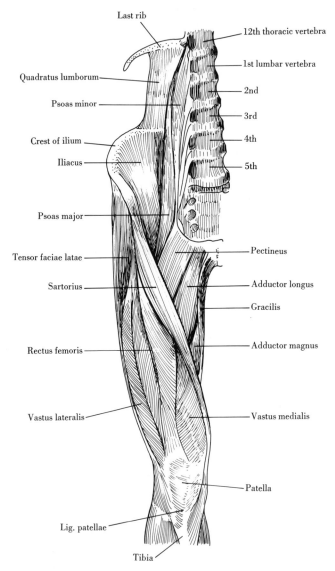

Figure 7–3.
Muscles in the iliac region and the front of the thigh. (*After Goss*)

MUSCLE	DESCRIPTION AND ACTIONS

MUSCLE

DESCRIPTION AND ACTIONS

on the lesser trochanter. It flexes and rotates the thigh laterally.

Sartorius
(Figure 7–3)

This long two-joint muscle attaches proximally on the anterior-superior spine of the ilium, and extends downward and inward to its distal attachment on the upper medial surface of the tibia. It flexes, abducts, and rotates the hip laterally, and flexes and rotates the knee medially.

Adductor
brevis
(Figure 7–5)

The proximal attachment is on the front and lower surface of the pubis bone. It extends diagonally downward and attaches on the medial-posterior surface of the femur about one-third of the way between the hip and knee joints. It adducts, flexes, and rotates the thigh laterally.

Adductor
longus
(Figure 7–5)

Attaches proximally on the front and lower surface of the pubis bone, extends diagonally downward and outward to its distal attachment on the medial surface of the femur about halfway between the hip and knee joints. It adducts, flexes, and rotates the thigh laterally.

Adductor
magnus
(Figure 7–5)

Attaches proximally to the lower portion of the pubis bone. It extends downward and outward to its distal attachment on the medial-posterior surface of the femur just below the neck. It adducts, flexes, and laterally rotates the thigh.

Gracilis
(Figure 7–3)

It attaches proximally on the lower front portion of the pubis bone and its distal attachment is on the medial surface of the tibia below the condyle. This muscle is very long. It runs the length of the upper leg on the medial surface. It adducts the leg at the hip and flexes the knee.

Hip extension

Hip extension is another strong movement. It is caused by six muscles, of which one is the gluteus maximus, often referred to as the strongest muscle in the body. Three of the muscles (hamstrings) cross over two joints and contribute to actions in both the hip and knee. Like hip flexion, hip extension is used in almost all performances, because it is one of the basic movements in running and walking. Some specific athletic performances in which hip extension is of prime importance are swimming, lifting, shot-putting, jumping, throwing, and several dance movements.

MUSCLE	DESCRIPTION AND ACTIONS
*Gluteus maximus (Figure 7–6)	This massive and powerful muscle lies diagonally across the buttock. The proximal attachment is on the crest of the ilium (lateral-posterior face) sacrum and coccyx. It extends downward and outward and attaches onto the back of the femur below the great trochanter. It extends and laterally rotates the thigh. Also, the upper fibers abduct and the lower fibers adduct the thigh.
*Semimem-branosus (Figure 7–4)	Attaches proximally on the lower surface of the ischium bone, extends downward and attaches onto the medial epicondyle of the tibia. It extends and medially rotates the thigh, and flexes and medially rotates the knee.
*Biceps femoris (Figure 7–4)	This powerful, two-joint muscle lies vertically down the back of the thigh. Its long head attaches proximally to the lower portion of the ischium bone, and the short head attaches to the middle-anterior surface of the femur. The distal end attaches onto the lateral side of the head of the fibula and the lateral condyle of the tibia. It flexes the knee and rotates it laterally. The long head also extends the hip.
*Semi-tendinosus (Figure 7–4)	The proximal attachment of this two-joint muscle is on the tuberosity of the ischium. It extends downward across the knee and attaches to the upper part of the medial surface of the tibia. It extends the thigh and rotates it medially. It also flexes and medially rotates the knee.
Gluteus medius (Figure 7–6)	Attaches proximally along the outside of the ilium near its crest, extends downward and attaches to the lateral surface of the great trochanter (top) of the femur. It is a strong abductor of the hip. Its posterior fibers also cause hip extension, while the anterior fibers cause flexion and medial rotation.
Gluteus minimus (Figure 7–4)	The proximal attachment is on the middle part of the outer surface of the ilium. It extends downward and attaches to the front surface of the great trochanter (top) of the femur. The posterior fibers cause extension of the hip, while the anterior fibers cause medial rotation and flexion. The whole muscle causes hip abduction.

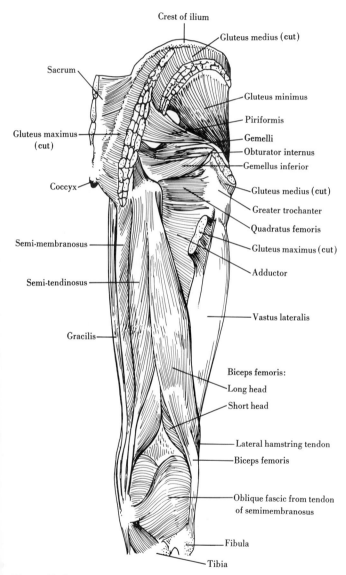

Crest of ilium

Gluteus medius (cut)

Sacrum

Gluteus minimus

Piriformis

Gluteus maximus (cut)

Gemelli

Obturator internus

Gemellus inferior

Coccyx

Gluteus medius (cut)

Greater trochanter

Semi-membranosus

Quadratus femoris

Gluteus maximus (cut)

Semi-tendinosus

Adductor

Vastus lateralis

Gracilis

Biceps femoris:

Long head

Short head

Lateral hamstring tendon

Biceps femoris

Oblique fascic from tendon
of semimembranosus

Fibula

Tibia

Figure 7–4.
Muscles in the back of the hip and thigh. (*After Goss*)

Hip abduction

Abduction of the hip is a very weak movement and one not frequently used. It is caused by relatively small muscles, and the mechanical ratio against which most of the muscles work in this movement is unfavorable to strength. The movement is used in such performances as side-stepping in the overhand throw, shot put, and javelin throw; side-stepping in court and field games; side-kicking with the outside of the foot in soccer and speedball; and the recovery phase of the frog and whip kicks in swimming. These muscles also function in supporting the pelvis during walking and running.

Gluteus medius (Figure 7–6)	See Hip Extension, page 98.
Gluteus minimus (Figure 7–4)	See Hip Extension, page 98.
Gemelli (Figure 7–7)	The proximal attachment is on the upper portion of the ischium bone. It lies horizontally and attaches to the medial surface of the great trochanter (top) of the femur. It rotates the thigh laterally and abducts it.
Sartorius (Figure 7–3)	See Hip Flexion, page 97.
Tensor fasciae latae (Figure 7–3)	Attaches proximally to the anterior crest and the spine of the ilium, extends down the outside of the thigh about one-third of its length, and inserts on the outside of the femur. It abducts and medially rotates the thigh.

Hip adduction

The six adductor muscles work against a much better mechanical ratio than the abductor muscles, and hip adduction is considerably stronger than abduction, but it is still a relatively weak movement. Adduction of the hip is used in such activities as side-stepping movements in various field and court games, side-kicking with the inside of the foot, and the frog and whip kicks in swimming.

Adductor brevis (Figure 7–5)	See Hip Flexion, page 97.

*Adductor longus (Figure 7–5)	See Hip Flexion, page 97.
*Adductor magnus (Figure 7–5)	See Hip Flexion, page 97.
*Gracilis (Figure 7–3)	See Hip Flexion, page 97.
Gluteus maximus (lower portion) (Figure 7–6)	See Hip Extension, page 98.
Pectineus (Figure 7–3)	See Hip Flexion, page 95.

Medial rotation at the hip

Medial hip rotation is a frequently used movement because it occurs in walking and running during the latter phase of each stride. It is also used extensively in dodging and turning actions, the frog and whip kicks, batting, and golf and tennis strokes. It is a relatively strong movement in spite of the fact that most muscles contributing toward it do so as a secondary function. Five muscles contribute to medial rotation.

*Gluteus medius (Figure 7–6)	See Hip Extension, page 98.
*Gluteus minimus (Figure 7–4)	See Hip Extension, page 98.
*Tensor fasciae latae (Figure 7–3)	See Hip Abduction, page 100.
Semi- tendinosus (Figure 7–4)	See Hip Extension, page 98.

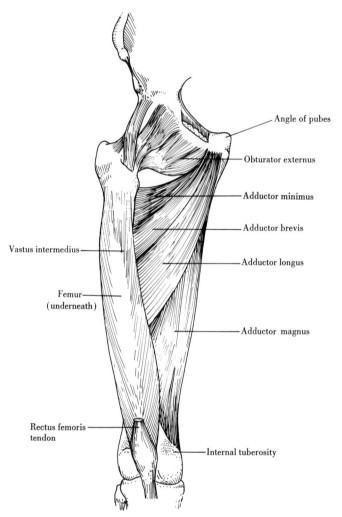

Figure 7–5.
Muscles in the medial side of the thigh, and the vastus intermedius muscle.

Semimem-   See Hip Extension, page 98.
branosus
(Figure 7–4)

Lateral rotation at the hip

More muscles (10) contribute to lateral rotation at the hip than almost any other movement. Yet it is a weak movement because the muscles contribute to it as a secondary function, and the muscles work against a poor mechanical ratio. The movement occurs during the recovery phase (forward swing) of running and walking strides, and it contributes to dodging and turning actions, certain swinging actions as in tennis, golf, and baseball swings, and in the final movement of the trail leg in high-jumping (roll).

*Obturator externus (Figures 7–5 and 7–7)	Attaches proximally onto the obturator foramen on the inner wall of the pelvis. It lies horizontally, and attaches onto the femur just below the great trochanter. It rotates the thigh laterally.
*Obturator internus (Figure 7–7)	Attaches proximally to the inner surface of the wall of the pelvis on the obturator foramen. It lies horizontally and attaches to the greater trochanter of the femur. It rotates the thigh laterally.
*Piriformis (Figures 7–4 and 7–7)	The proximal attachment is on the anterior surface of the sacrum. It passes in front of the pelvis and attaches onto the upper border of the great trochanter. It rotates the thigh laterally.
*Gemelli (Figure 7–7)	See Hip Abduction, page 100.
*Gluteus maximus (Figure 7–6)	See Hip Extension, page 98.

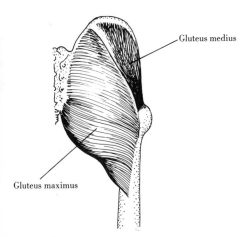

Figure 7–6.
Gluteus maximus and gluteus medius muscles.

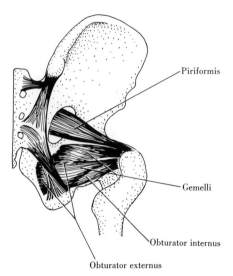

Figure 7–7.
Interior muscles of the hip.

Sartorius (Figure 7–3)	See Hip Flexion, page 97.
Pectineus (Figure 7–3)	See Hip Flexion, page 95.
Adductor brevis (Figure 7–5)	See Hip Flexion, page 97.
Adductor longus (Figure 7–5)	See Hip Flexion, page 97.
Adductor magnus (Figure 7–5)	See Hip Flexion, page 97.

Hip circumduction

The hip joint is another one of the few joints capable of circumduction. As described earlier, circumduction is the sequential combination of flexion, abduction, extension, and adduction. It is not frequently used.

Muscular actions in the knee

The articulation of the tibia and femur at the knee forms a joint which is usually considered capable of only two movements—flexion and extension. However, the lower leg can rotate slightly when the knee is in a flexed position. As the knee extends, the amount of possible rotation decreases, until when full extension is reached no rotation is possible. These rotating movements aid in changing direction during running, but otherwise they have little effect on performance.

Twelve muscles contribute to knee extension and flexion. Eight of these are two-joint muscles acting on either the hip or ankle joint in addition to the knee. Knee actions are relatively strong because the muscles causing them are mostly the large and powerful muscles of the upper leg.

Knee flexion

Flexion of the knee is caused by the actions of eight muscles. Even though they work against a poor mechanical ratio, knee flexion is still a strong movement. It is one of the important movements in walking and running (during the recovery phase of the stride). Therefore, it is one of our most frequently used movements. Also, it is used extensively in swimming, primarily during the recovery phase of the various kicks.

*Biceps femoris (Figure 7–4)	See Hip Extension, page 98.
*Semimem- branosus (Figure 7–4)	See Hip Extension, page 98.
*Semi- tendinosus (Figure 7–4)	See Hip Extension, page 98.
Gastrocne- mius (Figure 7–8)	This large muscle of the calf attaches proximally just above the knee on the medial and lateral condyles of the femur. It extends down the back of the lower leg and inserts on to the calcaneus bone by way of the Achilles tendon. It flexes the knee and plantar flexes the ankle.
Sartorius (Figure 7–3)	See Hip Flexion, page 97.

Gracilis
(Figure 7–3)
See Hip Flexion, page 97.

Plantaris
(Figure 7–8)
This two-joint muscle attaches proximally to the middle of the posterior surface of the femur and extends down the back of the leg to its distal attachment on the upper surface of the calcaneus bone. It flexes the knee and plantar flexes the ankle.

Popliteus
(Figure 7–10)
Attaches proximally to the lateral surface of the lateral condyle of the femur and extends diagonally downward across the posterior and upper part of the lower leg and attaches on the medial posterior surface of the tibia. It flexes and medially rotates the lower leg.

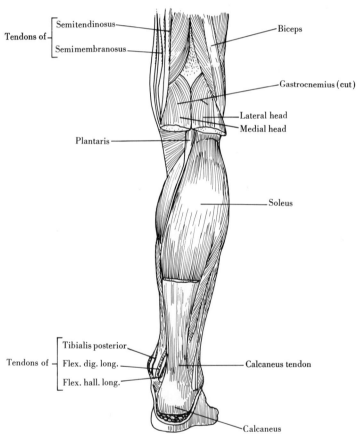

Figure 7–8.
Superficial muscles of the back of the lower leg. (*After Goss*)

Knee extension

The knee is extended by the contraction of four large muscles of the thigh known as the quadriceps group. The muscles work against a poor mechanical ratio, but they are very strong muscles, causing knee extension to be another powerful movement. This movement is very significant in locomotive activities such as walking and running, and it is of prime importance in specific skills such as jumping, swimming, lifting, kicking, skiing, skating, and dodging. Also, the knee extensors are principal postural muscles.

*Rectus
femoris
(Figure 7–3)

See Hip Flexion, page 95.

*Vastus
intermedius
(Figure 7–5)

This large muscle lies vertically along the front of the thigh, underneath the rectus femoris. Its proximal attachment is along the front of the femur, extending most of its length. The distal attachment is on the patella. It extends the knee.

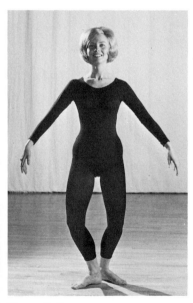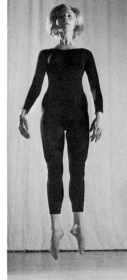

Figure 7–9.
Hip, knee, and ankle extension are prime movements in the jump following a plié.

*Vastus
lateralis
(Figure 7–3)

This muscle lies vertically along side the vastus intermedius. Its proximal attachment is on the upper portion of the lateral surface of the femur. The distal attachment is on the top of the patella. It extends the knee.

*Vastus
medialis
(Figure 7–3)

This muscle lies along the medial side of the vastus intermedius. Its proximal attachment is on the medial surface of the upper portion of the femur. It extends downward and attaches to the top of the patella. It extends the knee.

Lower leg rotation

When the knee is flexed, the lower leg may be slightly rotated medially and laterally. Because of the structure of the knee joint, these movements are not possible when the knee is fully extended. The movements are used in a few activities such as water and snow skiing. Following are the muscles which cause the lower leg to rotate when in a flexed position.

MEDIAL ROTATION

*Semimembranosus

*Semitendinosus

Sartorius

Popliteus

LATERAL ROTATION

*Biceps femoris

Muscular actions of the ankle

The ankle joint is a hinge-type formed by the articulation of the talus bone with the tibia and fibula. Like other hinge joints, the ankle is capable of only two movements, flexion (dorsiflexion) and extension (plantar flexion). Dorsiflexion is a relatively weak movement, whereas plantar flexion is a very strong movement, and one which is highly significant.

Plantar flexion (extension)

Eight muscles contribute to plantar flexion, and seven of these are multijoint muscles. One (gastrocnemius) extends beyond the knee joint and contributes to knee flexion, and five other muscles extend into the foot and contribute to foot movements. Plantar flexion is a powerful movement because it is caused by the strong muscles of the calf, and their mechanical ratios are reasonably good in this movement. This is one of the most significant movements because of its contribution to walking and running. It is also significant in jumping, lifting, and throwing, and these movements are used in a great number of physical education performances.

Gastrocne-mius (Figure 7–8)	See Knee Flexion, page 105.
*Soleus (Figure 7–8)	This large calf muscle lies underneath the gastrocnemius. Its proximal attachment is on the head of the fibula and medial border of the tibia. It extends down the back of the leg and attaches to the calcaneus bone, by way of the Achilles tendon. It causes plantar flexion.
Peroneus longus (Figures 7–10 and 7–11)	Proximal attachment is on the upper two-thirds of the lateral surface of the fibula and the upper tibia. It extends down the lateral side of the leg and attaches onto the first metatarsal and first cuneiform bones. It causes plantar flexion and eversion of the foot. It also helps to maintain the arch of the foot.
Peroneus brevis (Figures 7–9 and 7–11)	Attaches proximally on to the lateral surface of the lower two-thirds of the fibula, extends down the outside of the legs, and attaches at the fifth metatarsal bone. It causes plantar flexion and eversion of the foot.
Tibialis posterior (Figure 7–10)	This muscle lies vertically down the back of the lower leg, underneath the soleus and gastrocnemius. Its proximal attachment is on the upper posterior surface of the tibia and fibula. It passes diagonally downward across the inside of the ankle and attaches to the arch of the foot. It inverts the foot and assists in plantar flexion.
Flexor digitorum longus (Figures 7–10 and 7–13)	Proximal attachment is on the medial-posterior surface of the tibia about one-fourth of the way down from the knee. It lies vertically down the inside of the lower leg and attaches to the last phalanges of the four outer toes by way of four tendons. It flexes the phalanges and plantar flexes and supinates the foot.

Flexor hallucis longus (Figures 7–10 and 7–13)   Proximal attachment is on the distal two-thirds of the posterior surface of the fibula. It passes along the inside of the ankle and attaches to the base of the last phalanx of the big toe. It flexes the big toe and plantar flexes and supinates the foot.

Plantaris (Figure 7–8)   See Knee Flexion, page 106.

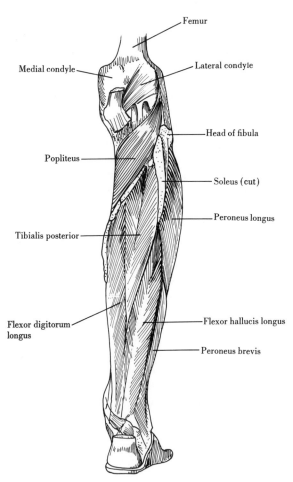

Figure 7–10.
Deep muscle of the back of the lower leg. (*After Goss*)

Dorsiflexion

Four muscles contribute to dorsiflexion, all of which are multijoint muscles extending across the ankle into the foot. This movement is relatively weak, but it is very important in swimming and in kicking. The dorsal flexors hold the foot in the desired position during kicking, and during walking and running they hold the swinging foot in position to clear the surface.

Peroneus tertius (Figure 7–11)	Proximal attachment is on the lower part of the fibula on the anterior-lateral surface. It extends down the outside of the leg and attaches onto the fifth metatarsal bone. It flexes the ankle and everts the foot.
Tibialis anterior (Figure 7–11)	Proximal attachment is on the lateral and upper part of the tibia. It extends down the front of the leg and attaches at the metatarsal bone of the big toe. It flexes the foot at the ankle and inverts the foot.
Extensor digitorum longus (Figure 7–11)	Attaches proximally to the lateral condyle of the tibia and upper anterior surface of the fibula. It extends down the outside of the leg and attaches onto the second and third phalanges of the four toes. It flexes the ankle, extends the toes, and everts the foot.
Extensor hallucis longus (Figure 7–11)	Attaches proximally to the anterior of the middle and lower fibula, extends down the anterior-lateral side of the leg, and attaches to the big toe. It extends the big toe and flexes the foot.

Muscular actions in the foot

The foot is a complex structure which is uniquely designed to play a major role in locomotion, balance, and cushioning of the force when landing. The foot includes many joints, and because of the actions of these joints it is able to invert, evert, abduct, adduct, pronate, and supinate. These movements occur mostly in the tarsal joints. The toes may be flexed or extended. Inversion and adduction combined result in supination, while eversion and abduction combined result in pronation of the foot. Some of the foot movements are not analyzed in this text because they are not significant enough in vigorous performance to warrant consideration. Only

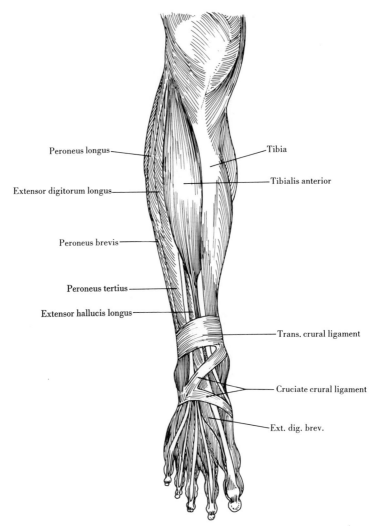

Peroneus longus

Extensor digitorum longus

Peroneus brevis

Peroneus tertius

Extensor hallucis longus

Tibia

Tibialis anterior

Trans. crural ligament

Cruciate crural ligament

Ext. dig. brev.

Figure 7–11.
Muscles of the front of the lower leg. (*After Goss*)

supination and pronation of the foot and flexion of the toes are discussed in this text.

There are twenty muscles contributing to foot movements which are worthy of mention here. Nine of the muscles extend from the lower leg, across the ankle joint, and attach to bones in the foot. The other eleven muscles are located totally in the foot.

Supination of the foot

Supination is not a strong movement, but it is frequently used in sports. The supinator muscles are used in running and walking where zigzagging and dodging are involved, and in side-stepping and other performances where body weight is shifted in a lateral direction. Such movements are frequent in field and court games—tennis, badminton, baseball, soccer, football, skiing, etc. Four muscles are important contributors to foot supination.

Tibialis anterior (Figure 7–11)   See Dorsiflexion, page 111.

Tibialis posterior (Figure 7–10)   See Plantar Flexion, page 109.

Flexor digitorum longus (Figures 7–10 and 7–13)   See Plantar Flexion, page 109.

Flexor hallucis longus (Figures 7–10 and 7–13)   See Plantar Flexion, page 110.

Pronation of the foot

Foot pronation is used with about the same frequency as supination. As one foot is used in supination, the other is generally used in pronation. Such is the case in dodging, side-stepping, and shifting the weight laterally from one foot to the other. For instance, if a field runner sidesteps to the right the supinators of the left foot and the pronators of the right foot are important contributors. Also, the pronators and supinators of opposite feet work effectively together when the body weight is shifted laterally, as in a tennis stroke, golf swing, and batting, skiing, and throwing actions or when the body is "set" to resist lateral force. Four muscles pronate the foot.

*Peroneus brevis (Figures 7–9 and 7–11)	See Plantar Flexion, page 109.
*Peroneus longus (Figures 7–10 and 7–11)	See Plantar Flexion, page 109.
Peroneus tertius (Figure 7–11)	See Dorsiflexion, page 111.
Extensor digitorum longus (Figure 7–11)	See Dorsiflexion, page 111.

Toe flexion

Toe flexion is one of the most important and frequently used movements. It is used extensively in locomotion, especially walking and running. And it is of prime importance in all performances where the body is thrust, as in jumping (Figure 18–1). Seven different muscles are important contributors to toe flexion.

*Flexor digitorum longus (Figures 7–10 and 7–13)	See Plantar Flexion, page 109.

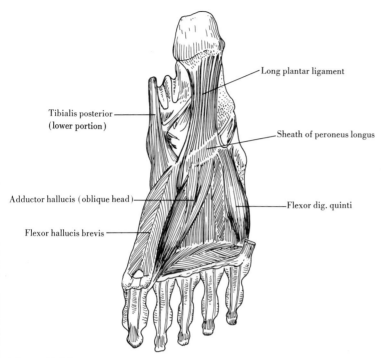

Long plantar ligament

Tibialis posterior
(lower portion)

Sheath of peroneus longus

Adductor hallucis (oblique head)

Flexor dig. quinti

Flexor hallucis brevis

Figure 7–12.
Deep muscles of the bottom of the foot. (*After Goss*)

*Flexor hallucis longus (Figures 7–10 and 7–13)	See Plantar Flexion, page 110.
Flexor digitorum brevis (Figure 7–14)	Proximal attachment is on the medial process of the tuberosity of the calcaneus. It extends along the middle underside of the foot, and attaches to the phalanges of the second, third, and fourth toes. It flexes the toes.
Flexor hallucis brevis (Figure 7–12)	Attaches proximally to the area known as the cuboid (under the arch of the foot) and extends diagonally to the lateral side of the foot. It attaches to the first phalanx of the big toe. It flexes the big toe.

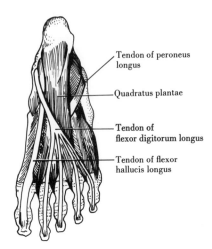

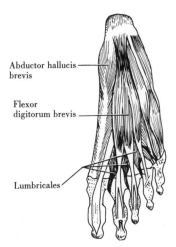

Figure 7–13.
Middle-layer muscles of the bottom of the foot. (*After Dawson*)

Figure 7–14.
Superficial muscles of the bottom of the foot. (*After Dawson*)

Adductor hallucis (obliquus) (Figure 7–12)	Attaches proximally to the second, third, and fourth metatarsal bones and ligaments (approximately under the arch), extends along the medial side of the bottom of the foot, and attaches to the medial side of the first phalanx of the big toe. It adducts and flexes the big toe.
Lumbricalis (Figure 7–14)	Attaches proximally to the tendons of the flexor digitorum longus (about 1 inch behind the toes). It splits into four small muscles, which attach to the phalanges of the four outer toes. It extends the last phalanges of the toes, and flexes the first phalanges.
Quadratus plantae (Figure 7–13)	Attaches proximally to the anterior surface of the calcaneus, and extends to the arch of the foot, where it attaches to the tendon of the flexor digitorum longus. It flexes the toes.

The toes are also capable of extension, and a very limited amount of abduction, adduction, and circumduction. But these movements are not significant contributions to performance.

Recommended supplementary reading

RASCH, PHILIP J., and ROGER K. BURKE: "Kinesiology and Applied Anatomy," 3d ed., chaps. 15–17, Lea and Febiger, Philadelphia, 1967.

THOMPSON, CLEM W.: "Kranz Manual of Kinesiology," 5th ed., chaps. 6–8, The C. V. Mosby Company, St. Louis, 1965.

WELLS, KATHERINE F.: "Kinesiology," 4th ed., chaps. 17–19, W. B. Saunders Company, Philadelphia, 1966.

Student projects

A. After carefully studying the muscular actions of the lower extremities, indicate on the following muscle action table which muscles cause each movement. Mark PM to indicate prime mover and AM to indicate assistant mover.

B. On the skeletal charts at the end of this chapter, place drawings of the muscles in the lower extremities discussed in this chapter. Trace additional charts if needed.

Muscle Action Table: Lower Extremities

				Hip		
	FLEXION	EXTENSION	ABDUCTION	ADDUCTION	MEDIAL ROTATION	LATERAL ROTATION
Rectus femoris						
Pectineus						
Psoas major						
Iliacus						
Sartorius						
Adductor brevis						
Adductor longus						
Adductor magnus						
Gracilis						
Biceps femoris						
Semimembranosus						
Semitendinosus						
Gluteus maximus						
Gluteus medius						
Gluteus minimus						
Gemelli						
Tensor fasciae latae						
Obturator externus						
Obturator internus						
Piriformis						

	Knee and Lower Leg			
	FLEXION	EXTENSION	MEDIAL ROTATION	LATERAL ROTATION
Biceps femoris				
Semimembranosus				
Semitendinosus				
Gastrocnemius				
Sartorius				
Gracilis				
Plantaris				
Popliteus				
Rectus femoris				
Vastus intermedius				
Vastus medialis				
Vastus lateralis				

	Ankle and Foot					
	DORSIFLEXION	PLANTAR FLEXION	SUPINATION	PRONATION	TOE EXTENSION	TOE FLEXION
Tibialis anterior						
Extensor digitorum longus						
Extensor hallucis longus						
Peroneus tertius						
Peroneus longus						
Peroneus brevis						
Gastrocnemius						
Soleus						
Tibialis posterior						
Flexor digitorum longus						
Flexor hallucis longus						
Flexor digitorum brevis						
Flexor hallucis brevis						
Adductor hallucis						
Lumbricalis						
Quadratus plantae						
Extensor digitorum brevis						

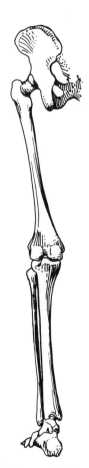

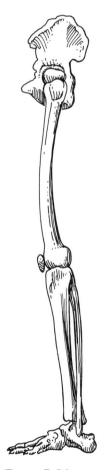

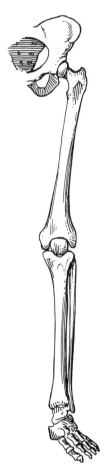

Figure 7–15.
Skeleton of the lower ex-
tremities (posterior).

Figure 7–16.
Skeleton of the lower ex-
tremities (side).

Figure 7–17.
Skeleton of the lower ex-
tremities (anterior).

8

Increasing the effectiveness of muscles

his chapter presents important facts about muscular strength, endurance, power, speed of contraction, and tone that are pertinent to the improvement of muscle use.

Strength

Strength is the ability of the body or a segment of the body to apply force. People often have the impression that strength is simply the contractile force of a muscle or group of muscles. But strength involves a combination of three factors: (1) the combined contractile forces of the muscles causing the movement; (2) the ability to coordinate the agonist muscles with the antagonist, neutralizer, and stabilizer muscles; and (3) the mechanical ratios of the lever (bone) arrangements involved. The first factor depends on the maximum contractile force of each muscle agonistic to the movement. This force can be increased significantly through progressive resistance training. The second factor depends on the ability to coordinate the contractions of the individual muscles. This coordination can be improved by practicing the particular movements involved (develop skill in the movements). The third factor depends on the relative length of the resistance and effort arms of the levers. Sometimes this ratio can be altered advantageously by changing positions of certain body parts.

Strength is basic to motor performance, and some leading educators and coaches claim it is the most important single factor in performance. Because almost all vigorous performances depend on ability to apply great force against a resistance, increased strength will often contribute to better performance.

The contractile force of a muscle is directly related to the cross-sectional measurement of that muscle. As muscle strength increases, the cross section of the individual muscle fibers increases, resulting in a greater cross-sectional area of the total muscle. Theoretically, this measurement is proportionate to strength. However, this is not always true because other factors are involved. For instance:

(1) Two muscles having equal cross sections may differ in strength due to varying amounts of fatty tissue. Fat not only lacks ability to contract, but it also causes friction and interference with the shortening of muscle fibers. (2) The proportion of active fibers in different muscles influences strength. And (3) the efficiency of contraction has an important influence on strength. Nevertheless, muscle size and strength are very closely related.

Conditions influencing strength development

Several conditions influence the rate that strength develops and how long it is retained. Following are brief discussions of the more important facts which affect strength.

Strength may be increased by training.   A muscle increases in strength when it contracts regularly against resistance greater than usual. If the rate of increase is to be rapid, the muscle must contract regularly against a heavy resistance, and the resistance must be increased as the muscle increases in strength. This is known as a *progressive resistance strength-building program.* Strength gains in certain muscles of over 100 percent in a week have been reported on rare occasions. But typically, strength gains of 5 percent weekly over several weeks are considered a fast rate of gain. Percent of gain is usually greater during the early part of training, especially if the muscles are weak in the beginning.

Not all muscles respond equally.   When the same training program is used, the amount of strength development varies among different people. Within each individual, certain muscles respond better to strength stimuli than other muscles. When put on a strength-building program of equal intensity, some muscles may increase at 5 percent weekly, while others increase only 1 percent. This results partly because some muscles are in better condition at the beginning of training; ordinarily, those in poor condition increase more rapidly than those in good condition.

When vigorous muscle use ceases, strength decreases.   Research results show that when a strength-building program ceases, the individual begins to lose strength almost immediately (five to ten days). Strength developed at a slow rate lasts longer than strength developed rapidly. On the average, after strength training ceases, strength is lost at approximately one-third the rate it was gained. But a small amount of the gained strength remains indefinitely. If a segment of the body is completely immobilized, as when placed in a cast, strength decreases very rapidly (20 to 30 percent per week).

Strength relates closely to age.   Strength increases at a rather steady rate from birth to about age twenty-five (18 for women), at which time it levels off and then begins to decline at a gradual rate. At age sixty-five the typical individual is approximately 70 to 80 percent as strong as he was at age twenty-five. Of course, the rate at which a person develops and loses strength is influenced by his rate of maturation and the amount and kind of activity in which he participates. As a result of training, a person can maintain near-maximum strength for several years beyond age twenty-five.

Contractile force varies with muscle length during contraction.   The contractile force of a muscle is greatest when the muscle is fully extended (on stretch). Force steadily diminishes as the muscle moves through contraction (shortens); when the muscle is fully contracted, its contractile force has been reduced to zero. This situation may be paralleled to a rubber band, which has its greatest tension when on stretch. It should be noted that contractile force does not reduce in the same proportion as the length of the muscle. During the early phase of contraction, force reduces much more slowly than muscle length; whereas during the late phase, force reduces proportionately faster than muscle length.

Strength differs slightly on the two sides of the body.   Even though right-handed people use the right side of the body considerable more than the left side (vice versa for left-handed people), the right side is only slightly stronger, and its musculature is only slightly larger than that of the left side. Physiologists generally attribute this to the cross transfer theory, which means that training of one side of the body will influence the development of like muscles on the other side.

With equal training, strength develops more slowly among women than men.   Research results on this topic are conflicting, but the available information favors that after the age of approximately twelve years, females respond slightly less readily to strength stimuli than males. When male sex hormones (testosterone) are injected into women during training, they develop strength at an increased rate. The main reason men are stronger than women is not that they differ in response to strength stimuli, but that men are larger than women. Per cubic unit of muscle, women are nearly as strong as men.

Reserve strength becomes available under great stress or excitement. The reserve strength theory is supported by observations of people who performed great feats of strength while under emotional stress or excitement and were unable to perform voluntarily the same feats after the emotional state had passed. This idea has little support from research, probably because the topic is difficult to treat experimentally. The excitement and stress cannot be provided under controlled conditions. Physiologists have explained reserve strength as a condition resulting from (1) increased secretion of adrenalin, causing the muscles to become more irritable, or (2) a stronger stimulus from the central nervous system and a reduction of inhibitions, causing more muscle fibers to respond.

Methods of increasing strength

To increase rapidly in strength, muscles must be contracted against heavy resistance, and the resistance must be increased as the muscles become stronger.

In other words, the overload principle is applied—meaning the muscles are loaded beyond previous requirements. There are several different approaches to developing strength. In fact, any form of exercise which applies heavier than usual resistance to muscle contractions will stimulate an increase in strength. Strength-building stimuli may be provided by:

1. Hard manual labor or vigorous athletic performance
2. Specific exercises against body weight, as in pull-ups or dips (additional weight may be added to body weight)
3. Exercises against external movable resistance, such as weight-training equipment and wall pulleys
4. Application of muscle tension against a fixed object or another body part

The first three methods result in isotonic (dynamic) contractions, meaning the muscles change in length and movement of body segments occurs. The fourth method results in isometric (static) contractions, meaning the muscles apply tension but do not shorten, and movements of body segments do not occur (small amount of movement may occur).

Isotonic (dynamic) strength-building methods.   Prior to World War II, strength-building programs were used very little in athletic training. In fact, it was generally believed that "muscle-boundness" resulted from such programs. They were taboo to those seeking to improve performance. During World War II, Thomas DeLorme experienced great success with heavy resistance exercises in the rehabilitation of hospital patients. Following his work, much research was done to determine the effectiveness of this type of training for improving athletic performance. It was learned that increased strength was highly beneficial to athletic performance and that heavy resistance exercise was the most expedient method of increasing strength. Hence, weight training gained popularity among athletes and coaches.

Strength can be increased most rapidly by exercising against very heavy resistance for a few repetitions. After much study and experimentation, DeLorme and Watkins (**21**) declared that strength can be increased at the most rapid rate by employing heavy resistance for 10 repetitions and three sets. They specifically recommended the following program to be executed every second day.

One set of 10 repetitions with ½ 10 RMs
One set of 10 repetitions with ¾ 10 RMs
One set of 10 repetitions with 10 RMs

(RM means repetition maximum. Ten RMs is 10 repetitions of an exercise using the maximum weight that can be lifted successively 10 times.)

Recently, other investigators have produced evidence that even fewer repetitions and heavier weight are more effective. For instance, Berger (**8**) found that strength increases most rapidly when four to eight RMs are used with three sets. Other studies have added support to Berger's findings. Currently there is lack of agreement among experts about the exact program that is best for building strength, but the following points are well established and universally accepted:

1. Exercises must be selected to work the specific muscles in which strength is to be developed.
2. Muscles should be contracted regularly (every second day) against heavy resistance.
3. Near-maximum weight for 10 repetitions (or less) should be used.
4. The weight must be progressively increased as strength increases, to provide continual overload to the muscles. (This is progressive resistance.)

Suppose you wanted to design a strength-building program for a shot-putter, who requires great strength and speed. In analyzing the putting action, it becomes apparent that the following muscle groups are major contributors:

Finger flexors	Trunk extensors
Wrist flexors	Trunk and hip rotators
Elbow extensors	Hip extensors
Shoulder flexors (horizontal position)	Knee extensors
Shoulder girdle elevators and protractors	Ankle plantar flexors

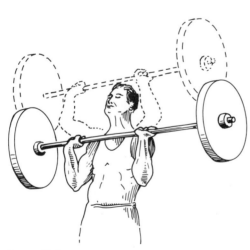

Figure 8–1.
Two-arm press exercise (isotonic).

By this time you know which muscles are involved in each of the above groups. You can now proceed to select exercises which apply heavy resistance to those muscles. A typical procedure follows:

1. Select the specific exercises to be performed every second day.
2. Determine the maximum amount of weight that can be lifted with each exercise, and start with 50 percent of maximum weight.
3. Perform 10 repetitions and three sets of each exercise with two to four minutes between sets.
4. Increase weight approximately 5 percent (more if possible) each week (progressive resistance).

Specific exercises for strengthening certain muscles can be obtained from weight-training charts and books. However, with knowledge of the actions of the major skeletal muscles, you should be able to design your own exercise program to suit your specific purpose. If in doubt, the exercise movement which most closely resembles the skill in which you are interested will probably be the correct choice. Be aware that the resistance must oppose the actions of the muscles you want to strengthen.

Isometric (static) strength-building methods.   Studies which support increasing strength through static muscular contractions were introduced by Hettinger and Muller of Germany in 1953. Since that time, coaches and athletes have been almost too enthusiastic about implementing isometric programs. Implementation has been more rapid than the development of knowledge about the effectiveness of static exercises. Since Hettinger and Muller's original study, numerous other studies have been published, most of which generally support the belief that strength can be increased at a rapid rate by use of isometrics.

Muller and Rohmert of Germany established evidence that strength will increase more rapidly by use of isometrics when (1) near-maximum muscle contractions are used and (2) five to ten repetitions are used. They also established the theory that strength will increase more evenly throughout the range of motion if the contractions are executed at various positions.

On the basis of presently available evidence, the following points are presented as guides for designing isometric strength-building programs:

1. Best results can be obtained by using near-maximum contractions of five to six seconds in length and repeating five or more times, with a few seconds' rest between contractions.
2. The exercises should be performed daily.
3. The contractions should be applied at varying points throughout the range of motion if maximum strength is desired throughout the full range. Where strength is needed only at the beginning of the motion, as in ballistic movements, the exercises should be designed accordingly.

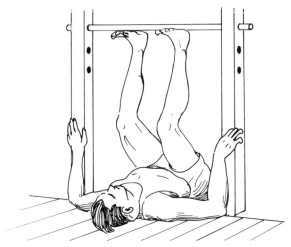

Figure 8–2.
Two-leg press exercise (isometric).

Comparison of isometric and isotonic methods.   When the programs described above are used, strength gains from isometric and isotonic methods appear about equal. However, each program has certain advantages, and final selection should be based on administrative feasibility and personal preference. Following are some guides:

> 1. For some individuals there is a psychological advantage in isotonic exercises because the performance of heavy work can be seen.
> 2. More muscular hypertrophy and, it appears, more muscular endurance result from isotonic exercises. Also, some experts claim that isotonic exercises have a more favorable influence on coordination because they require use of the muscles throughout the range of motion.
> 3. The greatest advantage of the isometric method is administrative economy and feasibility. It requires less time, less effort, less space, and much less equipment than the isotonic method. A reasonable amount of ingenuity can make a good isometric program possible with the equipment normally available in a gymnasium and by having students work in pairs to provide resistance for each other. However, when measures are taken to eliminate the disadvantages of this method, some of its advantages are lost.

Other strength-building methods.   In addition to pure isometric and isotonic methods, some programs combining the two methods have received limited attention. Reasonable success has been experienced with the following procedure:

> 1. Contract the muscles isometrically against a rope or cable arrangement. After tension has been held for five or six seconds, reduce the resistance which holds the

rope, allowing slow-motion isotonic contractions to occur. This exercise combines isometric and isotonic contractions.

2. Repeat each exercise five to six times, and do so daily.

Another method that has had limited use and experimentation is *intermediatory exercises.* Isotonic contractions are executed in slow motion to a 10-second count. The weight is lifted slowly over a 10-second period, then lowered at the same rate. Each repetition is followed by a 10-second rest, and 10 repetitions are executed daily. There is little evidence either for or against this method, but some successful athletes do employ it.

Still another method is *functional overload* in which the activity itself is performed under resisted conditions. Weighted vests, ankle weights, and other weighted objects and implements are used. This method has the advantage of closely coordinating the strength gains into the activity pattern, but some experts think that it reduces coordination and timing.

Endurance

Endurance is defined as resistance to fatigue and quick recovery after fatigue. This definition may apply to the body as a whole, to a particular body system, or to a local area of the muscle system. For instance, we sometimes refer to total body endurance, circulorespiratory endurance, muscular endurance, or endurance of a particular part of the muscular system. But regardless of how many different names we give to endurance, the loss of it (fatigue) always has the same result— the muscles discontinue to function effectively. The exact location of the fatigue which causes muscle failure is extremely difficult to determine.

A high level of endurance implies that the person can maintain a given level of performance. When endurance gives way to fatigue as a result of muscular work, several elements important for good performance diminish: strength, timing, neuromuscular coordination, speed of movement, reaction time, and general alertness. Increased endurance prolongs the onset of fatigue; therefore, endurance contributes to improved performance when fatigue is a limiting factor.

Conditions influencing endurance

Several factors influence endurance. Following are brief discussions of the more important factors.

Strength contributes to muscular endurance.   Suppose a man has a given amount of strength with which he is able to move a particular amount of resistance through the range of motion one hundred times. If his strength were increased 50 percent, he would be able to move the same resistance with greater ease; therefore, he could repeat the movement considerably more than one hundred times. Increased strength would result in increased muscular endurance.

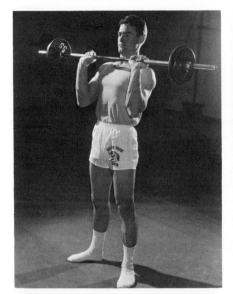
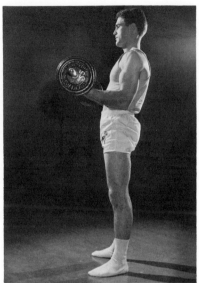
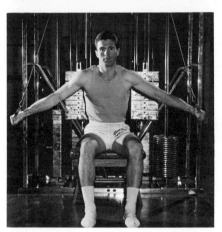
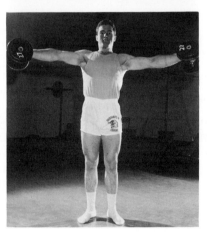

Neuromuscular skill influences endurance.   During performance, a certain amount of energy is wasted in unnecessary and uncoordinated movements. The skilled individual wastes less energy than the unskilled. It has been found that an unskilled swimmer may use more than five times as much energy as a skilled person to swim the same distance. Similar comparisons could be made between skilled and unskilled performers in other activities.

Fatty tissue within and surrounding the muscles decreases endurance. Fat lacks the ability to contract; therefore, it does not contribute to an individual's

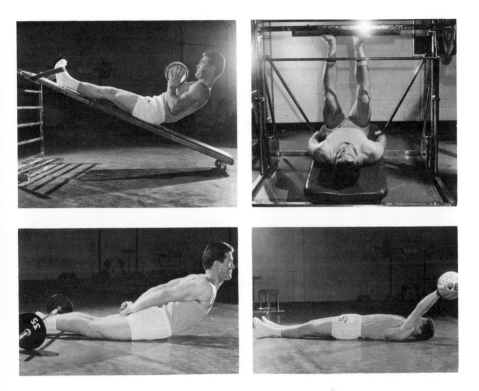

Figure 8–3.
Examples of isotonic exercises that work the major muscle groups. These groups may
be worked by isotonic exercises which employ the body's weight or some external weight
for resistance, or by isometric exercises.

performance. In fact, it hinders performance in three ways: (1) Fat within the
muscle causes friction and contributes to inefficiency in muscle contractions;
(2) fat within and surrounding the muscle adds dead weight, increasing resistance
against the movement; (3) fatty tissue places an overload on the circulatory
system. It is estimated that 1 pound of fat causes an increase in the vascular
system of 1 mile.

**Sustained muscular work is dependent upon the circulatory and respira-
tory systems.**   For a muscle to continue to function, the individual muscle
cells must receive nutrients and oxygen from the circulatory system, which also
transports waste products from the muscles. The respiratory system supplies
oxygen to the circulatory system and receives carbon dioxide and other waste
from it. If the circulatory and cooperating systems do not keep the muscles adequately supplied with nutrients and oxygen and free of waste products, fatigue
occurs.

Sustained muscular work is dependent upon the nervous system.   A muscle contracts only when it receives a stimulus, and the strength of its contraction is dependent partly upon the intensity of the stimulus. (A more intense stimulus causes more motor units to respond with each unit contracting to its maximum.) Therefore, under strenuous effort, if the nervous system does not continue to supply the muscles with intense stimuli, the muscles will not continue to contract strongly. In such a case, the muscles appear to be fatigued, but the actual location of fatigue may be in the nervous system. Classic experiments with frogs reveal that in the connections between neurons (synapses) and between the neuron and its motor unit, fatigue occurs more readily than either in the nerve or in the muscle tissue itself.

Muscular endurance is dependent upon one's ability to tolerate a high level of acid waste.   The process of muscle contraction results in acid waste products, primarily lactic acid. Muscular activity is greatly hindered, and in fact it usually ends, when the lactate level in the blood is between 0.032 and 0.140 percent. Therefore, a person's endurance is strongly influenced by his ability to dispose of lactic acid and to tolerate a high level of this by-product. Tolerance seems to increase as a result of training.

Endurance is related to body type, sex, and age.   The following relationships exist: (1) On the average, mesomorphs (heavily muscled athletic type) and ectomorphs (slight body type) are more durable than endomorphs (obese type) with mesomorphs slightly more durable than ectomorphs. (However, there are exceptions to these rules.) (2) Up to the age of approximately thirteen, boys and girls possess about the same amount of endurance. After age thirteen, the durability of girls increases very little, while that of boys continues to increase to at least maturity, and sometimes considerably beyond that. Some men have been known to increase in endurance until they reach their middle thirties. (3) The relationship between age and endurance varies. Endurance increases with age up to a certain point, at which time endurance begins to decrease as age increases. Peak endurance potential occurs somewhat later than peak strength potential.

The most economical pace is an even rate over the entire distance.   In walking, running, swimming, and other locomotive activities, stopping, starting, accelerating, and decelerating are very costly in terms of energy. Therefore, the most economical approach is to distribute evenly the available energy over the entire distance. Theoretically, a four-minute mile should consist of four 60-second quarters; however, this is not feasible because the quarters are influenced by the start and finish of the race and by the necessity of gaining and holding position during the race. The idea of even pace also has strong application to long-duration games, such as basketball, soccer, tennis, or handball. Playing in "bursts" requires much additional energy.

Methods of increasing endurance

Because endurance is a factor in almost all vigorous performances, methods of increasing endurance are of prime concern. We have already talked of the need to apply the overload principle for the development of strength—that principle must also be applied if endurance is to be increased. Overload for endurance simply means working the organism beyond previous repetition levels.

The most expedient method of increasing the *endurance of a particular muscle group* is to contract those muscles regularly against reasonably heavy resistance for near-maximum repetitions for three sets. Research results show that 20 to 30 RMs with three sets will increase endurance faster than 100 RMs with three sets. There is also evidence that 10 RMs with three sets will increase endurance as fast as a greater number. Ten RMs will increase strength and endurance simultaneously, while more RMs with less resistance increase endurance but have little influence on strength and muscle size. Hence, if increased endurance and strength are desired, a strength-endurance building program is preferred (10 RMs for three sets). If increased endurance without increased strength and increased size is desired, then more RMs (20 to 30) with lighter weight should be employed.

In *total body endurance* or *circulorespiratory endurance*, the main limiting factor is oxygen supply to the working tissues. The most effective method for increasing both general and circulorespiratory endurance is interval training, which consists of a number of short bouts of vigorous exercise with a brief recovery period following each bout.

Interval training for endurance makes very good sense from the physiological point of view because the prime objective of an endurance training program is to expose the person to the greatest work load before the onset of fatigue. This can be accomplished best through interval training. Research results (**22**) show that a work level which can be tolerated for an hour with the interval training technique will bring about exhaustion in nine minutes when done continuously. Thus, the total work accomplished before fatigue is more than three times greater when interval training is used instead of continuous training. This greater output of work during a particular training session results in a stronger endurance stimulus.

The interval training technique is used extensively for swimmers and distance runners and can be used successfully for total body conditioning of performers in activities such as wrestling, baseball, basketball, and various field sports. It has been found that interval training produce the best results when each exercise bout consists of approximately 30 seconds of vigorous work (running, swimming, or other forms of exercise), followed by light exercise or rest for two to three minutes or less. DeVries (**22**) states that the rest interval is adequate when the resting heart rate returns to 120 beats per minute. (This figure undoubtedly varies for different individuals.) He also points out that training can be hampered by working the organism to total fatigue. The person should be able to recover from a workout within a few hours.

Endurance overload may result from interval training by adjusting the program in any of the following ways:

1. Gradually increase the intensity of the work in each bout.
2. Gradually increase the duration of each work bout.
3. Shorten the interval between work bouts.
4. Increase the number of work bouts in a particular training session.

Suppose a workout consists of fifteen 220-yard runs at three-fourths full speed with a two- to three-minute rest between runs. In this case, overloading could be caused by increasing the speed of each run, by increasing the distance of each run, by shortening the rest period between runs, or by increasing the total number of runs in a single workout. For increased endurance, athletes must not be brought along too fast or too slow. It is important that the highest level of endurance be reached at the climax of the performance season—not before or after. To establish the correct rate of increase of endurance requires sound interpretation of the athlete's present state of condition and his potential for endurance development.

Muscular power

Muscular power is a combination of speed and strength. It is the ability to apply force at a rapid rate. Power is typically demonstrated in projecting the body (as in the long jump) or an object (such as putting the shot) through space, wherein the muscles must apply strong force at a rapid rate to give the body or object the momentum necessary to carry it the desired distance. When expressed by a formula,

Power = force × velocity

It is possible for a person to be extremely strong and still not be extremely powerful; also, he may be able to move with great speed against a very light resistance but lack the strength to move rapidly against heavier resistance. Thus, he may be strong but not powerful, and he may have great speed but not power. If, however, he possesses great strength combined with great speed of movement, he is powerful.

Muscular power is very important to vigorous performances because it determines how hard a person can hit, how far he can throw, how high he can jump, and, to some extent, how fast he can run or swim. Power can be increased by increasing strength without sacrificing speed, by increasing speed of movement without sacrificing strength, or by increasing both speed and strength. The best approach to increasing power is to increase strength (force). However, speed can also be increased a limited amount as a result of training. Both speed and force can be stressed by applying strong force through rapid (explosive) motion.

Speed of muscular contraction

In different species the rate of contraction of muscle tissue varies greatly, and, generally, the smaller the species, the faster its muscles contract. (However, there are several exceptions to this rule.) In addition, among individual members within a particular species, muscle tissue varies a limited amount in its rate of contraction. And within an individual, different muscles contract at different rates of speed. In the human being, for instance, postural muscles (which are red) are relatively slow contractors, while most of the other motor muscles (which are pale) contract rapidly. In addition, there is a relationship between the size of different muscles and their speed of contraction; the smaller muscles tend to contract faster than the larger ones. However, there are also many exceptions to these rules.

The relative speed of contraction of different muscles varies greatly among individuals. For example, person A may have faster leg actions while person B has faster arm actions. Moreover, person A's arm extensor muscles may contract relatively fast while his arm flexors contract relatively slowly. In other words, speed varies with the individual body movement. Although a person is a slow runner, he may have very fast arm and finger movements.

If all else is equal, a longer muscle will produce proportionately greater speed than a shorter one. Assume that muscle A and muscle B contract at the same rate of speed per linear inch of muscle and that muscle A is five times as long as muscle B. Muscle A will contract five times as far as muscle B in a given period of time simply because it is five times longer.

Increasing speed of contraction

A muscle almost always contracts against some resistance, even if the resistance is only the weight of the body segment being moved. Because of this, strength can influence the rate of contraction. If all else remains equal, as a muscle becomes stronger, the resistance has less retarding effect on speed of contraction. As the amount of resistance against which one performs becomes greater, strength has a greater influence on speed of contraction; where resistance is very light, it is doubtful that strength is a significant factor in speed of contraction.

Increased coordination of muscles (skill) can increase the speed of specific movements. As the several mover muscles become better coordinated, they can cooperatively overcome the external resistance with greater speed. When muscles are well coordinated, one contractile force arrives at the peak velocity of the previous force; consequently, the second force is more effective (Newton's law of inertia). Also, as the agonists and antagonists become better coordinated, the antagonists furnish less resistance to the contractile efforts of the agonists. If increased speed is desired in a particular performance, the skills should be practiced at rates equal to or exceeding those used in performance.

A. V. Hill (**38**) claims that speed of contraction can be increased by approximately 20 percent by raising body temperature 2°C. The magnitude of this claim lacks sufficient evidence, but it is well established that increased body temperature does increase rate of contraction to some degree. Apparently such increase is due to decreased viscosity of the muscles when body temperature is raised. Raising body temperature a measurable amount requires much work, which is one argument in favor of warm-up in preparation for explosive-type performances. The major problems with warm-up are to prepare the correct muscles (selective activities) and to exercise an amount which is adequate, yet not fatiguing. Another factor is to time the warm-up properly, so its effects are maximum.

The efficiency of muscle contraction can be increased by training, which may result in increased contractile speed. For example, if fatty tissue within a muscle is eliminated or if viscosity is reduced, then friction is reduced. This results in greater efficiency and a faster contraction. If flexibility of antagonist muscles is inadequate, an increase in flexibility will cause those muscles to furnish less resistance to the movement, resulting in greater speed. Also, reducing neural inhibitions as a result of training will allow the performer to call voluntarily upon greater numbers of available motor units. The more motor units involved, the greater the strength and the more quickly the resistance can be overcome.

Influence of speed on muscular power

When the mechanical ratio (leverage) of a body movement remains constant, the speed of movement is directly proportionate to the speed of contraction of the mover muscles. If the rate of contraction were increased by 5 percent, the speed of movement should increase by the same percentage. In turn, the increased speed of movement would contribute to increased power ($P = F \times V$). If other factors remain constant, power will increase in proportion to speed of movement.

Influence of speed on energy cost

The energy cost of a muscle contraction varies with the cube of the speed of contraction. For example, if muscle X contracts twice as fast as muscle Y, the energy cost of muscle X is eight times as great as that of muscle Y. Whereas if muscle X contracts three times as fast as muscle Y, the energy cost of muscle X is twenty-seven times as great as that of muscle Y. This factor has great significance because it explains why maximum efforts produce fatigue so rapidly. In determining one's pace in endurance activities, energy cost is the prime consideration. This explains why spurts of speed and unnecessary rapid movements are undesirable in endurance events.

Muscle Tone

Muscle tone is a condition which gives firmness and proper shape to muscles. It relates to the state of conditioning; that is, a well-conditioned muscle possesses good tone while a poorly conditioned muscle is poorly toned.

Traditionally, muscle tone has been defined as "a constant state of contraction of part of the muscle fibers." Supposedly, this constant contraction results from a steady flow of impulses from the nervous system. Recent evidence expands the traditional definition.

As a result of electromyographic study, Basmajian (6) found that there is both a *passive* and an *active* component which compose muscle tone. The passive component consists of constant electricity in muscles and connective tissues plus turgor, which is the pressure of body fluids tending to distend their surrounding tissues. Always present in muscles, this passive component varies in amount depending upon muscle condition. The active component consists of contraction of certain mucle fibers which are stimulated by the stretch reflex. This dependence on the stretch reflex makes the active component rely upon body posture for its existence. The reflex causes nervous stimulation of certain muscle fibers which contributes to muscle firmness.

Effects of exercise on tone

DeVries (22) reported results of one limited study which indicated that increased strength did not change muscle tone. However, practical experience and observation strongly support the idea that one of the benefits of exercise is increased muscle tone. Increased strength and muscle endurance resulting from exercise is generally accompanied by firmness and proper shape, the most obvious qualities of tone. Lack of exercise produces the opposite results. The loss of strength, endurance, and tone is especially noticeable when a body segment is totally immobilized, as when cast for a fracture. It must be concluded that muscular strength and endurance-building exercises do increase tone. The relationship between tone and other muscular qualities, such as speed, efficiency, and flexibility, is not established. But, highly toned muscles seem to have a degree of tension already available, so they should be better prepared to act.

Summary statement

By increasing *strength, endurance, power,* or *speed of contraction* of the muscles, one's ability to perform can frequently be improved. In fact, such increases are often the best approach to improving performance. Teachers, coaches, and athletes should not overlook these possibilities for improving performance. Increasing *flexibility* of the muscles antagonistic to the primary movements in a performance may help to forestall fatigue and avoid injury.

Recommended supplementary reading

CAPEN, E. K.: Study of Four Programs of Heavy Resistance Exercises for Development of Muscular Strength, *Res. Quart.,* vol. 27, pp. 132–142, 1956.

CLARKE, H. HARRISON: "Muscular Strength and Endurance in Man," Prentice-Hall, Inc., Englewood Cliffs, N.J., 1966.

DeLORME, THOMAS L., and A. L. WATKINS: Techniques of Progressive Resistance Exercise, *Arch. Phys. Therap.,* vol. 29, pp. 262–273, May, 1948.

deVRIES, HERBERT A.: "Physiology of Exercise," William C. Brown Co., Dubuque, Iowa, 1966.

HETTINGER, THEODOR: "Physiology of Strength," Charles C Thomas, Publisher, Springfield, Ill., 1961.

Student project

Select a specific skill which requires a large amount of strength, endurance, or speed. Describe in detail how to best increase muscle effectiveness to cause improvement of that skill. Give specific exercises and procedures to be followed. Do not include any exercise or procedure that you cannot justify.

9

Muscular analysis of a specific skill

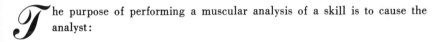he purpose of performing a muscular analysis of a skill is to cause the
analyst:

1. To become fully aware of the specific body actions involved in the performance
2. To become better informed of all the muscles involved in different roles and to
develop a greater insight into the complexity of their coordination patterns
3. To identify the specific muscles and muscle groups used, so that muscle-strength
and endurance-building programs may be designed to benefit those muscles
4. To identify the muscles in which flexibility is needed

The analysis should consist of three major phases. *First,* identify the objectives
and nature of the particular performance; that is, determine exactly what the
performer is attempting to accomplish and how he should proceed in his attempt.
Second, determine the specific body actions that are part of the performance and
identify their sequence. *Third,* identify the muscles which contribute to each action
and indicate each muscle's role in the performance. Following is an example of a
muscle analysis of a specific skill.

Muscle analysis of hurdling action

In hurdling (high hurdles), the objective of the performer is to clear the hurdle
as quickly as possible and come off the hurdle in good running position to sprint
rapidly to the next hurdle. Three running strides are taken between hurdles, and
the hurdle is cleared on the fourth stride. The barrier is not taken in three strides
and a jump, but rather in four running strides, the last of which is longer and
accentuated in action (a leap). The hurdler should leave the ground approximately 7 feet in front of the hurdle and land about 3½ feet behind it.

The pattern of specific body actions in hurdling is complex. In clearing the barrier, the forward leg, led by the knee, should be driven forward and upward to clear the hurdle. At the same time, the upper portion of the body is thrust forward and downward to meet the upward driven leg. The arm opposite the lead leg (or both arms if preferred) is extended forward, and the chest is dipped toward the knee of the lead leg. These movements are coordinated with the upward-forward push from the push-off leg.

As the lead leg clears the hurdle, it is driven downward with tremendous force. The upper body should still be well forward to aid in the downward drive of the leg. As the leg is driven downward, the upper body becomes more erect. At this time the trail leg is whipped forward into the next running stride.

To clear the hurdle as quickly as possible, the runner must thrust his body weight forward, much the same as a high-jumper thrusts his weight upward. This forward thrust of weight tends to pull the runner over the hurdle and to the ground in a minimum length of time.

In working for perfection in hurdling action, the athlete should keep these points in mind: (1) clear the hurdle in the shortest possible time and with as little vertical height as possible, (2) let the hurdle interfere as little as possible with running rhythm, and (3) maintain as near-perfect balance as possible and come off the hurdle into a good sprint position.

On the muscle analysis chart that follows (pp. 140–147) are (1) the more important specific body movements that occur in hurdling and (2) identification

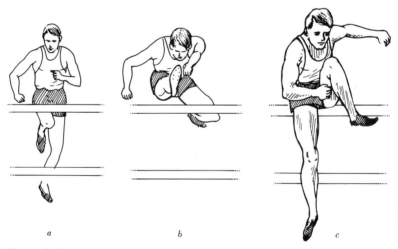

a   *b*   *c*

Figure 9–1.
Body actions in running the high hurdles. (*a*), (*b*), and (*c*) are front views of different phases of the hurdling action.

of the muscles which are involved in each of the movements and the specific role that each muscle plays in the movement. It is not practical to identify all body movements and all muscles that contribute to hurdling; therefore, only those actions and muscles which make major contributions to hurdling are identified.

Student project

Select a performance such as a track and field event, swimming stroke, or gymnastic skill, and write a muscular analysis of the performance similar to the one illustrated in this chapter.

SPECIFIC MOVEMENTS	AGONIST MUSCLES (MOVER)	MAIN STABILIZING ACTIONS	ANTAGONIST MUSCLES (MUST BE RELAXED TO ALLOW MOVEMENT)	MAIN NEUTRALIZING ACTIONS
Movements into the hurdle				
Hip flexion of lead leg (approximately 100°)	Adductor brevis Adductor longus Gracilis Rectus femoris Pectineus Psoas major Sartorius Iliacus (The gracilis and sartorius are probably only partially used in hip flexion in this case, because they also flex the knee. In this case knee extension occurs simultaneous to hip flexion.)	The obliquus abdominis externus and internus and rectus abdominis muscles contract to stabilize the pelvic region on which the leg moves.	Gluteus maximus Biceps femoris Semimembranosus Semitendinosus	The adductor brevis, adductor longus, pectineus, and gracilis muscles all adduct the thigh as they flex it. The sartorius abducts and flexes the thigh, tending to neutralize the adduction of the other four muscles. Probably other hip abductors contract slightly to assist the sartorius. The adductor brevis and longus and the pectineus also laterally rotate the thigh. This is a necessary movement in hurdling; therefore, it is not neutralized.
Knee extension of lead leg (100°)	Rectus femoris Vastus medialis Vastus intermedius Vastus lateralis	In this case the hip flexor muscles are the main stabilizers. While they are contracting to flex the hip, they also give the upper leg the stability it needs so the	Biceps femoris Semimembranosus Plantaris Popliteus Semitendinosus Gastrocnemius	No neutralizing actions occur in knee extension.

knee can extend. Several other muscles which control movements of the upper leg contribute to its stability in this case, but the hip flexors are by far the greatest contributors.

Movement	Muscles	Analysis	Antagonists	Notes
Trunk forward flexion (50°) and rotation toward lead leg (25°)	Rectus abdominis Obliquus externus Obliquus internus Psoas (These muscles all appear in pairs, and when both members of each pair contract, trunk flexion occurs. In order for the desired trunk rotation to occur simultaneously with flexion, one member of each pair of muscles contracts with greater force than the other member. See trunk rotation in Chapter 6 for details. Also, the deep spinal rotator muscles are probably active in this case.	Ordinarily the hip and leg extensors contract to stabilize the legs and pelvis to provide a base on which the trunk can flex. But, in this case, hip flexion and knee extension occur simultaneously with trunk flexion. The weight of the leg and trunk pulled toward each other provides most of the stability necessary for their movement.	Sacrospinalis Semispinalis Multifidus The small and deep posterior muscles of the spine.	The opposite members of each pair of active muscles neutralize each other's tendencies to laterally flex the trunk.
Shoulder flexion of opposite arm (90°)	Coracobrachialis Deltoid (anterior)	When the arm flexes on the shoulder girdle, the girdle	Deltoid (posterior head) Latissimus dorsi	The coracobrachialis and pectoralis major adduct the

SPECIFIC MOVEMENTS	AGONIST MUSCLES (MOVER)	MAIN STABILIZING ACTIONS	ANTAGONIST MUSCLES (MUST BE RELAXED TO ALLOW MOVEMENT)	MAIN NEUTRALIZING ACTIONS
(Cont.)	Pectoralis major (upper portion) Biceps (long head)	tends to depress and rotate downward; therefore, the main stabilizers are those muscles which cause the opposite movements, the elevators and upward rotators of the girdle. They are the levator scapulae, trapezius I and II, and the serratus anterior.	Infraspinatus Teres major Teres minor Triceps (long head)	arm as they flex it. The deltoid (anterior) abducts only slightly as it flexes the arm. Probably the deltoid (middle) and supraspinatus contract lightly to help nullify arm adduction. The pectoralis major also medially rotates the arm, but this action is apparently not neutralized because in hurdling the lead arm does rotate medially as it flexes.
Elbow extension of opposite arm (90°)	Anconeus Triceps Extensor carpi ulnaris Extensor digitorum communis	When the elbow extends, the shoulder tends to extend also. In the case of hurdling, the shoulder is flexed as the elbow extends. The flexion action of the shoulder provides the stability needed for elbow extension.	Biceps Brachialis Brachioradialis Pronator teres Palmaris longus Flexor carpi ulnaris Flexor carpi radialis Flexor digitorium	When the triceps brachii contract to extend the elbow, the long head also tends to extend the shoulder. This means the shoulder flexors must contract with enough force to overpower the shoulder extension action of the triceps.

Pushing off with the leg

SPECIFIC MOVEMENTS	AGONIST MUSCLES (MOVER)	MAIN STABILIZING ACTIONS	ANTAGONIST MUSCLES (MUST BE RELAXED TO ALLOW MOVEMENT)	MAIN NEUTRALIZING ACTIONS
Hip extension of push-off leg (20°)	Gluteus maximus Biceps femoris	The proximal ends of the hip extensors attach to	Adductor brevis Adductor longus	The gluteus maximus adducts and rotates the hip

Semimembranosus Semitendinosus	highly stabile bone structures (the back of the pelvis and the sacrum). Therefore, less stabilizing actions are needed for this movement than other comparable movements. Muscles that help to stabilize the pelvis and sacrum for this movement are the obliquus abdominis (internus and externus) and the quadratus lumborum.	Gracilis Pectineus Sartorius Iliacus (Ordinarily the rectus femoris and psoas muscles would be listed as antagonistic to hip extension. They are not listed in this case because here the rectus is active in causing the knee to extend, and the psoas is contracting to pull the trunk downward. Their tendency to resist hip extension simply has to be nullified by the hip extensor muscles.)	laterally in addition to extending it. The gluteus medius and minimus muscles must contract to nullify those undesired actions. The medius and minimus muscles also cause hip medial rotation, which is desired in this case. The hamstring group (biceps femoris, semimembranosus, and semitendinosus) tend to flex the knee as they extend the hip. Knee flexion is undesired in this case; therefore, the knee extensors contract with enough force to extend the knee, thus nullifying the knee flexion action of the hamstrings.
Knee extension of push-off leg (20°) Rectus femoris Vastus medialis Vastus intermedius Vastus lateralis	When the knee extends, the hip tends to flex because of the dual action of the rectus femoris. Hip flexion is not desired so the hip extensors must contract to stabilize the upper leg. Actually they are contracting with maximum force to cause hip extension.	Plantaris Popliteus (Ordinarily the gastrocnemius and the hamstring group would be listed as antagonistic to knee extension. But in this case the hamstrings must be active in hip extension, which occurs simultaneously with	In this case knee extension and hip extension are desired simultaneously. The rectus femoris is a prime mover in knee extension, but, at the same time, it flexes the hip. Therefore, its hip flexion action is overcome by the hip extensors which are contract-

SPECIFIC MOVEMENTS	AGONIST MUSCLES (MOVER)	MAIN STABILIZING ACTIONS	ANTAGONIST MUSCLES (MUST BE RELAXED TO ALLOW MOVEMENT)	MAIN NEUTRALIZING ACTIONS
(Cont.)			knee extension. The gastrocnemius is active in plantar flexion of the ankle.)	ing with maximum force here.
Plantar flexion of the push-off foot (40°)	Gastrocnemius Peroneus brevis Peroneus longus Tibialis posterior Flexor hallucis longus Flexor digitorum longus Soleus	Very little muscle contraction is required for stabilization in this case. The foot is firm against the surface, and the weight of the body rests upon it. In this case plantar flexion can bring about only one action, and that is the desired one.	Peroneus tertius Tibialis anterior Extensor hallucis longus Extensor digitorum longus	The peroneus longus and peroneus brevis contribute to foot pronation in addition to plantar flexion. The tibialis posterior tends to neutralize the pronation because it supinates and plantar flexes the foot at the same time.
Toe flexion of the push-off foot (30°)	Flexor digitorum brevis Flexor digitorum longus Flexor hallucis longus Adductor hallucis obliquus Flexor hallucis brevis Interossei plantar Lumbricalis Quadratus plantae	None necessary	Extensor digitorum brevis Extensor digitorum longus Extensor hallucis longus	None
Clearing the hurdle				
Hip abduction of trail leg (80°)	Gluteus medius Gluteus minimus	When one leg abducts, the pelvic region tends to tilt	Adductor brevis Adductor longus	When the abductors contract, three of them (glu-

	Gemelli (superior and inferior) Obturator internus Obturator externus Piriformis Quadratus femoris Sartorius Tensor fasciae latae	toward that leg due to the pull of the abductor muscles on the pelvis. The pelvis is stabilized from lateral tilt by the obliquus abdominis (externus and internus) and the quadratus lumborum muscle on the same side as the abducted leg. In turn, their contractions tend to tilt the upper portion of the trunk. This causes numerous other muscles to contract to keep the trunk aligned.	Adductor magnus Gracilis Gluteus maximus	teus medius, gluteus minimus, and tensor fasciae) rotate the leg medially. This action is neutralized by the other two abductors (piriformis and sartorius) which tend to rotate the leg laterally as they abduct it.
Horizontal flexion of trail leg (90°) *	Same as hip flexor muscles (see first movement listed)	Same as in hip flexion.	Same as in hip flexion.	Little if any neutralizing action occurs.
Knee flexion of trail leg (100°)	Biceps femoris Semimembranosus Plantaris Popliteus Semitendinosus Gastrocnemius	When the knee flexes, the upper leg tends to extend because of contraction of the hamstring group. In this particular case, the upper leg is stabilized against extension by the action of the hip flexors, which contract to flex the hip at the	Vastus medialis Vastus intermedius Vastus lateralis (The rectus femoris is antagonistic to knee flexion, but in this case it does not relax because it is active in horizontal flexion of the hip.)	In addition to flexing the knee, the biceps femoris rotates it laterally when it is flexed. The other three knee flexors rotate the knee medially when it is flexed. The rectus femoris overpowers the rotary actions of the other muscles, causing

* It should be made clear that hip abduction of the trail leg occurs simultaneously with the early phase of horizontal flexion of that leg. During the latter phase of horizontal flexion, hip adduction occurs. Most of the force for adduction results from gravity.

SPECIFIC MOVEMENTS	AGONIST MUSCLES (MOVER)	MAIN STABILIZING ACTIONS	ANTAGONIST MUSCLES (MUST BE RELAXED TO ALLOW MOVEMENT)	MAIN NEUTRALIZING ACTIONS
(Cont.)		same time the knee is flexed.		the toe to be turned outward so it will not hook the hurdle.
Coming off the hurdle				
Hip extension of the lead leg (100°)	Gluteus maximus Biceps femoris Semimembranosus Semitendinosus	The proximal ends of the hip extensors attach to highly stabile bone structures (the pelvis and the sacrum). Therefore, less stabilizing is needed for this movement than other comparable movements. Muscles that help to stabilize the pelvis and sacrum for this movement are the obliquus abdominis (internus and externus) and the quadratus lumborum.	Adductor brevis Adductor longus Gracilis Rectus femoris Pectineus Psoas major Sartorius Iliacus	In this case the hip extends while the knee is in a straight position. Three of the four hip extensors (the hamstrings) also flex the knee. Therefore, the knee extensors (except the rectus femoris) must neutralize knee flexion. The rectus femoris is probably not used here because it opposes hip extension. Medial hip rotators must neutralize the lateral rotation action of the gluteus maximus.
Trunk extension (30°)	Quadratus lumborum Sacrospinalis Deep posterior spinal muscles	When the trunk extends, the pelvic region and the legs must be stabilized to form a base on which the trunk can move. In this case, extension of the lead	Rectus abdominis Psoas (Ordinarily the obliquus abdominis muscles would be listed as antagonistic to trunk extension. But in	The opposite muscles on the two sides of the body neutralize each other's tendency to laterally flex the trunk.

		leg and trunk extension occur simultaneously, and the two moving segments equalize (stabilize) each other. In fact trunk extension happens primarily as a method of providing a stabile base on which to extend the leg with great force.		this case they are active in stabilizing the pelvic region for hip extension. Therefore, their trunk flexion actions must be overpowered by the trunk extensors.)
Shoulder extension of lead arm (100°)	Deltoid (posterior head) Latissimus dorsi Infraspinatus Teres major Teres minor	The shoulder girdle must be stabilized, and, in this case, the key stabilizer muscles are the rhomboids and trapezius III and IV.	Coracobrachialis Deltoid (anterior head) Pectoralis major Biceps	The latissimus dorsi and teres major also adduct the arm and rotate it medially. The deltoid also abducts the arm, and the infraspinatus and teres minor rotate it laterally. These muscles neutralize each other's abduction, adduction, and rotary action.

NOTE: As the runner comes off the hurdle and resumes his running action, the prime movements are hip flexion and knee extension of the trail leg, along with shoulder flexion of the arm opposite that leg.

Part 2

Contributions of other body systems to muscular function

It is well established that effective muscular function is strongly dependent upon other body systems which support the muscular system. The three body systems most directly involved are the circulatory, respiratory, and nervous systems. Therefore, these are the supporting systems whose efficiency we try to improve through training programs.

It is assumed that students of kinesiology have completed basic courses in human anatomy and physiology. So Part 2 of this book is written only by way of review, in an effort to expand and further emphasize certain information which has great significance in performance. Only information which closely relates to vigorous activity is included in this part.

Chapter 10 describes the important contributions the nervous system makes to performance. The interrelatedness of the nervous and muscular systems is emphasized. Chapter 11 consists of the important facts about how the circulatory and respiratory systems support muscular functions. After studying Part 2, the interrelatedness and interdependence of these body systems with the muscular system will be better understood. The limitations of muscle use, and the reasons behind those limitations, will also be understood better. The content of these chapters will give the reader additional insight into why certain training techniques are employed to improve performance.

10

Neuromuscular control of movement

*S*killed movement cannot be understood without a basic understanding of the function of nervous tissue. All body activity, both obvious movement and unseen internal movement, is coordinated by nerve impulses and/or chemical reactions. Normally, without nerve impulses, the muscles are unable to contract, and consequently, the organism is unable to function—or even survive. Other impulses (inhibitory in effect) prevent unwanted contractions or reduce the strength or length of contractions. The timing with which impulses arrive at particular muscles determines skill (coordination of movements). Physiologically, the establishment of coordinated movement patterns is a highly complicated process. Gaining insight into this process is difficult, but it is a mark of a well-prepared physical educator.

System divisions

The nervous system is conveniently divided into two parts according to function (Figure 10–1). The *autonomic system* is most aptly described by a similar word, automatic. There is no conscious control over autonomic functions. Mostly, this system governs vegetive responses which keep us alive, and while of utmost importance to us, it is beyond the scope of this discussion. The *voluntary system* is that part of the nervous system over which we can exercise conscious control, but which often operates below conscious level. The nerve impulses which control the functions of the skeletal muscles originate and travel in the voluntary system. This system and how it contributes to performance is discussed in the remainder of this chapter.

Structurally, the voluntary system is divided into the *central nervous system* (CNS) and the *peripheral nervous system* (PNS). The CNS includes only the brain and the spinal cord, and the PNS refers to all other nervous tissues in the

151

voluntary system. The tissue of the PNS is distributed in all areas of the body and connects with the CNS at various levels along the spinal column.

Functionally, the voluntary system may be subdivided into the *afferent system* and *efferent system*. The afferent system (also called *sensory*) conducts impulses which originate in the sensory organs and travel toward the CNS. It supplies information about both our internal and external environments. The efferent system (also called *motor*) carries impulses which move away from the CNS and terminate in the muscles.

The neuron

Each of the trillions of cells in the body is self-sufficient, able to live, grow, and reproduce its own. Cells can be grouped according to common functions, though they may be very different in appearance. Nerve cells are mostly diamond or star-shaped. Those cells that exhibit the properties of *irritability* and *conductivity* are nerve cells, or *neurons*. If a cell has irritability, it will respond to a stimulus, and if it then passes on the response to other cells, it has conductivity. The stimulus itself is not conducted, but the cell's response to the stimulus is conducted in the form of electrochemical impulses. The impulses provide information about the stimulus.

A neuron (nerve cell) consists of a cell body and appendages which are called *nerve fibers*. The fibers, which branch out from the cell body, are two types, *axons* and *dendrites*. Each neuron usually has several dendrites which conduct impulses toward the cell body. They serve as receptors. Each neuron has only one axon, which is the fiber that conducts impulses away from the cell body, usually to muscles or other neurons. Axons are bound together into bundles, and a bundle of axons (fibers) is called a *nerve*.

If a neuron of the afferent (sensory) system receives a stimulus, the information usually terminates in a specialized area of the brain. On the other hand, the stimulus may originate in the brain, travel the efferent (motor) system via a motor neuron, and terminate in a muscle, causing the muscle to contract. In addition, some afferent impulses may travel to the spinal cord, and there may transfer to the efferent system and arrive at the muscle without any brain involvement.

The sensory neurons are quite different from the motor neurons (Figure 10–2), but they both have the same basic components. Each has a cell body in which all of its life functions are centered, and each has its threadlike appendages which perform their specialized functions. There are about three times as many sensory as motor neurons in the human body.

Nerve tissue is either white or gray in color, with the cell bodies gray and the appendages to the bodies white. This difference is functional as well as structural,

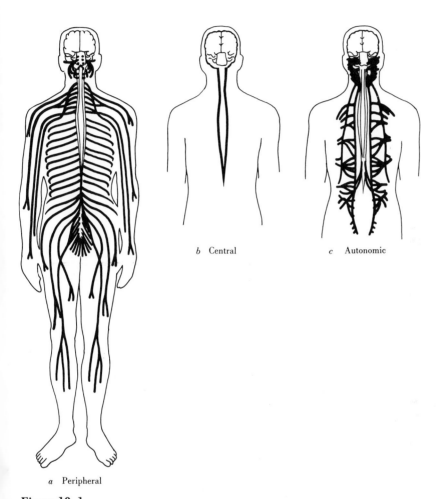

b Central

c Autonomic

a Peripheral

Figure 10–1.

Divisions of the human nervous system simplified. All these systems are inter-connected and integrated. (*a*) The peripheral nervous system reaches out to the end organs, such as the retina of the eye and nerve endings on the surface of the skin. As shown above, the nerve trunks originating from the central nervous system have been cut off before branching out and reaching the end organs to which they go. Many fine, complex branches are not shown. (*b*) The central nervous system includes the brain and spinal cord. (*c*) The autonomic nervous system, which parallels but lies outside the spinal cord, includes both sympa-thetic and parasympathetic nerves and their junctions (ganglia). This system "automatically" controls many body functions, such as breathing and digestion. (*After Schifferes*)

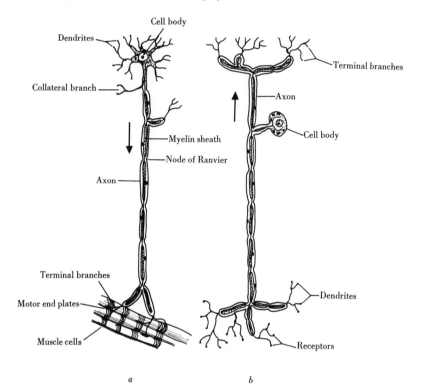

Figure 10–2.
Typical spinal neurons: (*a*) motor; (*b*) sensory.

for the white color of the appendages is due to deposits of a fatty material called *myelin*, which surrounds the appendages. The myelin covering (or *sheath*) serves two functions: (1) insulation, hence the prevention of the dispersion of the impulses to surrounding neurons; and (2) speeding the conduction process. *The larger the fiber and the thicker the myelin sheath, the faster is the conduction of the impulse.*

Impulses travel over white matter relatively fast. The PNS is almost exclusively white matter (either axon or dendrite nerve fibers), while the CNS, in which most of the cell bodies are located, has a mixture of white and gray matter (unmyelinated cell bodies combined with heavily myelinated nerve tracts of the spinal cord and the brain).

Incidentally, very little white matter is found in the autonomic nervous system, even on the nerve fibers, since speed of response is of limited importance. Also, an immature CNS will not yet have received its full complement of myelin. This hampers children in performance of intricate skills which require speedy and precise impulse patterns.

The central nervous system

The following discussion of the CNS includes only those parts and processes which are directly associated with skeletal muscle function.

Cerebral cortex

Most of the cranial cavity is occupied by the largest section of the brain called the *cerebrum* (Figure 10–3). The surface of the cerebrum is known as the cortex and is composed almost entirely of cell bodies of neurons. Because the nerve cell bodies are unmyelinated, the cortex is composed of gray matter. The function of the whole CNS seems to be based upon an arrangement where the more intricate the operation, the higher its location; the cerebral cortex, being highest (at the top of the CNS), is the most complicated. If the cortex is divided into front and back halves, the neurons in the front are mostly motor, and those in back are mostly sensory.

The cerebral cortex appears to be the seat of voluntary movement. It orders gross actions but relies on lower levels of the CNS to control the details. It is responsible for *consciousness, perception, memory* (including the memories of the patterns of past muscular actions), *interpretation,* and *reasoning.* Probably a combination of these functions result in two other functions, *judgment* and *will,* or *desire.* The mechanism by which motor impulses are originated in the cerebral cortex is unknown, but it is believed that the thought to move produces chemical secretions which stimulate the appropriate neurons.

When a situation occurs which has been encountered previously, the cortex makes a decision to initiate an impulse volley which will best meet the requirements of that situation. The exact response is based upon the success or failure of similar actions in the past. Successes are usually repeated and failures are rejected. The more extensive and well established its store of memories, the faster and more accurate will be its responses in terms of muscular action. The particular situation at hand may be a near duplicate of successfully handled situations of the past, in which case the response will probably be satisfactory. But if the problem is unique or only rarely experienced, the chances of responding quickly and correctly are considerably lessened. In the latter case, the judgment of how to respond will be based on the most nearly related experiences. All this indicates that children should be provided with opportunity for experience in a wide variety of basic movement patterns before their interests become specialized, or else overall skill development will be limited. Granted, a large amount of inherited neuromuscular capacity is needed to be judged a "natural athlete," but it must be recognized that "natural" motor responses are mostly the result of related past experiences. Certainly heredity sets the limits, but experiences set the level of development within those limits.

The parts of the cerebral cortex directly concerned with producing impulses which cause muscular contractions and receiving impulses which alert the organism to changing conditions can be separated into three rather large divisions, according to function. (Refer to Figure 10–3.) The three divisions are the *motor cortex, premotor cortex,* and the *sensory cortex.*

The motor cortex seems to provide stimulation to individual muscles and small muscle groups. The smallest sections of nerve tissue in this area control the largest areas of the muscular system. The nerve tissues in the motor cortex which control the thumbs, lips, and tongue are proportionately massive in size when compared with the size of the muscles involved. The reverse is true for the hips and thighs. Thus, it seems that gross, big muscle movements require less cortical nervous control than fine movements.

The premotor cortex produces innervation for complicated patterns of movement (complex coordinations). If the area of the motor cortex which controls the little finger is damaged, the little finger will not move alone; but the finger can receive impulses in coordination with other movements, such as clenching the fist, which is controlled by the premotor cortex. Coordinations are less complex when they are controlled by the cerebellum and other lower brain parts. Many coordinations are basically repetitious, so the performance of the premotor area is not as complex as it may appear. Perhaps the human being only uses several hundred relatively complicated coordinate patterns in his lifetime, many of which are repeated often. Loss of function of the premotor cortex destroys the sequence and timing of many

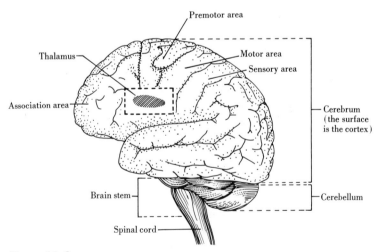

Figure 10–3.
Parts of the CNS which have major functions in the control of skeletal muscle actions.

movement patterns, but if the motor cortex is still intact, individual muscular movements controlled by the motor cortex are not impaired.

The sensory cortex is the final terminating area for most of the afferent information coming from the various sensory receptors. An interpretation of the sensory impulses takes place in this area. If impulses are spread to many cell bodies, and if the impulses arrive rapidly (high frequency of impulses), it means the stimulus at the receptor was intense.

Interior of the cerebrum

The interior of the cerebrum is composed largely of white matter. This white matter is actually a part of longer strands of white matter (nerve fibers) which link the cerebrum to all the levels of the spinal cord. This white matter serves the purpose of providing fast, and often direct, impulse conduction from lower levels of the CNS to the brain, and vice versa. These nerve fibers are bundled together according to common functions, and the bundles, called *nerve tracts*, are separated from one another. The afferent bundles are *ascending tracts* and transmit sensory impulses to be interpreted in the sensory cortex. The efferent bundles are *descending tracts*, and they conduct impulses which cause muscular contractions.

In addition to the white matter of the interior cerebrum, several clusters of gray matter are present. Little is known about the specific functions of these concentrations of gray matter, but the largest, and probably the most important, is the *thalamus*. The thalamus serves as an important relay center for both motor and sensory impulses. It has extensive connections with the cortex. Most authorities believe that the control of much of the voluntary muscular activity is a major function of the thalamus, and they claim that some of the activity of the thalamus is involved with feelings of pleasure and pain.

Cerebellum

The interior of the cerebellum is largely white matter except for permeations of treelike branches of gray matter. The gray matter seems to reach toward the exterior, or cortex, of this rounded brain section. The surface is essentially gray matter similar to the cortex of the cerebrum. The cerebellum is not in the "main line" of impulse travel but receives afferent information and sends *modifying* impulses mostly to the cerebral cortex by way of the thalamus. Only one line of direct control to the muscles exists, and it is used solely in response to incoming impulses concerned with equilibrium from the inner ear. All functions of the cerebellum are accomplished below the level of consciousness; outgoing impulses depend upon the stimulation of incoming sensory impulses. The cerebellum is not in the direct impulse line between the cerebral cortex and the muscles; therefore, paralysis will not result from its loss. Conversely, the thalamus is in the main line; therefore, if it were totally destroyed, all voluntary movement would cease. Nevertheless, the cerebellum is no less important to skillful performance than the thalamus, as will be illustrated soon.

The cerebellum receives afferent information (especially that information called proprioceptive), which originates in the receptors of muscles, tendons, and joints, and distributes impulses accordingly to modify motor acts. An individual with a malfunction of the cerebellum will not have the ability to refine a movement, nor will he be able to make needed adjustments as the movement progresses. He will exhibit extreme inaccuracy, overcompensation, and a marked jerkiness in movement. In fact, the cerebellum can *predict*, from the present state of the muscles and joints, what will occur as the movement progresses and will distribute signals which will prevent errors in the movement.

Brain stem

The functions of the brain stem are more directly concerned with autonomic responses than with the voluntary nervous system. The brain stem is obviously the direct connection between the brain and the spinal cord. Part of the gray matter of the brain stem (the medulla and the pons) governs the rates of respiration and heart contraction.

Some authorities place the origin of inhibitory impulses in the interior cerebrum, but others say they originate in the brain stem. Regardless of where these impulses originate, their importance is well established. The inhibitory impulses produce conditions which make it necessary for more faciliatory impulses to arrive to excite motor neurons in the spinal cord. If this phenomenon did not exist with a nominal degree of efficiency, we would experience unwanted contractions and an inability to stop contractions short of complete fatigue.

Brain and skill development

In general, the lower the involvement is in the CNS, the more gross, primitive, and stereotyped the movement will be. For example, a walking or running stride can probably be repeated over and over with an involvement of only the cerebellum, brain stem, and spinal cord. But if an abrupt change of direction or speed is required, the more involved coordinations and judgments would probably require the higher involvement of the cerebral cortex and/or the thalamus.

It has been postulated that as skill develops, the innervation is relegated to lower centers of the CNS. It is probably more accurate to say that the pathways of impulses within the cerebrum develop "ruts" by repeatedly traveling the same paths, and these ruts allow faster impulse travel with fewer detours from the etched pathway. The performance of the act then requires less conscious consideration to keep the impulses on the proper course. This action can develop to a point where the term "conditioned reflex" would apply.

Spinal cord

The spinal cord is actually an extension of the brain, encased within the vertebral column (backbone). It is composed of both gray and white matter. The central column of gray matter is butterfly-shaped, or roughly forms the letter *H* (Figure 10–4). The points of the *H* are referred to as horns, and the two horns on the anterior (front) side of the column are formed by motor neuron cell bodies. Called *anterior horn cells*, they conduct motor impulses. The chief function of the cell bodies forming the *posterior horns* is to serve as connectors from neuron to neuron. This intermediary action becomes important since the connectors may block signals, pass them on, or distribute them to several levels of the cord or to the brain.

The sensory neuron cell bodies (at times mistakenly thought to be the posterior horn cells of the cord) do not lie within the cord itself but just adjacent to the vertebral column. This collection of neuron cell bodies is called the dorsal root ganglion, and there is one pair of ganglia located at each level of vertebrae along the column.

The spinal cord has often been likened to a complex cable-type relay system to the brain, but it is more than that. It is capable of receiving sensory impulses and redirecting them to a level of the cord containing the anterior neurons which will evoke an appropriate motor response—an accomplishment entirely independent of brain involvement. Moreover, a sensory impulse may be transmitted to lower areas of the brain without involving any of the conscious thought associated with the cerebral cortex. Impulses are constantly traveling within the cord, both up and down simultaneously. Also, impulses may simultaneously leave and enter the cord from the peripheral nervous system (PNS) via the spinal nerves.

The peripheral nervous system

It is important not to confuse neurons and nerve fibers with nerves. In review, a neuron is a nerve cell which includes the cell body and all its appendages. Each appendage (usually one long one) is a nerve fiber. When nerve fibers are bound together side-by-side in a cablelike arrangement, the resulting bundle of fibers is a nerve. The larger nerves are those which connect to the spinal cord; they are called spinal nerves. Spinal nerves have many smaller collaterals (side branches) which become more numerous and smaller as the distance from the spine becomes greater.

All nerve tissue outside the CNS is classified as part of the PNS. Motor neurons originate at the spinal cord and terminate in the muscle tissue which they innervate. Sensory neurons arise in some specialized sensory receptor and terminate at the spinal cord. Both sensory and motor neurons make connection with the spinal cord, and the cord connects to the brain. Very near its entrance to the spinal

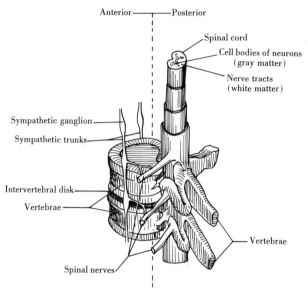

Anterior ——┬—— Posterior

Spinal cord

Cell bodies of neurons (gray matter)

Nerve tracts (white matter)

Sympathetic ganglion

Sympathetic trunks

Intervertebral disk

Vertebrae

Vertebrae

Spinal nerves

Figure 10–4.
Relationship of the vertebral column to the spinal cord, spinal nerves, and sympathetic trunks. (*After Anthony*)

cord, each spinal nerve branches into two connections (Figure 10–5). One branch goes to the front of the cord (anterior roots), and the other goes to the back of the cord (posterior roots). At this branch the mixed spinal nerve (impulses are conducted in both directions in a mixed nerve) is no longer mixed. The anterior roots conduct only efferent (motor) impulses away from the cord, and the posterior roots conduct only afferent (sensory) impulses toward the cord.

Spinal nerves

Man has 31 pairs of spinal nerves. One of each pair is on the right side of the body, and the other is on the left side. In general, the spinal nerves of the upper spinal cord innervate the neck and arm muscles, and those of the lower cord innervate the hip and leg muscles. Each of these spinal nerves is about as thick as a pencil and is composed of thousands of individual nerve fibers, each about as thick as a human hair. These fibers vary in length, with the longest ones several feet and the shortest hardly measurable. As previously stated, the larger the fiber and the thicker the myelin sheath, the more quickly the impulse will travel along the fiber. The larger fibers are capable of conducting over 2,000 impulses in one second.

All-or-none law of nerve impulses

At this point it is appropriate to state that the nerve fiber obeys the all-or-none law; that is, if the stimulus is intense enough to create a chemical environment which will excite the neuron, the neuron will generate an impulse of only *one magnitude* and *one speed of transmission*. The magnitude and speed of transmission are dependent upon only one factor: the physical makeup of the nerve fiber. A neuron has two alternatives: to conduct an impulse or to remain at rest. Since neurons carry one magnitude (strength) of impulse at one speed, how do the impulses to muscles vary in their effects? By increasing or decreasing the frequencies of impulses. More impulses per second will cause muscle fibers to contract with greater force. If the stimulus that originates the impulses becomes more intense, the result will be an involvement of more neurons *and* an increase in frequency of impulses over each neuron. This increase in number of nerve fibers conducting impulses means that a greater number of muscle fibers will receive impulses, thus a stronger contraction will result. (Refer to Figure 2–9.)

Different neurons vary in their response to stimulation (irritability) and the speed at which their fibers conduct impulses. The magnitude of impulses also varies from fiber to fiber, but an impulse produced in a particular fiber will maintain a constant intensity regardless of the distance it travels.

Remember, a spinal nerve, which consists of a bundle of many fibers of both afferent and efferent neurons, may have impulses conducted in both directions at the same time, impulses of various speed and magnitude, and impulse volleys of various frequencies.

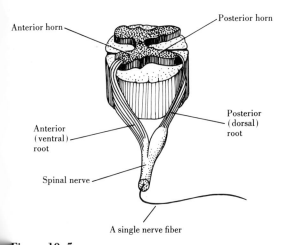

Figure 10–5.
Section of the spinal cord showing the anterior and posterior roots of a spinal nerve.

Neuromyal junction

The neuromyal junction is the place where a branch of a motor nerve fiber reaches the muscle fiber which it innervates. Each of the motor neuron cell bodies (located in the anterior horn cells of the spinal cord) has its nerve fiber (axon) that conducts impulses to a muscle. Although there is. only one conducting fiber (axon) per neuron, the end of this fiber is frayed into a large number of endings. Each of the endings (branches) will innervate one muscle fiber, and all the muscle fibers innervated by one neuron receive the same signal. Each ending of the nerve fiber makes a connection called the *motor end plate*. There are at least as many motor end plates in a muscle as there are muscle fibers (many thousands), and each muscle fiber has one, and sometimes several, motor end plates. The neuromyal junction is that junction between the end plate and muscle fiber (Figure 10–6).

The neuromyal junction should not be confused with a synapse, which is a junction between the appendages of two different neurons. It enables impulses to be transmitted from one neuron to another (see Figure 10–8).

Motor unit

A motor unit consists of all the muscle fibers that receive impulses from the same nerve fiber (Figure 10–6). This means that all fibers in a motor unit receive the same signal and contract in unison. However, some of the fibers are dormant because their thresholds are too high to be activated by the impulses. (A threshold is a minimum requirement necessary to achieve a response.) It is believed that strength training lowers the thresholds of muscle fibers, thus allowing more fibers to become active with a given level of stimulus. The threshold of a fiber is dependent on the nutrition and fatigue of the fiber. For a more detailed discussion of the motor unit, see Chapter 2.

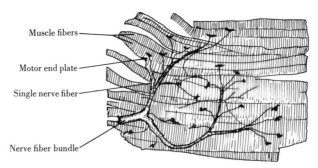

Muscle fibers —

Motor end plate —

Single nerve fiber —

Nerve fiber bundle —

Figure 10–6.
Motor nerve endings of intercostal muscle fibers of a rabbit. (*After Bremer: A Textbook of Histology, The Blakiston Company, New York.*)

All-or-none law of muscle contraction

The all-or-none law applies in a special way to the contraction of muscle fibers. If a single impulse reaches the motor unit, it will surpass the thresholds of certain muscle fibers. Those fibers whose thresholds are surpassed by the impulse will contract to their maximum present ability to respond to a single impulse. However, one impulse will cause each fiber to shorten only a small part of the total distance the fiber can shorten. Several impulses received in rapid succession will cause the fiber to contract more completely.

Motor units receive only one magnitude of impulses at a given time, but the frequency of impulses may vary considerably, depending on the strength of the stimulus. The frequency of the impulses is the most important factor in developing a full contraction of a motor unit.

Maximum contraction of a muscle at a given time requires impulses of adequate frequency to cause full contraction of each motor unit, and all motor units must receive stimulation simultaneously. To develop maximum contractile force in a muscle, contraction of all fibers in all the motor units must be prepared to contract, and certain structural changes must occur which allow each fiber to produce a greater tension. (Among the structural changes are more and tougher connective tissues and more protein and fluid in the muscle fibers.) For more detailed information about the all-or-none law and the strength of muscle contractions, see Chapter 2.

Sensory receptors

Sensory receptors are all located in the afferent (sensory) nervous system. They are divided into the three following general groups. *Exteroceptors*, which provide information about the external environment, are stimulated by temperature, pressure, light, vibrations, or chemicals. These receptors initiate the impulses for the interpretation of the classic five senses (touch, taste, smell, sight, and hearing). The impulses travel the cranial (within the skull) nerves. *Interoceptors* are mainly receptors which initiate sensory impulses in the visceral organs. Impulses from this group are conducted by the spinal nerves. *Proprioceptors* are of the most direct concern to this discussion. They provide the organism with information about skeletal muscle and joint awareness, which is called the *kinesthetic sense*. These impulses are also conducted by the spinal nerves.

All these receptors are very specific in nature, reacting only to the type of stimulation for which they were designed and rejecting all other types of stimulation under normal conditions.

Proprioceptors are of greatest concern in the study of kinesiology. They are sensory receptors located in the muscles, joints, and connective tissues, and they provide information based upon conditions existing in the areas of their location. These receptors provide information about position, direction, and rate of movement, as well as the amount of muscle tension in a locality. In truth, then, we have a muscle sense as real as the external five senses which can be demonstrated when one or more of the exteroceptive senses—sight, for example—are prevented from functioning. The organism is still aware of movements and positions of body and limb. *Kinesthesis* is the term given to this muscle sense. When a performer states that "it felt right" as he executes a skill, he is referring to his kinesthetic perception of the action. The sense becomes keener as the act is repeated a sufficient number of times. However, this does not necessarily mean that the skill is performed correctly; often the performer's mental picture of his action is incorrect, or his concept of a correct performance is erroneous.

The impulse: excitation and conduction

The nerve fiber is nearly cylinder-shaped. Under rest conditions, an electrical potential exists across the fiber from its outside to its inside. The fiber's outer area is electrically positive, and its interior is electrically negative. This condition results from an abundance of postively charged sodium ions located in the fluids on the outside of the fiber's membrane. The positive ions strive to enter the fiber through the membrane in an effort to establish equilibrium (neutral electrical state). It is as if a spring were compressed and its tension awaits release. The sodium ions are prevented from entering the interior of the fiber because of the impermeability of the fiber's membrane. Two other conditions, which may appear unimportant at this time, need to be noted: (1) a much smaller number of potassium ions (also carrying a positive charge), which are *not* restricted by the impermeability of the membrane, pass freely between the outside and inside of the nerve fibers but are incapable of causing an impulse (no resistance to passage—no tension); and (2) all points along the nerve fiber are electrically the same, meaning that no difference exists in potential between any two points along the length of the fiber.

Conduction of impulses

The nerve impulse is actually a reversal of the electrical charge of the nerve fiber. As the impulse progresses along the fiber, it somehow affects the permeability of the membrane to sodium ions, and a very minute amount of sodium quickly rushes in, providing a momentary change in electrical potential. At this moment, the outside of the fiber is electrically negative to the inside. The electrical difference between the nerve fiber at this point and at other points is called the *action potential*, and its strength is between 50 to 100 microvolts (100 microvolts = .0001 volt). The impulse moves along the fiber by removing the membrane's resistance to sodium ions, thus allowing some of them to enter the fiber at

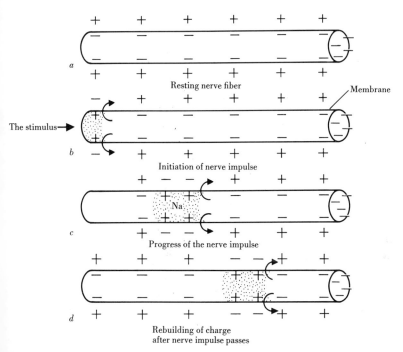

Figure 10–7.
The progress of the nerve impulse along the nerve fiber. (*a*) The resting nerve
fiber, with positive charge on the outside of the membrane and negative charge
within. (*b*) The initiation of the nerve impulse; for a fraction of a second the
charges on the membrane are reversed. (*c*) The nerve impulse passes rapidly
along the nerve fiber. (*d*) The charge on the membrane returns to normal after
a brief refractory period. (*After DeCoursey*)

another point. The passage from one point on the nerve fiber to the next is much
like a row of dominoes—when one falls, each adjacent one is knocked over in
succession. One impulse may travel as fast as 300 to 400 feet per second, depending on the particular fiber and its condition.

Repolarization

The positive sodium ions which enter the fiber are trapped, for the membrane
will not allow their passage to the outside. Potassium ions have been relatively
free flowing, and they proceed to "fill the void" left by the sodium ions. They
reestablish a positive ion concentration on the outside of the membrane. Within
a few thousandths of a second, potassium ions provide the equalizing effect which
sodium ions cannot accomplish, and the nerve fiber is again ready to conduct an

impulse. Repolarization trails directly behind each impulse. This process can continue for 100,000 successive impulses in some fibers because very few of the total number of sodium ions cross the membrane with each impulse, and many more are still available. When the fiber is no longer receiving impulses, the sodium ions are returned to the outside by a metabolic action called the *sodium pump*. The normal range of impulse frequencies is between 10 and 500 per second.

Excitation

Impulses result from a stimulus caused by environmental changes near or about (1) special sensory receptors, (2) free nerve endings, or (3) neurons located in various areas of the brain. Impulses can be initiated by temperature changes, pressure changes, and electrical or chemical stimulation. Such conditions produce disturbing effects on the membranes of the receptors, and impulses result. Initiation of a voluntary impulse within the brain probably results from chemical secretions (stimulus) associated with the thought process.

A weak stimulus will only produce excitation of receptors of low thresholds in the area of the stimulus. A more intense stimulus will excite more receptors, causing more nerve fibers to conduct impulses. If a larger surface area is stimulated, a greater number of more widely separated receptors becomes excited.

A stronger stimulus will not cause the impulses to travel faster but will cause more impulses to be produced per unit of time (frequency increase) on each conducting fiber. Frequency of impulses is limited by speed of recovery of the nerve fibers, which in turn depends upon the fiber's structure and condition.

Synapses

A synapse is a weblike relay junction between neurons (see Figure 10–8) which will relay impulses in only one direction, from axons to dendrites. There is no direct "jumping" of an impulse to the next neuron; each succeeding neuron in a pathway must become excited by a chemical stimulation acting on the neuron's gray matter. Different synapses offer different amounts of resistance to impulses. The resistance depends upon the threshold of the synapse. In effect, impulses follow the path of least resistance when they have several choices. From impulses repeatedly following the same path, a "neuro pathway" becomes ingrained, and movements and responses become more automatic and usually more skillful. Neurons are very difficult (nearly impossible) to fatigue, but at the synapses and motor end plates, lactic acid (a substance produced by muscular contraction) will accumulate and retard the passage of impulses. Therefore, the synapses and motor end plates are often the "seats" of fatigue. In general, stimulants aid transmission across synapses and end plates, and substances labeled "depressants" retard this transmission.

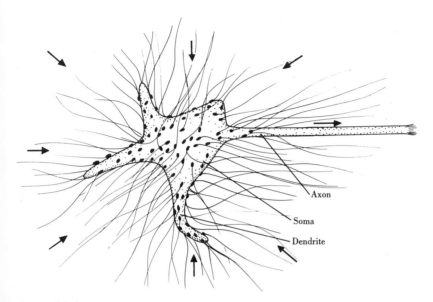

Figure 10–8.
A typical synapse, showing hundreds of terminals that originate
in other neurons.

Reflexes

An innate (inborn) reflex is a predictable response to a given stimulus which
is accomplished below the level of conscious control. Such reflexes must originate
in the afferent system, and the efferent (motor) response will occur before the
organism is consciously aware of the stimulus. If the organism is aware of the
stimulus, the reflex response may occur without interference, or it may be consciously inhibited or intensified.

Reflexes which are learned (not innate) are called *conditioned reflexes*. If the
performer learns to respond in the same manner to the same stimulus, this is a
conditioned reflex. A conscious movement can be superimposed on a reflex, either
innate or conditioned, by consciously adding nerve impulses.

Three innate reflexes seem most pertinent to human performances. The first and
simplest of these is the *stretch reflex*. It depends upon the muscle spindles to
initiate the impulse volley when the muscle is stretched. For the human to remain
erect, the posture muscles (mostly extensors) must be active to support against
the pull of gravity. If there were no muscular contraction, the body would collapse to the surface. An example of a stretch reflex occurs when one falls asleep
while sitting, and the head nods (the neck flexes), causing a stretch to be placed
on the neck extensors. The stretch reflex responds, returning the head to the erect
position with a jerk (see Figure 10–9).

The stretch reflex is primarily a postural reflex, but the principle of it is used to aid contractions in voluntary movements. If a performer wishes to throw, the muscles that will be used in the action phase are placed on sudden stretch from the windup. The result is that the throwing muscles receive impulses originating in their own spindles (stretch reflex), in addition to impulses initiated in the CNS. Thus, the contraction is stronger than it would be without impulses from the reflex.

Pressure on the bottoms of the feet initiates the *extensor thrust reflex*, which produces contraction of extensor muscles. This reflex results in a highly complicated pattern of extension at all the weight-bearing joints. This reflex is especially important in maintaining balance and in preventing too much flexion upon landing from a jump or landing while in locomotion. Its extension pattern can be altered at one or several of the joints by the stretch reflex or by voluntary impulses. The importance of this reflex is that it causes the performer to automatically dissipate the shock of landing, so conscious thought can be devoted to other problems at hand.

The *withdrawal* (flexor) *reflex* is somewhat more complicated than the stretch reflex. The flexor muscles ordinarily respond to pain stimuli. If a person touches a hot stove, for example, the receptors will send a sensory impulse volley to the spinal cord, where a synapse is made with an internuncial neuron. From here the impulse volley is distributed to the appropriate levels of the spinal cord (higher, lower, or both), which house the motor neuron cell bodies that connect to the flexor muscles, causing withdrawal of the injured part (Figure 10–10). Apparently, this response is accomplished before the impulse reaches the brain because spinal animals (brain destroyed) perform the task with the same ease as intact specimens.

Speed of impulse conduction

Reaction time is the interval of time between the signal to respond (stimulus) and the beginning of the response, not including the time it takes to accomplish the task. The latter is *movement time*. Reaction time reflects the lag in the functions of an individual's nervous system. Variations in this time occur as a result of the distance the impulse must travel, the number of synapses it crosses over, the irritability of the receptors and synapses, the intensity of the stimulus, the chemical state and composition of the innervated tissues, and perhaps other factors. When a reaction involves nothing more than an automatic reflex, the terms reflex time and reaction time are interchangeable. But often the reaction demands involvement of the cerebrum, in which case it may be desirable to call this "thought delay" and distinguish it from the time it takes for the signal to travel the rest of the system. This "thought time"—also termed *analysis, interpretation,* or *judgment* time—is separable from reflex time, but not from reaction time.

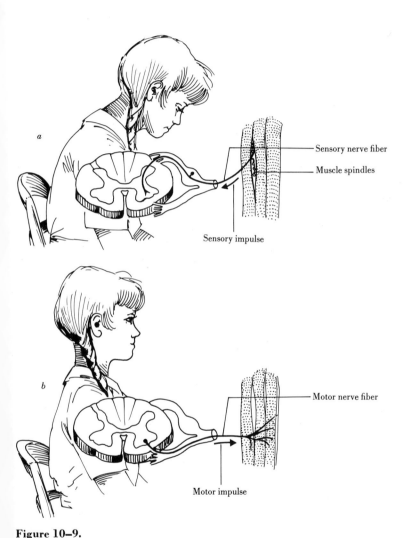

Sensory nerve fiber

Muscle spindles

Sensory impulse

Motor nerve fiber

Motor impulse

Figure 10–9.
A postural stretch reflex. (*a*) represents relaxation of trunk muscles causing
an increase in length of muscle fibers, which acts to stimulate the neuromuscular spindles (sensory receptor in muscles). The resulting impulse is transmitted to spinal cord by way of sensory neuron. (*b*) represents a motor impulse being transmitted to the muscle originally lengthened by relaxation. The
muscle contracts and regains its former length so that the posture is also
regained. (*After Grollman*)

Thought time means that the performer consciously analyzes the situation and then selects the proper response with the greatest haste. Reaction time includes a combination of reflex time and thought time, if thought is required. In most cases, the teacher or coach can have more influence on judgment (thought) time than on reflex time; however, it has been shown that reflex time can be improved somewhat in *specific* tasks. When a response is new to an individual, his reaction is usually slow, allowing great potential for improving reaction time. As the response is repeated many times, it becomes more automatic, reaction time becomes shorter, and the potential for improving reaction time is lessened. It should be remembered that a small change in reaction time may often have significant influence on performance. Reaction time is highly specific to a particular movement. Therefore, it seems that the current popularity of reaction drills, called *quick cals*, for increasing athletic quickness has little justification unless the movements duplicate those used in the contest, in which case both reaction and movement times may be reduced.

Neuromuscular integration

Now that the basic operations of the neuromuscular system have been established, the remainder of this chapter is devoted to additional concepts associated with

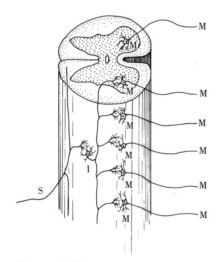

Figure 10–10.
An internuncial neuron of the spinal cord: S, sensory neuron; I, internuncial neuron; M, motor neurons. A flexor reflex is distributed in this manner.

the development of skills and to the practical applications of previously introduced concepts.

The establishment of skill patterns

It is generally agreed that skillful acts are accomplished without conscious thought, except for that needed to begin the act. Consequently, skillful acts are mostly conditioned reflexes. For example, we can perform the skill of walking while our conscious minds are occupied in deep thought or conversation. Actually, we may walk more skillfully under these conditions than if we concentrate on our movements. The movements involved in walking result from conditioned reflexes. During active contests, it is often essential that the performer concentrate on external cues, and any preoccupation with specific body movements will destroy his effectiveness. In such cases, while the general idea of the desired response is conveyed by the cerebrum, lower centers of the CNS work out the details. In the final analysis, the resulting movements are dependent upon three factors: (1) which neurons conduct impulse volleys, (2) the frequencies of the impulse volleys, and (3) exactly when these impulses reach the muscle fibers. Another important factor is which muscles are prevented from contracting because of neural inhibition.

As a certain skill develops, its specific movements tend to become less variable and more exact because the selected patterns of impulses have become more easily duplicated. This is so because the impulse volleys tend to follow previously followed pathways within the nervous system. As stated earlier, the impulses are conducted along the path of least resistance. Nerve pathway possibilities are inherited, but it is use that determines the development of the pathways. As certain synapses are used, their thresholds are repeatedly lowered, and the chance of repeating that path under like conditions is increased. Conversely, it is difficult to blaze new pathways for the same act once the pathways have been established. As in walking through deep grass, the more often a certain path is taken, the deeper the pathway becomes. Paths not repeated tend to become obscure, but they are never completely eliminated.

When one begins to learn a skill, inconceivable numbers of pathways are possible. But gradually, pathways are selected which have resulted in successful performances, and the pathways that have been less successful are rejected. The more often the pathway is repeated, the more firmly ingrained the pattern becomes and the more difficult to avoid. Gradually the path is used with greater ease and smoothness, and superfluous movements are eliminated. Unproductive paths are rejected, and the act becomes "skillful."

Certain obstacles exist; for example, (1) conditions, both of the internal and external environments, are never exactly the same from one time to the next; (2) most skills are complex enough to involve many joints and muscles, and even though the skill may appear correct, variations in only a few joints may detract from successful results; (3) the performer may incorrectly judge his performance as successful and continue to perform incorrectly. For instance, he may throw with the wrong foot forward and assume this is the proper procedure since he achieves a degree of success. Or a young basketball player, who is a head taller than his opposition, may use an undesirable shooting technique with much success until he meets an opponent of equal height. If he does not change quickly, the improper pathways will be established, thus making it difficult to develop a more desirable shooting technique.

One role of a teacher is to recognize improper performances and to prescribe training procedures to replace them with correct performance patterns. The younger the performer when he benefits from properly directed teaching, the easier, quicker, and more precise will be his development, assuming his nervous system is matured adequately to develop the skill in question.

The acquisition of refined skills necessitates prior learning of gross skill patterns (basic skills). Highly refined skills are usually only slight modifications of basic patterns. For example, if a child learns a basic throwing pattern by throwing objects of all sorts under a variety of conditions, the addition of a forearm rotation and a wrist snap in the direction of the little finger can result in a curve ball.

Effective performance requires sufficient amounts of many physiological qualities, such as strength, speed, muscular endurance, circulorespiratory endurance, agility, and flexibility; but performers possessing lesser amounts of these factors often outdo their stronger and faster opponents because of well-coordinated and well-timed neuromuscular patterns (specific skills). It has been estimated that as little as one-fourth of the energy is required for a highly skilled performer to accomplish the same act as an unskilled performer. Similarly, high levels of the aforementioned physiological qualities may be of little use if they are wasted through inefficiency. Of course, the excellent athlete will have an abundance of all the mentioned physiological qualities, combined with the exact neuromuscular control (specific skill) needed to assure success.

Coordination: sequence and timing

Coordination of an act is merely the result of each movement occurring in the correct sequence and time. When a highly coordinated movement occurs, it appears smooth and rhythmical. Of course, joint movements occur only as the result of muscular contractions, and the muscles respond only to nerve impulses. Therefore, when a coordinated movement occurs, it is because the nerve impulses reach the proper muscles with sufficient intensity at the correct time. The muscle contractions then cause movements which constitute the skilled performance.

Ideal timing is exhibited when each force is applied at the crest acceleration of the previous force. If a force appears too soon, the momentum gained by the preceding force is less than what could have been attained, since the body part did not reach full acceleration. If the force appears too late, the previous force is already beginning to decelerate, and again momentum is lost. For instance, in the baseball pitch, each movement must be in correct sequence, precisely timed to contribute the maximum possible amount to the subsequent movement. The final result (speed and accuracy of the pitch) will depend upon the effectiveness of each preceding movement and how well the many specific movements were coordinated with each other.

The total force that can be applied to an object depends partly upon the distance over which the accumulation of forces can be applied. Some forces act longer than others, some contribute more to the total momentum than others, but unless all forces have an opportunity to add their part to the total momentum, something less than maximum performance will be achieved.

When the "O'Brien style" of shot-putting was accepted, greater distances were achieved. The primary difference is that this style emphasizes beginning the action with the back, rather than the left side (right-handed performer), toward the direction of the put. This basic change in form allows a greater range of motion through which the rotational forces can act, and the result is a greater total momentum. This illustration simply indicates that accepted forms are not sacred. O'Brien dared to experiment, and he found success. But such success is not likely to occur unless the experimenter has a basic knowledge of the mechanical and physiological factors involved.

Reciprocal inhibition

The inhibition or blocking of nerve impulses to those muscles in opposition (antagonistic) to a desired movement is of utmost importance to the efficiency of that movement. It appears that the antagonist muscles are automatically inhibited. And if this is an automatic response, one may wonder why it should even be discussed. It must be recognized that with the practice of a movement, the inhibition of the antagonist muscles becomes quicker and more complete. Obviously, an antagonistic tension interferes with the effectiveness of a performance; by reducing tension in the antagonists, effectiveness is increased, and the onset of fatigue is postponed.

If an animal has its cerebrum destroyed, it will, for a period of time, assume a position of strong extension at all postural joints. This condition is called *decerebrate rigidity*, and it illustrates both the importance and the source of inhibitory impulses. The interior cerebrum continuously emits high levels of inhibitory impulses to limit the magnitude of our movements, thus accomplishing the inhibition by chemical action at the synapses of the motor neurons. Anxiety or other emotional involvement can limit the effectiveness of inhibition upon voluntary movement; these heightened emotions tend to hinder performances where fine muscular coordinations are required. A good example of an activity that is adversely affected by anxiety is golf. Neural skill pathways are altered, and antagonistic tension tends to destroy skill. Other activities, not requiring fine muscle control, may benefit from heightened emotions. The performance of a football lineman or a shot-putter may be enhanced by anxiety. But if the football player must handle the ball, his performance is likely to suffer. Many so-called sophomore mistakes are attributable to inability to contend with emotional stress because the emotional stress has a detrimental effect on *fine* neuromuscular coordination.

Application of chapter content

Because the nervous system is very complex and its functions are not visually obvious, people often fail to recognize its importance in performance. The strength, speed, and duration with which muscles contract all depend directly upon the nervous system. Following are some specific examples of how knowledge of the functioning of the nervous system may influence performance.

1. The preparatory stage of a throwing or striking action, such as the backswing in golf or tennis, exists only to achieve the most advantageous forward swing. It is known that if a muscle is stretched approximately one-third beyond its resting length, it is best prepared for a forceful contraction. This is partly because the muscle is under greater tension (like a towrope, the slack has been removed) and can effectively shorten through a greater distance and partly because impulses, in addition to the voluntary impulses, result from the stretch reflex, adding to the force of the contractions.

     To avoid stimulation of inhibitory impulses and to maximize the efforts of the stretch reflex, the backswing must be fairly rapid. This negates the use of an extremely slow backswing, especially stopping the action at the height of the back-swing. On the other hand, too fast a backswing generates a momentum in the direction *opposite the action*. This momentum must be overcome by contractions of the muscles which produce the forward swing.

     The conclusion is to select that speed of backswing which is fast enough to utilize the stretch reflex, but not too fast. Typically, a performer tends to select a back-swing which is too fast, in which case he should be taught to slow it down. How-ever, occasionally the backswing is too slow, resulting in loss of force application. Similar examples could be given in batting actions, jumping actions, and other performances where the stretch reflex contributes.

2. To improve flexibility in an area of the body, movement must be consistently performed to stretch the muscles and connective tissues which tend to resist the movement. In this case, inhibitory impulses to the muscles which resist movement are essential. It is wise to avoid jerky movements which cause the stretch reflex. Slow stretching results in the blocking of impulses and the release of tension in the muscles, consequently allowing a greater degree of stretch. Also, too fast an

action may produce enough momentum to stretch tissues too far and cause injury. Slow and steady stretching is safer and more effective for increasing flexibility, although some flexibility may be achieved by bouncing at the end of the range of motion.

Recommended supplementary reading

GELLHORN, ERNEST: The Physiology of the Supraspinal Mechanisms, in Warren R. Johnson (ed.), "Science and Medicine of Exercise and Sports," pp. 108–122, Harper & Row, Publishers, Incorporated, New York, 1960.

GROLLMAN, SIGMUND: "The Human Body," pp. 49–57, 78–136, The Macmillan Company, New York, 1964.

GUYTON, ARTHUR C.: "Function of the Human Body," 2d ed., pp. 215–279, W. B. Saunders Company, Philadelphia, 1965.

LOOFBOUROOW, G. N.: Neuromuscular Integration, in Warren R. Johnson (ed.), "Science and Medicine of Exercise and Sports," pp. 80–107, Harper & Row, Publishers, Incorporated, New York, 1960.

MOREHOUSE, LAURENCE E., and AUGUSTUS T. MILLER: "Physiology of Exercise," 4th ed., pp. 30–42, 50–58, The C. V. Mosby Company, St. Louis, 1963.

RASCH, PHILLIP J., and ROGER K. BURKE: "Kinesiology and Applied Anatomy," 3d ed., Chap. 5, Lea and Febiger, Philadelphia, 1967.

11

Circulorespiratory functions in performance

*C*irculorespiratory is a term used to include both the circulatory and respiratory systems. The major parts of this system are the lungs, heart, and blood vessels. The ability of the human organism to sustain work is highly dependent upon the efficiency of this system, which supplies the muscles and other body tissues with substances necessary to sustain life and produce work. This chapter is designed to provide insight into how this system makes a major contribution to performance and how, in turn, vigorous activity influences the functioning of this system. The content of this chapter includes:

1. Contributions of the circulorespiratory system to performance
2. Effects of vigorous performance on the circulorespiratory system

Contributions of the circulorespiratory system to performance

The primary functions of the circulorespiratory system are to provide body tissues with needed substances and to carry waste products away from the tissues. Mainly nutrients and oxygen are brought to the cells, which expel lactic acid and carbon dioxide. Pumped through the body by the heart, the blood carries these materials. The elastic qualities of the vessels allow the blood to be directed in sufficient amounts to the areas of greatest need. Both at the tissues and in the lungs a gaseous exchange takes place. In the lungs oxygen enters the blood, and carbon dioxide leaves the blood and is expelled through exhaling. The opposite movement takes place at the tissues; oxygen leaves the blood and enters the tissues, and carbon dioxide is the waste gas picked up by the blood and carried back to the lungs for elimination.

The efficiency of the circulorespiratory system in vigorous performance is related primarily to endurance. Skill and strength are direct functions of the nervous and

176

muscular systems. But fitness of the circulorespiratory system is very important in determining how long an organism can maintain a particular level of effort. Most of us can function under conditions of rest or moderate activity with the ease of the fit individual, but level of fitness becomes more apparent as activity is intensified.

Pressure gradients—key to gas exchange

The exchange of respiratory gases (oxygen and carbon dioxide) across membranes in both the lungs and at the tissues is dependent upon the concentration of each gas on both sides of the membrane at the point of exchange. Each gas moves across the membrane without influencing the movement of the other gas; that is, the oxygen flow is only dependent upon the difference in concentration of *oxygen* molecules on either side of the membrane. Both gases move simultaneously. The gases are said to "diffuse down their pressure gradient," that is, to pass through the membrane from the greater to the lesser concentration.

As the blood returns to the lungs from all body cells, it moves into the capillaries which engulf the alveoli, or air sacs (Figure 11-1), and the relative pressure across the membranes causes the movement of carbon dioxide from and oxygen into the blood. At the lungs carbon dioxide concentration is higher in the blood than in the inspired air, and oxygen concentration is higher in the air than in the blood. The gas exchanges are slowed or halted as the concentrations approach equilibrium, and the exchanges are speeded as the differences in pressure become greater. The same process occurs at the cells, but the pressure differences are reversed, causing carbon dioxide to leave the cells and oxygen to enter.

External respiration—provisions for capturing oxygen (exchange at the lungs)

The total apparatus extending from the nose and mouth to the alveoli functions in the breathing process only as a passageway and is of little consequence to this discussion. The alveoli of the lungs are thin-walled air sacs, microscopic in size, as are the capillaries, and very much like bunches of grapes. Air enters the lungs because an increase in size of the chest cavity (thorax) results in air pressure less than that of the atmosphere, so the outside air rushes in to equalize the pressure. The expansion of the chest cavity is accomplished by the contraction, and thus flattening, of the dome-shaped diaphragm along with elevation of the ribs caused by contraction of the external intercostal muscle (sometimes aided by several other skeletal muscles). In expiration (if it is not forced), the diaphragm relaxes and "humps," thus reducing the thoracic space, increasing the pressure within, and causing the air to expel (Figure 11-2). In forced expiration, the contraction

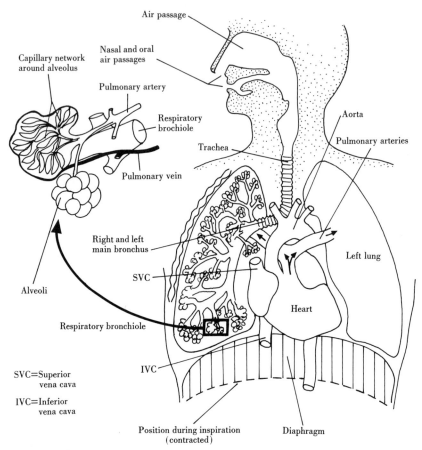

Figure 11–1.
Interaction of the respiratory and circulatory systems.

of the internal intercostal and the abdominal muscles further reduces the size of the thorax.

Vital capacity.   The total amount of air that can be forcibly expired after a complete inspiration is called *vital capacity*, which has been used frequently as a measure of adequacy of the respiratory system. Although it measures the approximate capacity of the lungs, it is of little use in predicting one's abilities to perform tasks of endurance. Obviously, other factors are involved which are more significant than vital capacity; for example, any limitation of the oxygen delivery system to the cells would reduce the effectiveness of the delivery, regardless of vital capacity.

The practice of hyperventilation (voluntary overfilling of the lungs by successive deep inhalations) is most often ineffective in aiding performance because the amount of oxygen transferred to the blood stream is not usually limited by the amount entering the lungs, but rather by the available area of contact between the alveoli and the capillary bed. If the blood is already fully saturated with oxygen,

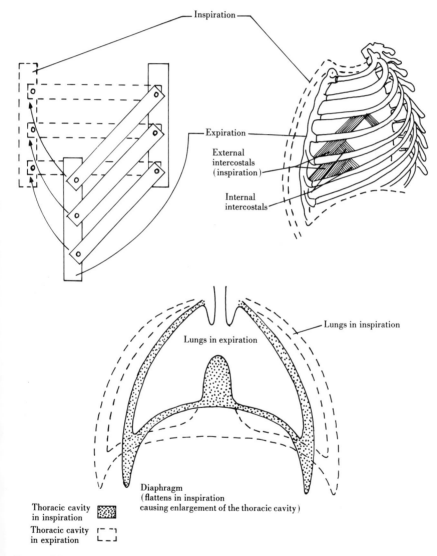

Figure 11–2.
Change of size of the thoracic cavity and lungs in breathing.

the excess oxygen in the lungs will only be expelled in normal expiration, because oxygen cannot be stored.

The only advantage of a greater vital capacity is the ability to take in more air per unit of time with *fewer*, but *deeper*, inspirations, thus prolonging the onset of fatigue in the muscles of respiration. A large vital capacity is more important during very intense exercise when a lack of oxygen may be found in the alveoli, but it is of little value when the exercise is less demanding.

Rate and depth of respiration.   The total amount of air inspired in one minute is called the minute volume, which is the product of the rate and depth of respiration. For the average adult at rest, the amount of air per normal respiration (500 cc) times the rate of breathing (about 17 per minute) equals an average minute volume (8,500 cc). This average volume varies in adults from 3,000 to 10,000 cc of air. Incidentally, rates of breathing of up to 75 per minute have been observed in athletes performing intensive swimming and running.

The ultimate control of the muscles of respiration is in the respiratory centers of the medulla of the brain (the pons also plays a significant role). These centers are part of the autonomic (automatic) nervous system; therefore, we breathe involuntarily. However, we may stimulate nerve receptors that generate impulses which will either increase or decrease the rate and depth of breathing. The factors influencing the stimulation of the nerve receptors, which alter rate and depth of breathing, are *muscular activity, emotions, carbon dioxide concentration, oxygen deficiency*, and *heart rate*. For example, voluntary control, such as breath holding, can be imposed for short periods of time until carbon dioxide excess causes stimulation of receptors which send impulses to the medulla, or until the medulla itself senses this condition in its arterial blood supply. The medulla then sends volleys of impulses to override the voluntary impulses which are holding the thorax immobile; thus inspiration begins involuntarily. Conversely, the stretching of lung tissues when an overabundance of air is in the alveoli, as after hyperventilating, stimulates pressure receptors, and the medulla will then send inhibitory impulses to the muscles which control breathing.

The most apparent and significant control of breathing results from excessive carbon dioxide in the venous blood flow. Oxygen deficiencies do not seem to exert as much influence until the lack becomes critical.

Factors governing external respiration.   The exchange of oxygen and carbon dioxide through the membranes of the alveoli and lung capillaries is dependent upon the following five factors:

1. *Pressure gradients of each gas.* As muscular work increases, the used blood traveling to the lungs becomes lower in oxygen content and higher in carbon dioxide content, thus enhancing the exchange of gases at the lungs.

2. *Amount of surface area of contact between capillaries and alveoli.* New capillaries are produced with endurance training, and perhaps alveoli also increase in surface area and, possibly, in number. Obviously, more surface area will allow

greater opportunity for exchange of gases. Amount of surface area becomes especially important during intensive exercise, when a faster rate of blood flow through a given surface area will allow less time for gas exchange.

3. *Thickness of the membranes.* Even though this is an important factor, it seems that little can be done to alter it. It is possible, although not confirmed, that the tars deposited on the membranes of the alveoli from smoking may restrict the gas exchange by adding thickness to the membranes and plugging available openings, thus reducing permeability. Negative effects of smoking on performance are more evident in endurance activities than in nonendurance performances.

4. *Capacity of the blood hemoglobin for oxygen.* Only a small amount of oxygen can travel in the blood plasma; most of it moves in loose compound with the blood hemoglobin. Thus the composition of the blood can limit the amount of oxygen the blood absorbs and carries.

5. *Respiratory minute volume.* The supply of air in the lungs becomes greater as the rate and depth of respiration increase. Under conditions of heavy work, a greater supply of air increases the amounts of gas entering and leaving the blood.

Blood—the circulatory vehicle

An adult's body contains 12 to 13 pints of blood. Blood that contains a high level of hemoglobin can transport more oxygen because oxygen travels through the blood in the form of oxyhemoglobin, a loose chemical combination. Each red blood cell (erythrocyte) is jammed with millions of molecules of hemoglobin. Each cell has a life span of about three to four months, and the younger cells have better gas-carrying properties, due to a greater hemoglobin concentration. If the replacement of cells lags, anemia results. Carbon dioxide also travels in combination with hemoglobin.

Blood transports other substances in addition to the respiratory gases. Among them are:

1. Nutrients, such as glucose, amino acids, and fats, which are carried to the cells
2. Regulatory substances, such as hormones, enzymes, and mineral salts, which are distributed to various locations
3. Metabolic wastes, such as urea, uric acid, creatinine, and lactic acid, which are carried away from the cells
4. Protective substances which continually circulate within the blood

Heart—the force for circulation

The heart is a hollow muscular organ divided into four chambers (Figure 11–3). The two upper chambers, atria or auricles, receive the blood and, by gentle contraction of their walls, aid the passage of the blood to the two lower chambers, the ventricles. Subsequently, the thick ventricle walls contract powerfully, squeezing the blood within them with such force that the blood is propelled out through the arteries and circulated to all body tissues.

For functional purposes, the left and right sides of the heart should be considered as two separate pumps, although their contractions are synchronous; both atria contract at the same time, followed closely by simultaneous contractions of both ventricles. The right side receives used blood in its atrium from all body tissues. The blood passes to the right ventricle from which it is ejected (upon the ventricle's contraction) to both lungs via the pulmonary arteries. The blood is oxygenated in the lungs and then returned to the left atrium via the pulmonary veins. It then proceeds to fill the left ventricle (extremely thick-walled and powerful) from which it is ejected through the aorta and circulated throughout the body. **Coronary system.**   The heart, an active working muscle, needs nourishment as does any other organ, but it cannot receive it from the blood which passes through it. The heart has its own circulatory system, the coronary system, which is a sort of feedback of 4 to 5 percent of the total supply of blood. An occlusion of this system results in a deprivation of blood to the heart muscle, called a heart attack. If the blocking is extensive, death results. All people develop a degree of heart disease (at least the loss of tissue elasticity) as they age, so those past thirty-five years should treat themselves accordingly.

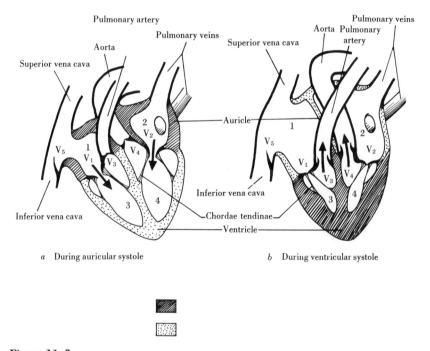

a   During auricular systole   b   During ventricular systole

Figure 11–3.
Valve actions and blood flow during auricular and ventricular systoles. (*After Amberson*)

Cardiac cycle and valve actions.   A cardiac cycle consists of all the actions of the heart, and in any one cycle no action is repeated. In adults, a complete cycle lasts about $\frac{8}{10}$ second (72 per minute). The blood flow within the heart is directed by the action of four valves. Each valve opens and closes as the result of pressure changes. The two cuspid valves (V1 and V2 in Figure 11-3) separate the upper and lower chambers on either side of the heart. The semilunar valves (V3 and V4) separate each ventricle from its arterial exit. Valves allow blood to flow in only one direction. Valves V1 and V2 allow it to flow from the atria downward to the ventricles, and valves V3 and V4 allow it to flow from the ventricles upward and out through the arteries.

Leakage of any of these valves is referred to as a murmur and results in an unwanted backflow, which reduces the effectiveness of the pump. Many murmurs are functional and do not interfere with operation of the heart.

Heart beat and blood volume.   The full cardiac cycle allows the atria to rest about 75 percent of the cycle and the ventricles to rest about 60 percent of the cycle. No other rest time is possible for these tissues; so the importance of rest during the cycle is great. Any increase in heart rate is made at the expense of the rest time, thus increasing the demands on the heart muscle.

The amount of blood ejected from the left ventricle with each contraction of the ventricles is called the *stroke volume* (SV). The SV multiplied by the number of contractions per minute (heart rate) is called the *minute volume* (MV). The output of both ventricles in a minute is referred to as the *cardiac output* (CO). The CO is equal to twice the MV. Under conditions of rest, an average SV is about 75 milliliters, and the average heart rate is about 72, resulting in an average MV of (75 × 72) 5,400 milliliters of blood, 5.4 liters, or 5.1 quarts, and a CO of twice that amount.

To summarize, CO may be altered by a change in either SV or heart rate, or *both*. If either SV or heart rate increases as the other decreases, the CO may increase, decrease, or not vary at all. In normal functioning, the activity of the body cells will determine the needed blood flow. The heart will respond to this need, and the heart rate will be adjusted accordingly. Changes in SV are not achieved immediately, and, consequently, an increased output (resulting from increased heart rate) results in a reduction of rest time for the heart muscle. This condition is not detrimental for relatively short periods of time, but if it is prolonged, it strains the heart. An intensive training program over a sufficient period of time will increase the SV. For a like amount of work, the heart with the greater SV will contract less often, and, as a result, it gets more rest. An increase in SV is an economical development in terms of heart function, but an increase of heart rate is not.

Overloading.   The CO depends upon the pumping effectiveness of the heart and the ease of blood return to the heart. An increase in the venous return will produce a greater filling of the heart, which in turn produces a stronger contraction. The stretching "overloads" the heart. A gradual overloading will strengthen the contractile force. Thickening (hypertrophy) of the heart tissue, especially the ventricle walls, results from the gradual overload. The stronger heart can then increase the SV, mostly because it causes a more complete emptying of the chambers.

Excessive stretching (especially over a long period of time) will elongate the fibers of the heart muscle, resulting in a condition called *dilation*. A heart usually is overextended (dilated) when blood is forced through the vessels despite excessive resistance. For example, hardening, or lack of elasticity, of the arteries (arteriosclerosis) or the deposits of materials on inner arterial walls (atherosclerosis) are conditions that produce resistance to blood flow. A dilated heart cannot contract with the force of a healthy heart because the chamber walls have grown thinner, similar to a balloon that is blown up. Continuation of this condition leads to an inability of the fibers to contract, which is called heart failure.

Hypertrophy and excessive stretching result in a heart whose exterior size is larger than average. The dilated (stretched) heart is a diseased heart, whereas the hypertrophied heart is more efficient and stronger than the average nonconditioned, disease-free heart. Endurance training produces a hypertrophied heart which can achieve a greater CO coupled with a slower heart rate for a given task. **Control of heart rate.**   The heart is dependent upon a great variety of sensory stimuli transmitted to the medulla of the brain. Impulses either to the accelerator or to inhibitory centers in the medulla may influence the heart rate. Two examples follow:

1. When a blood pressure increase is detected by the sensory pressure receptors, the rate of inhibitory impulses is increased, and the vagus nerve carries information to slow the impulses. This results in a decreased CO and thus reduced blood pressure.
2. The hormone *epinephrine* (adrenalin) works on the accelerator and increases the heart rate in time of emotional upheaval.

Although nerve receptors send information that causes heart rate to vary, the origin of the heart beat is within the heart itself. It can continue to perform at its own rate without other nervous control. However, this constant rate cannot meet the changing needs of the cells, so the changes in rate, accomplished by the autonomic nervous system, are vital to body functions, especially during performance.

Blood vessels—routes of circulation

The blood, after passing through the heart, leaves the left ventricle and enters the aorta, the main vessel of supply to the whole body. The movement of the blood from the aorta involves passage through vessels that progressively diminish in size and become more numerous, until finally the blood enters larger vessels called veins, which carry the blood toward the heart. The blood passes from smaller to larger veins until it finally enters the main veins, which return used blood back to the heart.

All vessels carrying blood away from the heart are called arteries. Arteries are encircled by smooth muscles which allow changes in size; thus the amount of blood that the arteries will carry varies. When the blood flow is greater than usual, the arteries dilate or enlarge their caliber; when the flow is less than usual, they constrict or narrow their openings. Constriction is due to contraction of the smooth muscles in the walls of the arteries whereas dilation results from relaxation of the muscles, thus allowing the force of the blood to expand the vessels. Additional blood can be "borrowed" from inactive areas and directed to areas of greater needs by varying the vessel openings (size).

Functionally, the capillaries are the most important vessels, for they deliver substances to cells and collect substances from cells. An adequate blood supply must be maintained in the capillaries because here the purpose of the circulatory system is finally realized. It is estimated that 1 cubic inch of muscle tissue contains several million capillaries. Some are so small that a single red blood cell is passed through them with great difficulty. Capillaries enlarge with greater blood pressure; they reduce in caliber with lesser pressure; and when not regularly forced to carry blood, they disappear.

The veins return blood to the heart, and compared with the arteries, they are relatively thin-walled. The numerous small veins near the capillaries tend to feed larger and larger veins until the blood enters the mainstream of return, the vena cava, which empties into the right atrium of the heart. The main pressure necessary to keep the blood moving through the veins is provided by the heart's pumping action, but auxiliary aids to venous flow come from (1) rhythmic pressure changes resulting from increased respiration action, and (2) the squeezing actions of skeletal muscles. Backup of blood in the veins is prevented by a series of pocketlike valves found on the interior walls of the veins. Surface veins appear blue in color because of the blood's high carbon dioxide concentration.

Blood pressure—maintaining the force for circulation

Blood flow is dependent upon the difference in pressure from one point to another along the length of the vessels. The flow is always from the point of higher pressure to the point of lower pressure. Pressure readings at any point are largely dependent upon the following factors:

1. *Heart pumping action,* which governs the amount of blood pumped in a given time (this is pushing pressure—pressure from behind). If the blood volume (CO) increases and all other factors remain constant, the pressure from behind increases.

2. *Resistance,* which is afforded by the vessels and the viscosity or composition of the blood itself (this is resisting pressure—pressure from ahead). If the caliber of the vessel increases and all other factors remain constant, the pressure from ahead decreases.

3. *Distance* from the heart. As the distance from the heart increases, and all other factors remain constant, the pressure decreases.

These factors are the same as those which affect water passing through a garden hose. Assuming the nozzle is at the point where pressure is measured, then (1) if less water comes in, less pressure is available to force water through the nozzle; (2) if the opening at the nozzle is increased, there is less pressure to resist passage of water through the nozzle; (3) the longer the hose, the greater the water force must be for effective pressure at the nozzle. Whereas the composition of the water is fairly constant, blood may be thicker or thinner depending upon several factors. The thicker the blood (greater viscosity), the more resistance there is to its flow.

Ideal blood pressure.   Ideal pressure is enough pressure to maintain the flow needed in the capillaries, but not so much that undue stress is placed upon the heart and vessels. Consequently, ideal pressure differs for each individual, since the integrity of the tissue differs from one individual to another. But certain blood pressure ranges have been found to be "safe" while extremes are indicative of malfunctions. Furthermore, because of changing conditions of the body tissues, what may have been safe at one time may now be cause for concern. For example, a slightly higher pressure reading in young adults may be advantageous in maintaining a constant and plentiful blood supply to the tissues, and the resilient young vessels may be under no undue stress. As the individual ages, the same pressure may produce strain to the point of rupture as the elasticity of the tissue lessens. The antithesis of this situation is blood pressure so low that blood supply to vital areas is insufficient.

Rerouting to active areas.   The control of blood pressure is involuntary, and changes in pressure occur in response to changing body conditions. The responses are directed toward insuring a constantly adequate blood supply. A common response to increased skeletal muscle activity in a local area can proceed as follows:

A certain local area may need more blood. To carry more blood, the vessels in that area must dilate. If all else remains constant, the dilation will reduce blood pressure in the area. The pressure may be retained at the needed level through an increase in heart action and/or constriction of vessels in less active areas.

The active area now gains more blood and an increased pressure, which speeds the flow of the blood through the area. The medulla concerns itself with overall needs of the body, so if the muscles are using so much blood that the function of any vital process is impaired, stimulation from the medulla will step up the cardiac output to meet the additional demand for blood.

Measurement of blood pressure and some interpretations.   Blood pressure, the outward pushing force of the blood at any point along a vessel, is measured in millimeters of mercury by the indirect method over the brachial artery wall. Although the pressure at this point is not the same as that at any other point, it is representative of the whole arterial system. The pressure becomes a lesser value as the measurement is taken a greater distance from the heart.

The pressure at the brachial artery reaches its greatest value soon after the ventricles of the heart have contracted (systolic pressure), and it reaches its lowest value immediately prior to the next contraction (diastolic pressure). These values are recorded by placing the systolic reading over the diastolic, and the average for the young adult is 120/80 mm. The average venous pressure at that point is only 5 mm. The systolic pressure provides direct information about the force of contraction of the left ventricle and indirect information about the elasticity of the vessels. The diastolic pressure provides direct information about the resistance of the vessels, thereby indicating the constant strain upon the vessels.

There are certain asumptions about one's physical condition that can be made from pressure readings, but none are clear-cut. Much depends upon whether readings are taken under conditions of rest, moderate exercise, or severe exercise, or when a state of disease exists (the latter can severely confuse readings).

Further complications in using blood pressure as a measure of fitness arise because of considerable unreliability of readings, chiefly caused by apprehension and other emotions. Difficulties in interpreting readings taken during exercise, as well as immediately after exercise, also contribute to unreliability of blood pressure measures. At best, blood pressures can be only rough indicators of fitness, and then only when the individual is assumed to be free of disease and emotional stress.

The pulse.   A pulse (such as at the radial artery in the wrist or the carotid artery in the neck) is produced by the alternating expansion and recoil of the arteries as the blood spurts from the left ventricle and progresses in wavelike fashion through the arteries. Pulse strength is influenced by the SV and the elasticity of the vessels. The pulse itself is the blood spurting through the point of the artery. Losing intensity as it gets farther from the heart, the pulse is nonexistent in the veins and capillaries.

Internal respiration—exchange at the tissues

The use of oxygen at the tissues is true respiration (biological oxidation). The oxygen take-up at the tissues is dependent upon (1) surface area of contact (this can be altered when more capillaries are produced through training), and (2) the pressure gradient. The pressure gradient will vary with the activity of the tissues and the oxygen content of the blood at the point of exchange. As the tissues become more active, they use more oxygen. It should be noted that under rest conditions the tissues extract only about 20 to 25 percent of the available oxygen in the blood. Therefore, venous blood remains about 75 to 80 percent oxygen saturated. The efficiency of the gas exchange between the capillaries and tissues will greatly influence the work capacity of the organism, especially its capacity to endure.

Use of oxygen by muscles—aerobic processes.   The chemical processes that produce energy for muscular contraction are highly complicated and are beyond the scope of this discussion, but one point usually misunderstood should be clarified. *Muscular contraction does not require the presence of oxygen.* Actually, it is best to think of oxygen as necessary for the recovery rather than for the contractile process. Certain chemical changes are accomplished without the presence of oxygen (*anaerobic*), whereas other changes require the presence of oxygen (*aerobic*). Anaerobic contractions may continue for about 40 seconds at maximum effort without any involvement of aerobic processes, though both processes are normally carried on simultaneously. Most products produced in the anaerobic processes at some time must be reconverted to the state in which they existed before contraction; mainly, lactic acid is reconverted to glycogen. This reaction depends upon the presence of oxygen. It is the anaerobic conversion which will cause blood lactate levels to rise significantly; high blood lactate has long been suspected as one of the prime causes of fatigue.

Steady state and oxygen debt.   If oxygen is delivered to the cells in sufficient quantity, the resynthesis keeps up with the anaerobic processes; and it is said that a *steady state* has been reached. Steady states for well-conditioned athletes occur under moderate work levels. During heavy exercise respiratory functioning often lags several minutes behind the increased need for oxygen, and oxygen deficit occurs. The organism may work for a duration of the effort without the respiratory system catching up. Of course, if the rate of work is so great that the respiratory system cannot provide sufficient oxygen, the steady state will never be established, and an oxygen deficit will continue to build up throughout the effort. The recovery, then, must take place after the exercise, and the amount of oxygen needed to restore the body to its prework status is called the *oxygen debt.* The oxygen debt that one accumulates depends upon:

1.   Physiological reserves, the availability of necessary substances within the body
2.   The efficiency of oxygen delivery during work
3.   The performer's tolerance to lactic acid accumulation

The lighter the exercise, the more quickly the steady state is attained; for very light work, little, if any, oxygen debt is noticed. Lactic acid is removed as it is produced. On the other hand, a maximum effort of brief duration may be completed before significant repayment of any oxygen debt can begin, as in running and swimming sprints. In such cases, nearly all the debt is repaid after the completion of the effort. The repayment is characterized by prolonged rapid and heavy breathing, and the contribution of the effort to improved endurance is proportional to the intensity and duration of the breathing.

Few, if any, performers have respiratory mechanisms which can exceed 5 liters per minute of oxygen delivery (most provide less than 2 liters). The capacity for oxygen debt is rarely more than a total of 10 to 15 liters. In general terms, the length of time an effort can be sustained can be estimated for an individual if the total debt capacity and the volume of delivery per unit of time are known. For example, if an individual who can deliver 3 liters per minute has a debt capacity of 15 liters and is working at a rate requiring 6 liters per minute, he is working at a deficit of 3 liters per minute and can continue at this rate for five minutes.

Alternate bursts and reductions of speed are uneconomical because the bursts incur unnecessary debt, and running at less than the steady state does not fully utilize the oxygen inhaled. Also, if the rate is too fast early in a distance run or swim, the limits of the oxygen-debt capacity will be approached quickly, after which the performer must slow down or possibly stop. Each of the foregoing statements emphasizes the importance of proper pace. Thus, we find that the best mile runs are accomplished with a relatively constant pace, in excess of the steady state. The last 200- to 300-yard sprint will bring on maximum oxygen debt.

A great deal of the oxygen debt is paid quickly after exercise, but a small amount of the accumulated lactic acid seems to linger for longer periods of time, probably because the body attempts to reestablish a reasonably comfortable condition quickly but then proceeds leisurely to complete the resynthesis.

Effects of vigorous performance on the circulorespiratory system

The fit individual has a circulorespiratory system which is capable of meeting the demands of the tissues under conditions of intense exercise. As the exercise increases in intensity, the following must occur:

1. External respiration keeps up with the increase of gas exchanges in order to help delay fatigue.
2. Amount and rate of blood flow increase, and blood pressures are adjusted to ensure that the blood supply to the tissues is adequate at all times.

External respiration

During both rest and exercise, the well-conditioned individual displays a slower rate and a greater depth of respiration. When hard exercise is performed, breathing becomes intense, and the respiratory muscles are worked much harder than usual. Excessive work is fatiguing to these muscles. Overexertion of the respiratory muscles produces a condition known as a "stitch in the side" (side ache). In poorly conditioned performers, this condition often produces pain levels that the performers cannot or will not tolerate. It has been shown that less oxygen intake is needed and less carbon dioxide is expelled for a given work load as an individual becomes more fit, and under a maximal load, a greater exchange of air is possible in the fit person. The specific results of conditioning on external respiration are:

1. A slower breathing rate under all conditions (the rate may sometimes be reduced by one-half).

2. Deeper breathing, which gives more assurance of enough air in the alveoli.

3. A lesser oxygen intake per work load, which probably results from increased neuromuscular efficiency.

4. A more extensive capillary bed in the lungs, providing a greater area for gas exchange (may increase up to 50 percent). Incidentally, this growth of capillaries is also evident, and no less important, in the area of the muscle tissues.

5. An increase of alveoli in both size and number, which provides a greater area for gas exchange (physiologists disagree on this point).

6. A faster return to resting levels of rate and depth of breathing after a *given work load*.* (This indicates less oxygen debt and greater efficiency in repaying the debt.)

A very well-conditioned individual can produce approximately three times as much gas exchange as a poorly conditioned person.

Circulation

Because the tissues utilize the materials needed for metabolism more rapidly during exercise, the blood (acting as the carrier) must be delivered more rapidly and in greater quantity to the tissues. Training increases the capacity of the circulatory system to transport blood, but this increase must be accompanied by respiratory improvements which will allow adequate time for the blood to become oxygen saturated. This is partly accomplished by dilation of the capillaries in the alveoli (bringing more blood to the area) and the expansion of the contact area between the alveoli and capillaries.

As the intensity of exercise increases, the circulatory system must keep up by providing more blood output and by maintaining correct blood pressures under changing conditions, thus assuring adequate delivery of blood to the tissues and removal of metabolic wastes. The specific characteristics of the well-conditioned circulatory system can be understood best when they are arranged under the topics of blood, heart, and blood pressure.

---

* It should be made clear that a "given work load" refers to equal loads for all individuals considered and not maximum loads for each individual.

Blood.   The following characteristics of blood accompany improved condition (fitness) :

1. The blood of well-conditioned individuals contains a reduced amount of lactic acid for a given amount of work. This indicates less reliance on anaerobic processes and greater efficiency of aerobic processes.

2. Well-conditioned individuals can mobilize blood sugar more rapidly and in greater quantities, and often they can maintain a high blood sugar level even after 30 minutes of intensive work. Significant reductions may not register until after three or more hours of constant work. In addition, more fuel (glycogen, phosphocreatine, and myoglobin) is stored in the muscle tissues themselves.

3. The exchange of materials between the blood and the tissues becomes more efficient, thus less blood needs to be provided to the working muscles for a given amount of work. This frees greater amounts of blood to provide for vital organs (kidneys, heart, brain, etc.) during exercise.

4. An increase of red corpuscles and a loss of water content, resulting from even small amounts of exercise, may increase blood viscosity up to 10 percent. This causes an immediate increase in pressure and gas-carrying capacity.

Heart.   A greater stroke volume is noted in the well-conditioned performer. It follows, then, that there is a greater minute volume or cardiac output without the expense of an increase in heart rate. Through conditioning programs, resting heart rate can be reduced as much as 10 to 20 beats per minute, thus providing a good indication of training progress. In summary, the more fit individual will show lower heart rates for a given amount of work and a faster return to resting rate. The latter is related to oxygen debt repayment.

Blood pressure.   There are several important general facts about blood pressure as it relates to exercise:

1. Chronic high blood pressure (not temporary strain) is considered detrimental, but even the highest temporary pressure rises resulting from exercise will not exceed physiological limits of a healthy vascular system.

2. No evidence exists to indicate that a healthy young circulatory system can be harmed as a result of exercise. However, it still seems prudent to increase amounts of exercise gradually during training in order that the system will not be severely overtaxed.

3. If blood pressures adjust well under various levels of exercise, it is logically assumed that tissues in need are receiving adequate blood supply, in terms of both volume and rate of flow.

The following *systolic pressure* changes result from exercise:

1. Little change in systolic pressure is noted in *moderate* exercise bouts, probably because vascular adjustments are adequate to maintain pressure or to produce slight pressure increases.

2. *Very moderate* exercise, such as a slow walk, may actually produce a slight pressure drop. Capillaries in the area of activity dilate and thus reduce overall pressure; under such conditions the heart may not receive any acceleration impulses. Most likely, a pressure rise, resulting from increased heart action, is not needed, since the active tissues are probably extracting greater amounts of oxygen from the available blood. Remember, the tissues will extract only about 20 percent of available oxygen under rest conditions, so plenty is still available for slight increases in effort.

3. Invariably *vigorous* exercise, at or near maximum, results in greatly increased pressure.

4. Generally, the more intensive the exertion, the greater will be the systolic rise. Incidentally, under high pressure the force of the blood through the capillaries provides the stimulus for more capillary growth, which is most important to greater endurance. Explosive efforts, however, do not hold pressure levels long enough for maximum effects.

5. Little change in resting blood pressure occurs, even when great improvements in conditioning are achieved.

Changes in *diastolic pressure* resulting from exercise are not as evident as changes in systolic pressure, but the following responses have been observed:

1. A fairly high resting diastolic pressure, though not too high, is characteristic of a well-conditioned circulatory system. An even more encouraging sign is near maintenance of the resting level of pressure under conditions of increased demands.

2. The rapid return to resting pressure is a further indication of good condition.

Changes in venous pressure are not measured so easily. It should be noted that if venous flow does not increase in velocity and volume, it will not be possible to achieve a greater stroke volume. Thoracic pressures and skeletal muscle contraction either aid or detract from venous flow. In general, sustained isometric exercises pinch the vessels and retard blood flow and, eventually, reduce heart output. Isotonic contractions are an aid to circulation. The resistance to flow caused by excessive isometric contractions may be too much for the heart to overcome, and fainting will result. When venous flow is retarded by a pinching of vessels, higher arterial pressures will reflect the effort to overcome this increased resistance.

Internal respiration

Training probably increases the number of capillaries at the muscle tissues, and this increases the gas exchange area (for oxygen and carbon dioxide) at the tissues, thus contributing to increased endurance.

Approaching fatigue

Fatigue may be general or local. Limited movements in local body areas may cause local oxygen debt without being extensive enough to bring about circulorespiratory adjustments needed to overcome the debt. This local fatigue will then concentrate anaerobic wastes, even when the total effort is well within the bounds of the oxygen delivery system. Despite boosts in oxygen supply, the rapidity of the movement may be so great that the area cannot be supplied quickly enough with sufficient blood.

As general fatigue approaches, a progressive systolic pressure drop is observed. The trained performer can maintain an effective pressure level for a longer period of time. This pressure drop seems to be associated with the inability of the heart to sustain adequate blood levels. Soon after exercise, or often during exercise, a drastic pressure drop indicates a loss of muscle tone in the vessels. Low levels of blood sugar, along with high lactic acid levels, may develop. When these signs of fatigue become evident, varying degrees of nausea and tendencies toward loss of consciousness are probable. Tolerances toward higher blood lactate concentrations are achieved only when the performer is continually subjected to these high concentrations.

Training for circulorespiratory endurance

Limited information is available on comparison of endurance training methods. But the information that is available seems to support the following:

1. Top speed of an individual performer is not dependent upon the circulorespiratory system, but *maintaining* a certain speed for longer distances is strongly dependent upon this system.

2. To increase circulorespiratory endurance, overload must be applied. Overload in this case means overloading of intensity rather than duration. Even though *muscular* endurance may be improved by efforts of long duration at slow rates, *circulorespiratory* endurance, which is usually the limiting endurance factor, is influenced little by long duration exercise at a slow rate.

3. When a training program of a certain intensity is used, the significant improvements are usually made in the first three weeks, with practically no improvement thereafter. This indicates that a *progression* must be imposed in order to continue to overload the system. The progression must be in terms of intensity of work. For a description of how to apply overload by use of interval training, refer to the section on endurance, Chapter 8.

4. If after about three weeks of the same program additional durations of exercise are imposed, but the same intensity of effort is retained, little additional improvement occurs. Conversely, if the intensity of the work is increased, then new levels of endurance result.

5. A reduction in length of rest between exercise bouts equally increases both circulorespiratory endurance and the intensity of each bout. In either case, progression of overload is applied.

6. Significant improvements are noted in 7 to 14 days at each level of training intensity. It takes close to 7 training days in the early season and close to 14 days as performers reach higher fitness levels. About six weeks of intensive progressive

training are needed to achieve near-maximum *respiratory* efficiency, after which little more can be achieved. No limit, however, has been established for circulatory improvements.

7. If training is halted for 10 days, no change in endurance is evident in performers who have moderate endurance levels, but those who have high endurance levels show some deterioration in about five days.

"Burning out" due to overtraining

An often-used term that appears to be a misnomer is "burning out." The assumption is that if a performer starts early in life and trains too intensively, somehow his physiological systems will exhibit decreased function, and performances will suffer at a later age. The human machine will not wear out as will a man-made machine. Not only is there no evidence to support such a contention, but the opposite has been shown to be true. Physiological systems only improve with use; in fact, *lack of use* will produce less efficiency and other detrimental effects. Demands placed upon the systems of youngsters produce stimulation which seems to enhance growth and development.

The inability of some performers to reach anticipated potentials is probably due to a variety of factors, two of which are noted:

1. Young performers who achieve strength and size advantages associated with puberty sooner than their peers often excel in competition (especially contact sports) for several years. At this time predictions of potential are made, but advantages disappear when the slow developers catch up.

2. The high success attained at very early ages in certain competitive activities (especially among women swimmers) may reduce the desire to continue intensive training. Additional honors and awards often mean little. Furthermore, the aims and desires of performers change considerably at different ages.

Recommended supplementary reading

BEST, CHARLES HERBERT, and NORMAN BURKE TAYLOR: "The Living Body," 4th ed., pp. 115–209, 225–252, Holt, Rinehart and Winston, Inc., New York, 1965.

BROUHA, LUCIEN: Training, in Warren R. Johnson (ed.), "Science and Medicine of Exercise and Sports," pp. 403–416, Harper & Row, Publishers, Incorporated, New York, 1960.

DeCOURSEY, RUSSEL MYLES: "The Human Organism," 2d ed., pp. 314–398, McGraw-Hill Book Company, New York, 1961.

TUTTLE, W. W., and BYRON A. SCHOTTELIUS: "Textbook of Physiology," 15th ed., pp. 136–241, 303–308, The C. V. Mosby Company, St Louis, 1965.

Part 3

Application of mechanical laws and principles to performance

Part 3 deals with important principles derived from the fields of physics, mechanics, and mathematics which influence performance. As these chapters are studied, the reader will become more aware of how modern techniques of performance evolved from basic scientific laws and principles. The simplified statements of the laws and principles, along with the many practical examples, make the content easy to understand and apply. The content of this part forms the basis for mechanical analysis of performance.

Chapter 12 deals with the principles of motion, which are derived from Newton's three basic laws of motion. In Chapter 13 important factors relative to force are identified and discussed. Chapter 14 covers the important principles governing projections; Chapter 15 deals with balance, stability, and posture; and Chapter 16 is an example of the practical application of the content of the previous four chapters.

After studying Part 3 the reader should be well prepared to analyze performances from the mechanical point of view. This will assist him greatly in becoming a better teacher and performer.

Motion

*M*ost athletic performances require the performer either to move himself or to impart motion to an external object; therefore, motion is basic to athletic skills. It is impossible for a movement to occur unless a force produces it. The forces most often used in athletics are those produced by muscular contractions in combination with the ever-present force of gravity.

There are two kinds of motion: *rotary* and *translatory*. Rotary (or angular) motion does not transport an object from place to place; it is simply a turning of the object about an axis, or fulcrum. Appropriate synonyms for rotary motion are spinning, twisting, and turning. In rotary motion any point on the object describes the arc of a circle with the axis of the movement being at the center of that circle. Translatory motion, on the other hand, is movement over a distance from one point to another. *Linear* translatory motion takes place when the path of movement is a straight line; *curvilinear* translatory motion occurs when a curved pathway is followed. Curvilinear motion is distinguished from rotary motion in that while curvilinear motion may be in a perfectly circular path, the axis of rotation is not within the mass of the moving object. An object often experiences both rotary and translatory motion simultaneously, as does the earth when it spins about its axis (rotary) and follows a curvilinear (translatory) path around the sun. An object often experiences linear and curvilinear motion (both translatory) successively. For example, when an object is hurled through space, it starts its flight in a linear path but immediately changes to a curved path as a result of the forces of resistance. When a baseball pitcher throws a curve ball, the motion of the ball appears to be linear, but almost immediately after release, the ball follows a curvilinear path (rotation continues). The curvilinear path is governed by the direction and intensity of the spin, which usually causes a left or right movement, and the force of gravity, which causes a downward movement. The curved path the ball travels is dependent upon the combined magnitudes of the linear and rotary forces applied to the ball.

197

Translatory motion

Following are facts which contribute to understanding the role of linear motion in human performance. Curvilinear motion is discussed further in Chapter 14.

    1. An object will move in a straight line when:

       a. The object is freely movable, and the force is applied off-center. As the force is applied at a point farther from the center of gravity, the object will rotate around its center of gravity at a faster speed.

       b. Regardless of where the force is applied, the object is free to move only in a linear path. Example: a sliding door or window.

    2. The human body experiences linear motion when it is pushed or pulled by an outside force or glides over a smooth surface. Examples: skiing (straight) or sliding down a slide.

    3. In many instances, the body experiences linear motion due to rotary motion of some of its segments. Examples: swimming, walking, running, and vertical jumping.

    4. In some instances a distal segment may experience linear motion due to rotary motion of the proximal segments. Examples: the hand in fencing and the foot in pushing, as in the vertical jump.

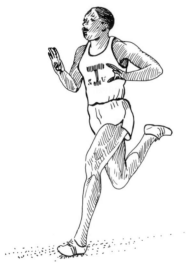

Figure 12–1.
Running illustrates linear motion of the total body and angular motion in the legs and arms.

Rotary (angular) motion

Following are important facts about rotary motion:

1. An object will rotate under the following conditions:
    a. If the object is freely movable, and the force is applied off-center. As the force is applied at a point farther from the center of gravity, the object will rotate around its center of gravity at a faster speed.
    b. If force is applied to any part of the object, and it is free to move only in a rotary path. Examples: swinging door, arm moving around the shoulder joint, and leg moving around the hip joint.
2. The human body as a whole experiences rotary motion under the following conditions: .
    a. When it is unsupported and revolves around its center of gravity. Examples: diving stunts, trampoline stunts, tumbling stunts, and certain gymnastic movements.
    b. When it is supported and revolves around the point of contact. Examples: cartwheel and handspring (both rotary and translatory). Giant swing (only rotary).
3. Individual body segments experience rotary movement by causing the segment to revolve around an axis which passes through the joint. Examples: arm rotates around the shoulder joint, lower leg rotates around the knee joint. Rotary motion may also occur around an axis which passes through the length of a segment. Examples: inward or outward rotation of the upper arm at the shoulder, pronation or supination of the forearm.

Speed of motion

The amount of distance an object travels in a given period of time represents its *velocity*, or speed. Usually an expressed velocity represents the average speed of movement and does not take into account the speed for any portion of the total distance. However, it is important to be aware that velocity of an object is seldom constant. Increase in the rate of speed is referred to as *acceleration*. The opposite of acceleration is *deceleration*. Acceleration may be uniform or varying, but, as with velocity, acceleration is seldom constant. When the weight (mass) of a moving object is combined with its velocity, the object is said to have *momentum*. $m V.$ Momentum is the product of velocity and mass. Therefore, an increase of either velocity or mass will cause an increase in momentum.

In explosive athletic events, one of the real concerns is the *final velocity* of the object in motion, which is the velocity at the climax of the action. For instance, when an object is thrown, the speed at which it is traveling when released (along with the angle of release) is the primary factor influencing the distance it will travel. The same is true of the human body when jumping. The velocity over the

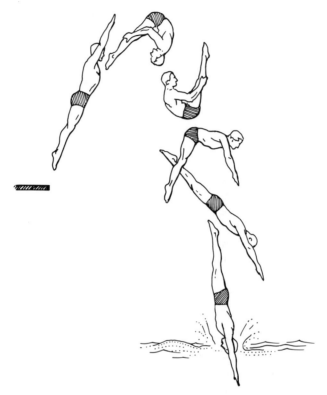

Figure 12–2.
The forward 1½ somersault illustrates rotary motion of the total
body as it moves through a curvilinear path of flight.

total effort (average) is of little concern, whereas the final velocity is of utmost
concern. If velocity climaxes at the correct instant, it is invariably the result of
muscular forces producing a sequential acceleration toward that climax. This
calls for precise timing, and its achievement is often the difference between the
skilled and unskilled performer. Obviously, greater force is necessary to produce
the same final velocity in a heavier object than in a lighter one. Therefore, an
increase in the body weight of a high-jumper could seriously reduce his final
velocity and thereby decrease the height he is able to jump. This principle also
applies to the jumping ability of a basketball or volleyball player.

In striking activities the greatest concern is *final momentum*, of which final
velocity is one important part. The same concepts apply to final momentum as
apply to final velocity, except in final momentum the weight of the striking implement is important as well as its velocity. This may cause a baseball batter to
select a heavier bat, but unless his muscular forces are sufficient to attain adequate

final velocity with the heavier bat, the final momentum may actually be less than it would have been with a lighter bat. If a football player can develop greater momentum with his moving body, he can strike a more forceful blow, which may mean that he should gain weight to be more effective. However, unless he can attain nearly the same velocity at impact that he had prior to the weight gain, his momentum may be either unchanged or less.

Basic laws of motion

Many teaching hints and coaching tips related to skill are derived from a number of principles of motion. These principles, in turn, are derived from just three basic laws of motion developed by Isaac Newton (1642–1727). If the teaching technique cannot be traced back to a basic newtonian law, assuming the technique has to do with motion, its soundness should be viewed with serious doubt. It is important to understand that some performance techniques may have evolved from ideas of performers who have been successful *in spite of* the unsoundness of their techniques. Furthermore, at times performers are convinced they do something in a certain way when actually it is done quite differently. For example, few divers are aware that most twisting movements are initiated while they are still in contact with the board.

At times, one law must be violated in order to observe another, if the latter produces effects of such magnitude that the effects of the former are made inconsequential. Following are Newton's three laws of motion:

Law of Inertia. A body at rest tends to remain at rest, whereas a body in motion tends to continue in motion with consistent speed and in the same direction unless acted upon by an outside force.

In effect, the first law refers to *resistance to any change* in motion. It takes force to begin motion, to retard motion, to accelerate an object, to change its direction, or to stop its motion. The greater the change is to be in the existing condition, the more force will be needed to produce the change. Resistance to change of motion is called *inertia*.

Law of Acceleration. The velocity of a body is changed only when acted upon by an additional force. The produced acceleration (or deceleration) is proportional to and in the same direction of force.

Obviously, if the body is at rest, it will have its greatest resistance to a force attempting to move it; the same amount of force will develop a greater acceleration after the body is in motion. To make this idea more applicable, let us say that if a performance calls for maximum acceleration, successive forces by body segments should be applied to the object, allowing no deceleration between forces.

If an applied force is directly opposite the movement of an object, then (1) it will tend to decelerate the object if the force is less than that of the object (air resistance, gravity, water resistance, etc., oppose the body with a small amount of force over a long period of time), (2) it will stop the object if the magnitude of the force is equal to that of the object, or (3) it will reverse the direction of the object if the magnitude is greater than that of the object. If a force is applied to a moving body at an angle (neither directly with nor against the path of motion), the resulting change in both velocity and direction of the body depends upon the magnitude and the angle of that force (determined by a parallelogram of forces).

Law of Counterforce. The production of any force will create another force which will be opposite and equal to the first force.

The effects of this law depend upon whether the body is supported or nonsupported. If the body is supported by a firm surface, the effects of a counterforce will be maximum. In the broad jump, for example, the resistance of the earth makes possible the thrust. The muscular force that is directed backward and downward against the earth is insufficient to overcome the inertia of the earth, and the counterforce of the earth pushing back is effective in propelling the performer. If the same action is attempted under conditions of improper foot contact, due to a slippery surface or a "giving" surface such as loose sand, the counterforce is reduced. To compensate for such conditions, the performer will automatically redirect the force of the thrust to a more vertical direction, thus preventing slippage. The counterforce will then be improved, but the direction of it will be more vertical, resulting in a takeoff angle which will not be conducive to maximum distance.

Another example of counterforce is in swimming, where the hands are directed backward against the water, and the water produces the counterforce necessary to propel the body. It is the *counterforce* which makes it possible for the performer to propel himself.

When the body is unsupported, the action of one of its parts will provide a counteraction of another part but will not alter the flight path because the air does not provide sufficient resistance to generate a counterforce, as does a solid (earth) or a liquid (water).

Principles of motion

Derived from basic physical laws, principles of performance are generalized statements which govern the technique of sound performance. It is difficult to separate principles of motion from those of force, but for convenience, the attempt is made herein, despite some evident overlaps.

Principles related to the law of inertia

If the following principles are observed, the law of inertia will not be violated, and performance will be aided rather than retarded.

Combining translatory and rotary motions. Successful performance often calls for effectively combining translatory and rotary motions.

Example A: An effective discus throw results from several movements. The performer moves the total body linearly from the back to the front of the circle, and in doing so he overcomes the inertia of the discus to that motion. He rotates the total body with ever-increasing velocity as he moves forward. Then, near the end of the total body rotary movement, he thrusts the discus by use of upper body rotation and rotary actions of the throwing arm. These combined motions, if performed correctly with proper sequence and timing, will produce maximum final velocity of the discus in the desired direction at release. *Example B:* A jumper uses both the translatory motion of the approach and rotary motion of his body segments at the takeoff. The approach overcomes the inertia to forward progress while the vertical thrust overcomes the inertia to vertical progress. The relative emphasis on each kind of motion depends upon the objective of the jump (vertical or horizontal). *Example C:* Shift of body weight is a movement common to many activities, especially throwing and striking actions. It is commonly referred to as "getting your body into the act." This means transferring the body weight from one foot to the other in the direction of the action and is another example of linear motion of the total body combined with rotary motion of the body segments. Batting a baseball, executing a tennis stroke, throwing an object, and changing direction in running are all examples in which the weight shift is valuable.

Continuity of motion. When performing activities in which two or more consecutive motions contribute to movement in the same direction, there should usually be no pause between the motions. The accomplishment of the first motion represents the overcoming of a certain amount of inertia. Any hesitation prior to the next motion will result in loss of some or all of the advantage gained by the previous motion. A force applied to an object already moving in the desired direction will be more effective in producing acceleration, because the object offers less resistance.

Example A: When a pole-vaulter pulls himself upward, then reverses and pushes himself farther upward, there should be no pause between the pull and the push (except as influenced by the reaction of the pole). Both motions contribute to movement in the same direction. *Example B:* During the kip, the gymnast pulls has body upward and then pushes himself farther upward. Again there should be no pause between the pull and the push. *Example C:* The tumbler requires less muscular force to execute a backward roll if he starts from a standing position and allows the force of gravity to begin the movement, thereby overcoming some of the resistance to his backward rotary motion. He accomplishes this by moving backward and downward to a sitting position. If he stops in the sitting position, he gains nothing because the next movement must continue immediately after the previous one. *Example D:* If the shot-putter hesitates between his movement across the ring and the final thrust, he loses the value of the former movement. This principle also applies to swimming, running, kicking, throwing, and other basic motor skills.

Effects of momentum.   If two objects are moving at the same velocity, the heavier of the two will possess the greater momentum, and the greater the momentum of an object, the greater resistance (inertia) it will present to a change in direction or velocity. If the motion of the object becomes a force (as it contacts another object), the greater its momentum at impact, and the greater will be its force.

Example A: As a football player moves with greater momentum, he becomes less susceptible to forces which attempt to alter that momentum. Therefore, weight is advantageous if it does not reduce speed. To completely stop the player's momentum, a body possessing equal or greater momentum must hit him head on. If that body has less weight, it can develop greater momentum only by attaining greater speed. If the contact is made from any direction other than straight on, the result will depend on the principle of multiple forces (discussed in Chapter 13). *Example B:* The basketball or football player who wishes to change his direction of movement quickly will find the change more difficult with greater momentum. He will also find the change more difficult as the degree of change in direction increases. Change of direction requires that a retarding force and a redirecting force be applied, and these forces, which overcome momentum, must be increased as momentum is increased. *Example C:* The selection of a heavier baseball bat, or any striking implement, provides opportunity for developing greater momentum, but only if sufficient muscular force is available so that the speed of the swing is not decreased. More momentum can be produced with a longer implement because if angular velocity is the same, the end of a longer implement will move faster than a shorter implement. (A more thorough explanation of this point may be found in the section on leverage, page 212.)

Transfer of momentum.   Momentum developed in a body segment may be transferred to the total body, but only while the body is in contact with the supporting surface. The longer and heavier the body segment is, and the greater its speed, the greater will be its contribution to total body momentum. This principle is applied in all jumping actions.

Example A: In jumping, the swinging action of the arms and the free leg transfers momentum to the rest of the body. *Example B:* If the swinging leg or arm is straight, it contributes more to momentum (if angular speed of the swinging limb is held constant) than if it is not straight. *Example C:* In the track start, the forward driving actions of the arms contribute momentum to the total body.

Note: Any movements of body parts after contact has been broken with the surface, such as swinging the arms or "running in the air" by the broad jumper, will not change the flight of the body as a whole.

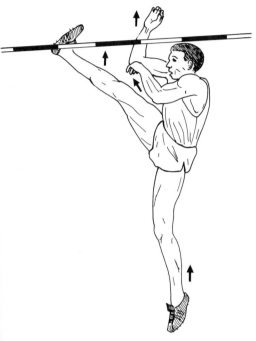

Figure 12–3.
The high-jumper swings his arms and free leg
vigorously, using them to pull the total body upward.
This is known as transfer of momentum from swinging body parts.

Principles related to the law of acceleration

Application of the following principles results in acceleration or conservation
of velocity and momentum.

Acceleration is proportional to force.   Acceleration is proportional to the
force causing it, providing the mass is held constant. Therefore, if the force is
doubled, the rate of acceleration is also doubled (except for effects of air or water
resistance which vary with the theoretical square law [Chapter 13]).

$f = ma$

Example A: A sprinter can increase acceleration by increasing the force that he
applies backward and downward against the surface on which he is running. If
he were able to reduce the mass (body weight) and keep the force constant, then
he would increase acceleration. *Example B:* A swimmer can increase acceleration
by increasing the force that he applies against the water with his stroke and kick.

Regarding acceleration, it must be realized that in body movements muscle
contractions provide the force, and more forceful contractions expend more

energy. The energy cost of a muscle contraction varies with the cube of the speed of contraction. If muscle X contracts twice as fast as muscle Y, then its energy cost is eight times as great as that of muscle Y. If muscle X contracts three times as fast as muscle Y, its energy cost is twenty-seven times a great as that of muscle Y. This fact has much application in determining the rate at which a performer should accelerate. It has great application especially in endurance activities.

Maximum acceleration and efficiency of motion.   To achieve maximum acceleration, all available forces should be applied sequentially with proper timing and as directly as possible in the intended line of motion. Body actions extraneous to the desired movement should be reduced to a minimum.

Example A: A swimmer performing the crawl stroke should attempt to increase the forces which propel the body in the desired direction and decrease all other actions, such as lifting the body upward or weaving it from side to side. *Example B:* Watching the head of a runner or hurdler from the side reveals whether or not the forces are properly directed forward rather than upward. In either case, the objective is to move forward, and excessive up-and-down head motion indicates misdirected force.

In some cases maximum acceleration (and thus maximum speed) is not the prime objective of the performance. Acceleration may be sacrificed for quickness of release, such as many throws in baseball other than pitching, or it may be sacrificed for greater accuracy, as in the basketball free throw. In these cases, usually fewer joint actions, and thus fewer forces, are used.

Effects of the body's radius on rotational (angular*) speed.   If a constant force causes a body to rotate, lengthening of the radius slows the rotation, whereas shortening of the radius increases the rotation. This results because the resistance against the rotating force is less effective when its radius is shorter.

Example A: In springboard diving, the rate of rotation (and thus the number of turns) is increased as the tuck is tightened, causing the body's radius of rotation to shorten. A pike position produces a slower rotation, and a lay-out position allows a still slower rotation. *Example B:* A skater or dancer may increase the speed of his spin by bringing his arms close to the body, or he may decrease the spinning speed by reaching outward. *Example C:* Pole vaulting involves several rotational movements. The two primary ones are the pole rotating about the box and the total body rotating about the handgrip. By lowering the grip on the pole the speed of the pole rotating about the box is increased, but the height to which the body is raised is decreased. By pulling the body toward the grip at the correct time, the rate of body rotation about the grip is increased, and the momentum resulting from the early phase of the swing is conserved.

---

* The terms *angular* and *rotational* are interchangeable. *Angular* is the term usually used when the rotating body has a point of contact with some surface, and rotational is the term usually used for freely moving bodies.

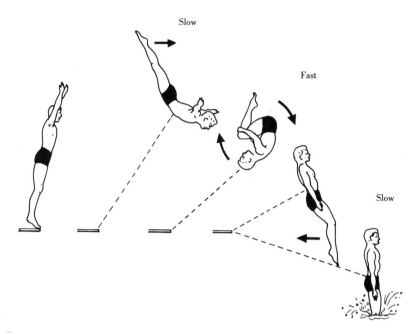

Figure 12–4.
When a performer, who is rotating, moves from the layout to the tuck position, his rate of rotation increases. In a tight tuck he will rotate about twice as fast as in a layout position. This principle is also apparent in turning movements in ice skating, dance, and gymnastics.

Conservation of momentum in swinging movements. To build or to conserve momentum in any swinging movement, the radius of rotation should be shortened on the upswing and lengthened on the downswing. The object is to maximize the effects of gravity when moving with it and to minimize gravity's effects when moving opposite it. This principle is especially applicable to swinging activities in which it is desirable to maintain rotational velocity.

Example A: In doing a giant swing on a high bar (or other circling movements), the performer shortens the radius of rotation during the upswing to reduce the effects of gravity. He lengthens the radius on the downswing to enable gravity to exert maximum effects. Shortening during the upswing is achieved by adducting the scapula, depressing the shoulder girdle, and slightly flexing several joints (within the limits that good form will allow). Opposite movements cause lengthening during the downswing. *Example B:* In the pole vault, the vaulter swings on the pole, with the handgrip serving as the center of rotation. He extends the body away from the grip during the initial phase of the swing, then pulls toward the grip during the middle and latter phases, thus conserving the momentum he has gained to carry him forward and upward. If the vaulter shortens the radius from the box to the grip, he will gain speed, usually at the expense of height. If this radius is lengthened, he gains height at the expense of speed (and distance). With the fiber-glass pole, the vaulter usually desires to delay the forward momentum in order to allow time for the energy stored in the bend of the pole (the same as that energy stored in a diving board) to be returned to him at just the right time. Holding the body behind the pole (seated hang position) and delaying the swing accomplishes the desired effects. *Example C:* On either a child's swing, the flying rings, or a trapeze, the technique of swinging remains essentially the same. Performers move their weight away from the point of rotation on the downswing and pull toward the point of rotation on the upswing. **Movements while unsupported.**   When the body is unsupported, movements may occur, and the body may rotate about its center of gravity, but its flight path will be unaffected by the movements. Such movements are useful in controlling rotation and balance, and they are especially useful in preparation for landing. While the body is unsupported, if a segment moves on one side of an axis of rotation, it causes movement of an equal magnitude on the opposite side of that axis.

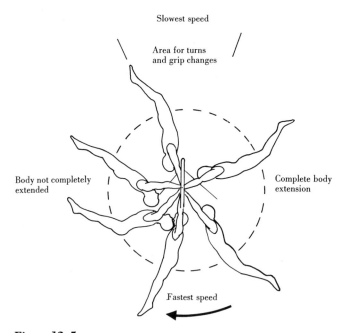

Figure 12–5.
When the body performs swinging movements, its center of gravity is moved away from the grip on the downswing and toward the grip on the upswing. Radius of the circle is greater on the right side than on the left side.

Example A: In the straddle roll high-jumping technique, the sequence of move-ment of body parts over the bar may determine the success of the jump, providing the center of gravity is projected high enough to clear the bar. The problem usually involves the trailing leg not clearing the bar. Downward-backward move-ment of the head, trunk, lead shoulder, and lead arm after they have crossed over the bar will aid in producing a lift of the trail leg. Conversely, a common fault is a "bucking" or hypertension of the neck. Although a beginning performer may feel this motion gives a lifting action, it produces a downward response of the part which has yet to clear the bar, the trail leg. *Example B:* When hurdling, the arm opposite the lead leg must be thrust forward and slightly toward the lead leg to enable the performer to keep balance in a straight forward direction. If this is not done, the body tends to rotate away from the lead leg, and the performer does not land in the direction of the run. Furthermore, the trunk should be well-flexed forward, because as the lead leg is snapped down to make early contact with the supporting surface after clearing the hurdle, the upper body tends to straighten. If too much straightening occurs, the runner loses his forward lean, which is necessary for driving toward the next hurdle.

In many common activities, such as running, the countermoves of body seg-ments in maintaining balance are automatic, and although the performer is unaware of them, they are essential to the performance. This principle applies at least partially to bodies in water as well as in air. However, bodies in water do not follow this principle entirely because the movement of a part does result in the displacement of the center of gravity. Water provides adequate support for pushing or pulling, but air does not.

Twisting movements.   No new principles are stated here, but it is useful to emphasize principles which have already been discussed and which apply to twisting actions.

Example A: Most twisting movements are based on the principle of the transfer of momentum. Usually a body segment is "thrown" in a given direction while the body is still in contact with the supporting surface. The body then follows by twisting in the same direction which the segment was thrown. *Example B:* If the body segment is thrown after the body is airborne, the effects will follow the principle of unsupported bodies. This means a rotation of segments will occur around an axis of rotation in an opposite direction. For example, if the right arm is thrown forward in a horizontal plane across the chest (motion to the left), the remainder of the body will twist to the right (toward that arm). *Example C:* Regardless of how the twist is initiated (from the surface or in the air), the speed of rotation is controlled by the principles governing conservation of rotational momentum. *Example D:* The longer and heavier the body segment is which initiates the twisting movement, the greater will be the resulting rotational motion (all other factors being equal).

Principles related to the law of counterforce

The following principles depend upon the performer applying muscular forces against a surface or object:

Surface variations and the amount of counterforce.   When a force is applied to a stable surface, a counterforce is returned to the body from which the force came. The less stable the surface, the less will be the counterforce.

Example A: When running or jumping, the surface pushes back to propel the body. If the surface "gives," as in the case of sand, much of the counterforce is dissipated, and the performer receives less propulsion for the amount of force applied. This results in more energy to achieve the given task. *Example B:* If the surface is slippery or if footwear is inadequate to cause proper friction, the results are the same as those described in Example A. *Example C:* Water offers less resistance than a solid surface; therefore, the propulsive force returned to the body is less for swimmers than for runners if equal energy is expended.

Direction of the counterforce.   The direction of the counterforce is directly opposite that of the applied force. These forces are most effective when they are perpendicular to the supporting surface, because then slippage or "give" is minimized.

Example A: To achieve maximum height in jumping, the force must be applied almost directly downward, meaning that to get best results, the center of weight must be almost immediately above the takeoff point. *Example B:* If a person runs or jumps while assuming too wide a stance, forces are poorly directed resulting in inefficient movements, and some surface slipping may result. *Example C:* In water the body moves directly opposite to the applied force. If the force is downward, the counterforce propels the body upward; if the force is backward, the body moves forward. Only those forces which propel the body forward should be emphasized. *Example D:* Track starting blocks change the angle of the supporting surface, so that the surface is more perpendicular to the desired direction of propulsion. For this reason the performer should be sure to get as much of the foot on the block as possible.

Counterforces in striking activities.   The amount of force a striking implement imparts to an object depends upon the combined momentum of the implement and the object at the moment of impact. Any give in the implement or the object at impact reduces the propulsive force (unless the implement or object is highly elastic, in which case propulsive force may be increased).

Example A: If the implement is held in the hands, the grip must be as firm as possible at impact to eliminate any give at the grip. All clubs, bats, paddles, and rackets used in sports should be gripped in this manner if the objective is to impart maximum force. *Example B:* If an object is struck by a body segment (foot in kicking, fist in boxing, hand in volleyball and handball, etc.), then all joints not actively moving should be firm in their positions in order to reduce give.

Temporarily stored counterforce. If a surface or implement used in a performance has elasticity (ability to respond from disfigurement), then an applied force produces bend or compression which represents an amount of stored energy. This stored energy increases the propulsive force over what it would be if elasticity were not present; the amount of energy depends upon the amount of disfigurement of the object, combined with its ability to spring back to original shape.

Example A: When contacting the bed of a trampoline, the legs must be stiff in order to depress the bed a maximum amount, thus causing it to respond with greater force. In fact, the technique used to dissipate the force provided by the bed is to sharply flex the supporting joints at the moment of contact. *Example B:* After the vaulting pole (fiber-glass) has been inserted in the planting box, the amount it will bend depends upon the final momentum the vaulter develops against the pole as a result of his approach and takeoff. Excessive give in the arms and shoulders of the vaulter reduces the force transferred to the pole. The more limber the pole is, the less force required to bend it, but also the less propulsive energy produced by it as it springs back to original shape. Other examples of stored energy can be observed when the diving board is depressed or when the golf club is swung forcefully, causing the shaft to bend during the early phase and to straighten during the middle phase of the swing.

Surface contact while applying forces to external objects. In throwing, pushing, pulling, and striking activities, one or both feet must be kept in firm

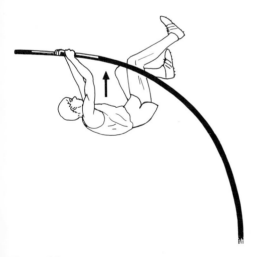

Figure 12–6.
The excessive bend of a fiber-glass vaulting pole represents stored energy which becomes available to the vaulter when the pole responds.

contact with the supporting surface until the force providing motion is complete. Otherwise maximum force is reduced. However, it must be recognized that when applying force to objects, greater momentum may be gained by developing maximum total body momentum (with a running approach) in the desired direction. In order to maintain this momentum, it may be impossible to comply with the "firm contact principle"; however, even then the principle holds true to some extent and cannot be ignored. The influence of the firm contact principle increases as the external object becomes heavier.

Example A: If a football lineman removes his feet from the ground before his maximum momentum is complete, the force of his block or tackle will be reduced. *Example B:* If a shot-putter breaks contact between the back foot and the ground before the main force-providing movements are complete, the force will be reduced. The same is true for a baseball batter and golf driver.

Use of leverage in human motion

A lever is a rigid bar revolving around a fixed axis known as the fulcrum F, with an effort E to move it, and a resistance R to be overcome by it. (The effort is sometimes referred to as the force.) A lever is useful for various purposes depending upon the relative positions of the fulcrum, effort, and resistance.

Motor movements in the human body result from the actions of body levers. The following points will help to explain the role of levers in human movement:

1. In the human body, a bone or combination of bones composes a rigid bar known as a lever.
2. The joint is the fulcrum, the point around which the lever moves.
3. The application of force (effort) is at the attachment of the muscle(s) producing the force.
4. The force (effort) is caused by the contraction of muscles which contribute to the desired movement.
5. The point of resistance is the center of gravity of the body segment being moved, plus the center of gravity of any external weight. The resistance may be either the weight of the body segment alone, the weight of the segment plus an external weight, or the application of an external force.

Classes (types) of levers

Levers are of three types, each one determined by the relative arrangement of the fulcrum F, point of effort E, and point of resistance R.

A *first-class* lever has an arrangement of *EFR*. An example of this type of leverage is extension of the arm at the elbow joint.

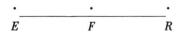

E   F   R

A *second-class* lever has an *ERF* arrangement. This type of leverage is seldom used in body movement. An example of this type is plantar flexion as when raising onto the toes.

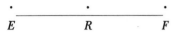

E   R   F

A *third-class* lever consists of an *FER* arrangement. Examples of this type of leverage are flexion of the arm at the elbow and shoulder and flexion of the leg at the knee and hip joints. This is by far the most common type of leverage used in human movements.

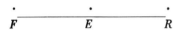

F   E   R

Each of the foregoing illustrations could have the points on the two ends of the lever reversed without a change in the lever class. For example, the first-class lever could just as well read *RFE* from left to right. As long as the *F* is between the *E* and *R*, it is a first-class lever. In other words the *middle* component determines the lever class, and a convenient tool to remember is the word *free* (*FRE*). This order corresponds to the order of middle components for first-, second-, and third-class levers.

Lever arms

Regardless of its type (class), a lever results in two separate arms, known as the *effort* or *force arm* (EA) and the *resistance arm* (RA). The effort arm (EA) is the distance from the fulcrum *F* to the point of effort *E*, and the resistance arm (RA) is the distance from the fulcrum *F* to the point of resistance *R*. The exact relationship between the effort and resistance arms varies with each class of lever. This can be readily understood by identifying the two arms for each lever.

1.   First-class lever

E   F   R

     EA   RA

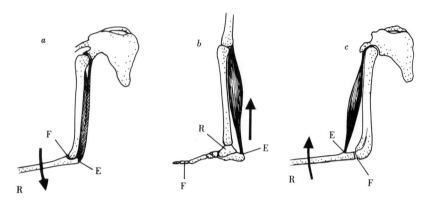

Figure 12–7.
The three classes of leverage used in human movement.
(*a*) Triceps muscle causes first-class leverage as it extends the elbow.
(*b*) Gastrocnemius muscle causes second-class leverage as it plantar flexes (extends) the foot.
(*c*) Biceps muscle causes third-class leverage as it flexes the elbow.

2. Second-class lever

3. Third-class lever

In first-class leverage, either arm (RA or EA) may be longer than the other, depending upon the location of *F* along the lever; in second-class leverage, the EA is always the longer; and in third-class leverage, the RA is always longer.

Moments

The effectiveness of a force in producing movement of a lever is called the *moment of rotation*, or *torque*. The following statements will help in understanding the meaning and significance of the moment of rotation:

1. The effectiveness of a force in producing movement against a given resistance depends upon the amount of the effort E, its perpendicular distance from the axis (EA), and the perpendicular distance of the resistance from the axis (RA).

2. In mechanics, the moment of rotation (torque) is defined as the product of the effort E times its perpendicular distance from the axis (EA). The moment of resistance is the product of the resistance R times its perpendicular distance from the axis (RA).

Moment of force $= E$ (pounds) $\times$ EA (feet)

Moment of resistance $= R$ (pounds) $\times$ RA (feet)

3. When force and resistance are in balance (lever is in balance), then $E \times$ EA $= R \times$ RA.

4. If $E \times$ EA exceeds $R \times$ RA, then muscular effort overcomes the resistance, and movement of the lever occurs.

5. If $R \times$ RA exceeds $E \times$ EA, then the resistance is not overcome, and movement of the lever either does not occur or occurs in the direction of the resistance.

6. If the effort arm becomes proportionately shorter, then the amount of effort necessary to cause movement is increased, but the linear speed with which the lever will move is also increased. In this case, ability to apply force against resistance is sacrificed to gain speed and distance of movement.

7. If the effort arm becomes proportionately longer, the amount of effort necessary to cause movement is reduced, but the speed with which the lever will move is also reduced. In this case speed is sacrificed to increase the application of force.

Range and speed of motion of points on a moving lever

When a lever revolves around its fulcrum F, all points on the lever move in an arc about the fulcrum. The distance through which a point on the lever will move is directly proportional to its distance from the fulcrum F. For example:

1. Point y is twice as far from the axis as point x, and z is three times as far as x. When the lever revolves, if point x moves through a distance of 1 inch, then point y will move 2 inches, and z will move 3 inches.

2. In the above example points x and z move through their arcs of 1 and 3 inches, respectively, in the *same amount* of time. This illustrates that a point which is farther from the fulcrum not only moves through a proportionately greater distance, but it also moves with proportionately greater speed.

From the facts that have been stated about leverage, several important conclusions can be stated:

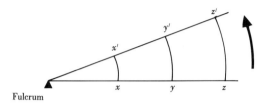

Fulcrum

Figure 12–8.
The length of a lever influences the linear speed and distance it will travel when the angular speed and distance are constant. Point y moves twice as fast and twice as far as x. Point z moves three times as far and three times as fast as x.

1. A relatively long effort arm with a shorter resistance arm is useful for moving heavy resistance through a short distance at slow speed. To produce this movement, a relatively light force (effort) is exerted through a long distance.

2. A long resistance arm with a short effort arm is useful for producing movement of great speed and distance against a light resistance.

3. Third-class levers are useful for producing movements of great range and speed at the expense of great force. (Note: In the third-class lever the resistance arm is always longer than the effort arm.)

4. Second-class levers are useful for producing movements of great force at the expense of speed and distance. (Note: Second-class levers always have a longer effort arm than resistance arm.)

5. First-class levers may produce either kind of advantage depending on the relative position of F. If the F is closer to E than it is to R, then the EA is shorter than the RA. If the F is closer to R, then the opposite situation exists.

6. Most of the levers of the body have short effort arms and long resistance arms. They are especially designed for movements of speed and distance against relatively light resistance.

Practical application

Nothing can be done in the human body to change the length of effort arms; but much can be done to change resistance arms, and thus the proportionate length between the two. Variations occur by extending or flexing the acting joints by various amounts during a performance, thus increasing or decreasing the length of the lever. The length of the RA changes with the length of the lever, whereas the EA usually remains constant. As levers are lengthened by extending at certain joints, greater potential for speed and range of motion occurs at the end of the lever, or at any point along it. When the lever is shortened by flexing at certain

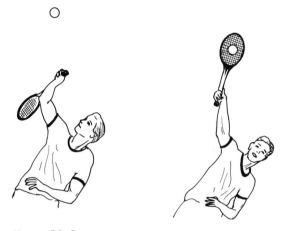

Figure 12–9.
Tennis serve demonstrates a long resistance arm to gain
speed at the end of the lever. The tennis racket adds length
to the moving levers, causing the racket face to move considerably faster than the hand.

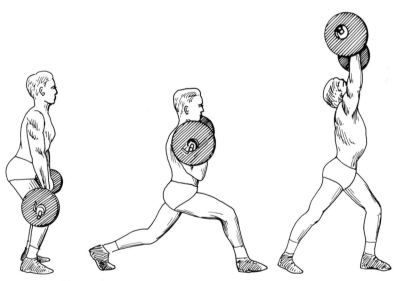

Figure 12–10.
Lifting maximum weight demonstrates the need for a short resistance arm (weight is
kept close to the body) so maximum force may be applied against the resistance.

joints, greater potential to exert force occurs. We use implements to increase the length of resistance arms, and we vary the point of grip to suit our convenience and purpose. The balance, center of gravity, and weight variations of implements also affect levers.

Sometimes the objective is not gaining linear speed at the end of a lever, but rather the objective is moving the whole lever through a range of motion quickly. The shorter resistance arm can be moved through a given range more quickly than a longer one, assuming that equal force (effort) is employed. Therefore, in some cases the lever is shortened (joints flexed) in order to accomplish the act better.

Building additional strength enhances the effectiveness of all our body levers, because greater muscular force (effort) adds to the force of movement and to the speed at which we can move against a resistance. This is true regardless of the class of lever or the proportionate length of the EA to the RA.

Recommended supplementary reading

BROER, MARION R.: "Efficiency of Human Movement," 2d ed., chaps. 5 and 6, W. B. Saunders Company, Philadelphia, 1966.

BUNN, JOHN W.: "Scientific Principles of Coaching," chaps. 1 and 3, Prentice-Hall, Inc., Englewood Cliffs, N.J., 1955.

RASCH, PHILLIP J., and ROGER K. BURKE: "Kinesiology and Applied Anatomy," 3d ed., chaps. 7 and 8, Lea and Febiger, Philadelphia, 1967.

13

Force

orce is described as push or pull, but it is more exactly defined as the product of the *mass* and *acceleration* of an object. The motion of a body never truly becomes a force unless it contacts another body (object). Usually one body exerts force, and the other receives it, but in some cases both bodies exert force against each other. A force is not effective in producing motion unless it is of sufficient magnitude to overcome the inertia of the body receiving the force.

Principles have been formulated which apply to all activities in which the development of force is desired. Although most of the principles are based on the *assumption* that the objective is to produce maximum force, one must be aware that such a result is not always desired. The golf putt, football pass, toss to initiate a baseball double play, and baseball bunt are examples in which less than maximum force is desired. Principles of force are logically grouped under the following headings: (1) general principles, (2) self-produced and other positive forces, (3) resistive forces, and (4) force dissipation.

General principles of force

In striking activities, *final momentum* is the most important factor in producing speed and distance. *Final velocity* is the prime factor in jumping and throwing, and *average velocity* is the prime consideration in locomotive activities where the objective is to cover a distance in the shortest time. Any human motion arises from the cooperation of muscular and gravitational forces acting on the body in a state of either motion or rest. If the body already possesses momentum in the correct direction prior to the force application, the force will be more effective.

Total force

A total force (or velocity) is the sum of the forces (or velocities) of each body segment contributing to the act, if the forces are applied in a single direction and in the proper sequence with correct timing.

Example A: At the moment of release, a ball which is thrown is traveling at a velocity approximately equal to the sum of the velocities of all the body movements contributing at the time of release. *Example B:* At the moment of release, the discus is traveling at a velocity approximately equal to the sum of the velocities of all the contributing forces. This includes the linear movement across the ring, the rotary movement of the total body (spin), and the angular movements of the different body segments contributing to the throwing action. *Example C:* In *any* explosive performance, the next force in sequence contributing to velocity should be applied at the peak of the prior force. To accomplish this, maximum coordination of specific movements is required. If the second force is applied too late, momentum from the first force is lost; if the second force is applied too soon, superimposing the force reduces the possible total effect of the two forces.

Constant application of force

Application of force should be constant and as even as possible so that maximum force is used to overcome the resistance of gravity and air or water, and minimum force is used to overcome inertia.

Example A: When pushing a car, less force is required to keep the car in motion at a constant rate than to increase the velocity of the car. The cost of running a car is more economical (less energy required) when driven at a constant speed as opposed to varying speeds. Frequent starting and stopping expends additional energy. *Example B:* A distance runner or swimmer moves more efficiently and economically when he travels at a constant speed, in which case he utilizes a minimum amount of energy to overcome inertia.

Direction of force application

In general, all forces should be applied as directly as possible in the direction of the intended motion. Forces applied in other directions either retard motion in the desired direction or result in wasted energy.

Example A: A swimmer or runner should reduce to a minimum all forces which do not directly contribute to forward progress. Unproductive muscular contractions are characteristic of unskilled performers. *Example B:* If a runner points his toes outward ("duck-footed") with each stride, he cannot direct his forces straight ahead. Only part of the lever (foot) is used, and the muscles that would otherwise contribute are ineffective; thus the force of the push is reduced. *Example C:* When the pole-vaulter makes his final push from the pole, it is necessary for the pole to be close to his body, with the center of his body weight generally above his hands. Otherwise, the pushing force will add momentum toward the horizontal rather than the vertical direction.

Distance of force application

If a constant force is applied to a body, the body develops greater velocity as the distance over which the force is applied increases.

Example A: In the shot put if the performer begins with his back instead of his side toward the direction of the put, he gains the advantage of another quarter of a turn over which to apply force. The same idea applies to the discus throw. *Example B:* Most throwing and striking events (performed right-handed) should terminate with the striding foot slightly to the left of the intended line of flight. This slightly "open" stance at the completion of the action permits a greater distance over which to apply the force. Also in throwing, the greater the range of motion of each contributing body segment, the greater will be the velocity resulting from that segment.

Multiple forces

When two or more forces act upon a body, or two or more forces act upon each other, the resulting movement is determined by the direction and magnitude of the acting forces. If two forces act in the same general direction, the direction of the resulting force is somewhere between the two, and the magnitude of the resulting force is more than either, but not as much as the total, of the two contributing forces. The magnitude and direction of the resulting force can be determined exactly by constructing a parallelogram of forces.

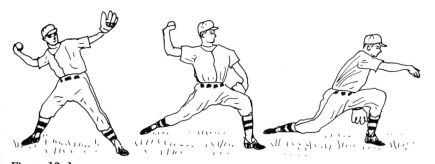

Figure 13–1.
Baseball pitch illustrates the application of force over a long range of motion, thus allowing more time to increase the velocity.

Example A: The *gather* in the high jump or broad jump means to "ready" the body just at takeoff to apply a vertical force with the least possible loss of horizontal momentum, which has already developed in the approach. The resulting magnitude and direction of flight are dependent upon the relative contributions of both the horizontal and vertical forces. *Example B:* If two football opponents make contact, each will change direction and speed, depending upon the momentum of each at the time of contact and the angle at which they collide. If they collide exactly head on with equal momentum, then both players will totally lose their momentum. If they collide at an angle (not head on), then they both maintain part of their momentum, but it will be transferred to a new direction. *Example C:* A high-jumper applies force to the surface with the push-off leg, adds force in the vertical direction with the swinging leg, and adds more force with the extension of the trunk and the arm swing. All these contributing forces are in the same general, but not the exact, direction. Therefore, the total vertical force is less than the sum of all contributing forces.

Self-produced and other positive forces

Muscular contractions are the only self-generated forces available to human beings. However, environmental forces, especially gravity, can often be used effectively in conjunction with muscular contractions. The following principles must be observed in order to gain maximum results:

Correct muscle selection

The performer must select (unconsciously in skillful actions) the muscles which are most effective for the task at hand. In a maximum effort the stronger the muscles and the more muscles that are brought into the action, the greater will be the force, and the less likely that muscle strain will occur.

Example A: When lifting heavy objects, the muscles of the legs provide greater strength than the extensor muscles of the back; therefore lifting with the legs is more effective and much less hazardous. *Example B:* In boxing, the force of a left hook is greatest when it is initiated from hip and torso rotations, whereas the force is minimal when developed only from shoulder and arm actions. The same can be said of throwing or striking an object with arm action only as opposed to total body action (involvement of more and stronger muscles).

Stability and the loss of effective force

Certain muscles must be "set" in performance of certain skills, especially those skills which involve heavy resistance. Also, a firm base of support, which contributes to stability of the body and its parts, helps to reduce loss of force.

Example A: The thrusting (putting) action against a shot is most effective if all joints not used in the development of force are stabilized, and contact of the back foot with the surface is firm. The follow-through or reversal occurs after the propelling forces have contributed all they can to the final velocity of the shot. *Example B:* Striking forces are more effective if all joints are either stabilized or moving in the direction of the action at the time of contact.

Effect of the angle of application on the force produced

In angular movements of body segments, the maximum effective force (and velocity) occurs when the limb is at right angles to the direction in which the object is moved. The same applies to the angle of muscle pull (see Example C).

Example A: A swimmer using the crawl stroke is able to apply the maximum force and move the limb with maximum velocity in the direction opposite body movement when the hand is directly below the shoulder, in other words, when the limb is at right angles to the direction of body movement. In this position the effect of the stroke is the greatest. *Example B:* When batting a baseball, the position of greatest possible force occurs when the bat is in front of the body. At this point, the bat is approximately at right angles to the flight of the ball. *Example C:* More pulling force is available at the elbow when the lower arm is at right angles to the upper arm. At this point, all the available force of the elbow flexors is directed at right angles to the lower arm (which is a lever). Consequently, the difficult phases of a chin-up occur when the arm positions deviate farthest from the right angle (either straight or greatly bent), never at the midpoint of the movement.

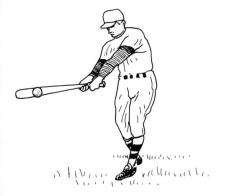

Figure 13-2.
The momentum of a baseball bat will have maximum effects when it meets an oncoming ball at right angles to the direction the ball is moving.

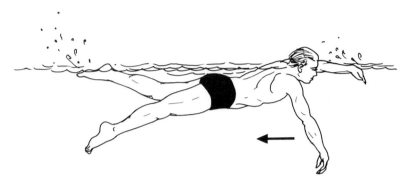

Figure 13–3.
A swimmer can apply the greatest amount of effective force when his arm is at right angles to the direction of movement and the body.

Initial muscular tension

The force of muscular contraction may be increased by increasing the initial tension on the muscle (putting the muscle on stretch). The nearer a muscle is to complete contraction, the less force it can apply. Usually it is not possible to adhere completely to both this principle and the previous one at the same time. Often a compromise is necessary.

Example A: Drawing the arm backward in preparation to pitch a ball places the mover muscles on stretch thereby increasing their initial contractile force. *Example B:* Although the legs are bent initially in preparation for a vertical jump, an additional slight dip prior to extension provides increased stretch of the extensor muscles and adds to the force of their contraction. *Example C:* Backward lean of the trunk prior to kicking places the rectus femoris muscle on stretch, enabling it (and other muscles) to extend the knee with greater force. (See section on stretch reflex, Chapter 10, for additional information about this principle.)

Striking force

When the angular velocity at the point of rotation remains constant, the velocity at which a lever moves is directly proportional to its length. This principle is based upon the system of levers, meaning that when a body lever is lengthened by extending it, or by adding an implement such as a ball bat or tennis racket, velocity is increased, and distance of movement and striking force are also increased.

Example A: When a tennis racket is added to the length of the human lever which rotates around the shoulder joint, the length of the original lever is almost doubled. If the angular velocity at the shoulder remains constant, then the velocity at the end of the lever (racket face) will be approximately twice what it was before the lever was lengthened. *Example B:* When a golfer holds a golf club in his hands, the length of the swinging lever is increased. When he strikes a golf ball, the velocity at impact is increased in proportion to the increased lever length, providing the angular velocity remains constant.

Follow-through

Emphasis on correct follow-through eliminates the tendency to decelerate a throwing or striking action prior to its completion. In addition to this, two other purposes exist for follow-through: (1) to maintain balance and (2) to protect the joints by gradually slowing the body parts. In any case, once contact is broken with the object, follow-through actions have no influence on the flight of the object.

Example: In putting a shot or throwing a discus or javelin, the reversal (follow-through) allows the performer to maintain balance and prevent fouling. If the reversal were eliminated and fouling were to be avoided, the performer would have to discontinue force application sooner, thereby reducing the total force because it would be applied over a shorter distance.

Environmental forces

Many external forces must be confronted. Often they can aid in performance; in such cases their influence should be maximized. But frequently, they are detrimental and must be regulated to exert minimum influence.

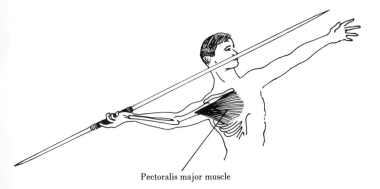

Pectoralis major muscle

Figure 13–4.
The powerful pectoralis major muscle is on stretch in preparation for the thrust of the javelin. Numerous other muscles are also on stretch in the above body position.

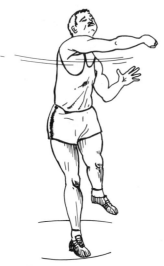

Figure 13–5.
Follow-through is essential to maximum force in throwing, putting, and striking performances. The discus throw is an example.

Contending with external forces

Among the forces with which we must commonly contend during performance are (1) water resistance, (2) friction, (3) gravity, and (4) air resistance. We should attempt to utilize these forces to our advantage. In some cases we will want to minimize and in other cases maximize their effects.

Example A: A swimmer should attempt to increase the water resistance against the power phase of the stroke and kick, in order to increase the propelling force. But at the same time, he should decrease to a minimum the water resistance against his forward movement, which is done by using the correct body positions and correct techniques of recovery from the stroke and kick. *Example B:* A water-skier purposely increases the water resistance during the pull-up phase. Then after he is up on the skis, he attempts to reduce the resistance to a minimum. *Example C:* While performing in basketball, tennis, track, soccer, and other activities where increased traction adds to stability, the athlete should attempt to increase friction between himself and the surface on which he performs by wearing a special type of footwear. But dancers, skiers, skaters, and swimmers all attempt to reduce friction to some degree in order to improve their performances. The extent to which friction is purposely increased or decreased is determined by the task to be accomplished. *Example D:* The force of gravity on a given amount of mass remains constant, and the wise performer utilizes this force to maximum advantage whenever possible. Gravity is one of the forces which pulls the sprinter forward, especially during the momentum-gaining phase. The gymnast utilizes gravitational force during swinging movements, whereas divers and trampoline performers take advantage of the force of gravity to increase the spring they get from the bouncing surfaces. *Example E:* Air resistance is a force which the performer must reduce to a minimum whenever speed or distance is the goal, as in throwing, running, or jumping.

Theoretical square law

Air and water resistance vary approximately with the square of the velocity, meaning that if the velocity at which a body travels is increased by two, the air or water resistance against it will be increased by four; if velocity is increased by four, the resistance will be increased by sixteen.

Example A: If a swimmer pulls his arm through the water at the rate of 10 feet per second, he meets a given amount of water resistance, used to propel him forward. If he increases the rate of pull to 20 feet per second, then the resistance is increased four times, resulting in four times as much propulsive force from the stroke. *Example B:* A ball is projected through the air at a speed of 50 feet per second and, therefore, meets a given amount of air resistance. A second ball projected at twice that velocity (100 feet per second) will meet four times the amount of air resistance. Even though the second ball leaves the hand at twice the velocity as the first ball, it will travel less than twice the distance because the air resistance is four times as great as that against the first ball. Similarly, in Example A, four times the propulsive force will not increase the swimmer's speed through the water by four times, because the water's resistance against his travel also increases proportionately.

Centrifugal force

Centrifugal force is experienced only in rotational (angular) or curvilinear motion, never during linear motion. It creates a tendency for an object to continue momentum in a straight line instead of in a curved path. It is counteracted by forces (usually muscular) which, if effective, exceed the centrifugal force and tend to maintain the object in its curved path. This counteracting force is centripetal force. In the case of a freely moving body, such as a sprinter running around a curve, as velocity increases, centrifugal force increases. Additional weight also increases centrifugal force. In angular movements, the longer the radius of rotation, the greater the centrifugal force with the same angular velocity and weight. More centrifugal force demands more centripetal force to counteract it. In human performance, body lean and/or banked surfaces counteract centrifugal force.

Example A: A 220-yard sprinter running around a curve must lean in the direction of the curve. The faster he runs, the more he must lean. *Example B:* As the slalom skier increases his velocity, he must also increase his body lean in the direction of his turns, in order to compensate for the increased centrifugal force. *Example C:* In gymnastics or diving stunts involving angular or swinging motions, the effects of centrifugal force must be considered. Centrifugal force (1) is used to help the performer clear the apparatus by properly timing the release in apparatus dismounts; (2) is nonexistent at the ends of pendulum-type swings, thus allowing maneuvers without danger of flying off the apparatus; (3) tends to straighten the body during a somersault in a tuck, demanding that the performer increase the forces holding the tuck as the rotational velocity increases. *Example D:* The objective in the discus throw is to achieve a maximum velocity of the discus in a curvilinear direction prior to release. The release eliminates centripetal force, allowing the centrifugal force to take over and propel the discus in a straight line.

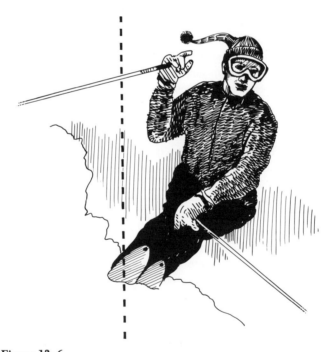

Figure 13–6.
When moving at high speeds, the skier must lean excessively
into the turn to compensate for the centrifugal force. This
also applies to turning movements while running.

Force absorption

In certain activities it is important to dissipate the force of impact. The impact becomes greater as the moving object has more weight and moves at a greater velocity; in other words, impact is determined by the amount of momentum. If momentum is reduced gradually, the performer's chances of incurring injury are decreased. Therefore, when *landing* from a fall or a jump or when *catching* an object, it is important to absorb the force. This becomes increasingly important as the momentum of the moving object becomes greater. But, recall, it has already been established that in activities such as diving and trampolining (rebound tumbling), the objective is to cause the body to rebound, and, consequently, force absorption must be avoided.

In general, the performer prepares for an impact by placing all shock absorbing joints in extension. As contact is made, the extended joints flex, due to the force of impact. This force must be gradually reduced ("apply the brakes") by an opposing force, provided by the extensor muscles. The joints move through flexion, but the extensor muscles contract eccentrically and control the action by gradually increasing their contractile forces, thereby dissipating the momentum of the moving object and absorbing the force.

Absorbing a blow

A force from a blow can be diminished by distributing the force over either a greater time (and distance) or area, or both.

Example A: As a person lands after jumping from a table, the shock-absorbing joints move through flexion in order to distribute the force over a greater time (and distance). *Example B:* When a person falls to the ground, he attempts to distribute the impact over the hands, arms, and larger fleshy areas of the body as opposed to the point of the elbow. Distributing the force over a greater area results in less force per square inch of surface. *Example C:* When a boxer is struck with a 16-ounce glove as opposed to an 8-ounce glove, the blow is distributed over a larger surface, resulting in less force per square inch. The increased ability of the larger glove to compress causes the blow to be distributed over a longer time; therefore, the effects of the blow are decreased in two ways.

Landing with balance

In general, the center of gravity must be kept above the supporting levers in order that each lever makes its greatest contribution. Each lever must bear weight as it moves through flexion.

Example A: A gymnast must cushion his fall when dismounting, but as he does so, he wants to maintain his upright position. His center of gravity must stay

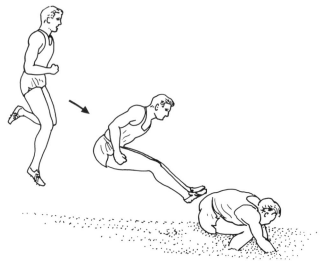

Figure 13–7.
Controlled flexion of the joints during landing absorbs the force over a longer time, thus reducing the chance of injury. A soft landing surface, such as a sand pit, also causes absorption of force over a longer time.

within the base of support. *Example B:* A long-jumper makes contact with the surface while his center of gravity is well behind the feet, but he must be sure the center of gravity is within, or in front of, the base of support after all the momentum has been dissipated; otherwise, he will fall backward. *Example C:* If a person falls from a height, and the center of gravity is outside the base of support, even though the feet make initial contact, the levers cannot be fully effective in absorbing the shock. The further the displacement of the center of gravity, the less effective the joints can be in cushioning the blow, and the more the force of contact is transferred to the next body part contacting the surface.

Transferring momentum from vertical to horizontal

After achieving all absorption that the levers can provide, transferring the momentum from the vertical to the horizontal can reduce the momentum over a longer time and a greater surface area.

Example A: When thrown from a fast-moving car, falling during fast locomotion, or falling from a great height, a rolling action is necessary to prevent injury. *Example B:* The football coach tells his players to "fall and roll," which simply means absorb the momentum over a longer time (and distance).

Catching objects

Catching objects is accomplished by following many of the principles already presented. Regardless of the object being caught, the sequence of catching follows a similar pattern: (1) a body part, such as the palm of the hand, makes initial contact; (2) the object's momentum is dissipated by eccentric muscular contractions allowing the joints to move through controlled flexion; and (3) while momentum is being reduced, body parts (usually fingers, sometimes arms) flex to grasp the object securely.

Example A: The "cradling" action often used to catch a football which passes over the receiver's shoulder involves the use of shoulder, elbow, wrist, and finger flexors working in eccentric contraction in order to dissipate momentum. This action is opposite the usual catching action and uses the opposite muscles, but the principle is the same. Finally, the ball is secured by finger, wrist, and elbow flexion (concentric action of flexors) to pin the ball to the catcher's torso. *Example B:* When the catching action is continuous with a throwing action, such as the quick release of the ball by the second baseman in a double play, the force dissipation and the preparation for the throw can be accomplished in the same motion. In baseball an infield grounder is often handled this way. *Example C:* If no "give" takes place, and the object has sufficient momentum, it will rebound. The football receiver who allows the first contact of the ball to be on his chest

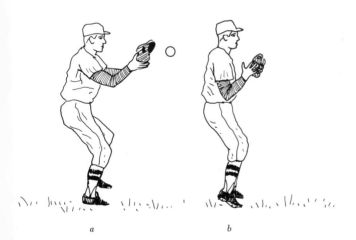

a　　　　　　　　　　*b*

Figure 13–8.
Absorbing the force of a fast-moving object (baseball) allows the receiver more time to grasp the object and reduces the chance that it will rebound from his hands.

must move his arms with great accuracy and speed to trap the rebounding ball. He has reduced the chances of a successful catch by not cushioning the ball.

Recommended supplementary reading

BROER, MARION R.: "Efficiency of Human Movement," 2d ed., chap. 7, W. B. Saunders Company, Philadelphia, 1966.

BUNN, JOHN W.: "Scientific Principles of Coaching," chaps. 1 and 4, Prentice-Hall, Inc., Englewood Cliffs, N.J., 1955.

14

Projections

*O*bjects are projected through space in athletic activities by throwing, striking, or kicking actions of the human body, and the body itself becomes a projectile in jumping and leaping activities. Obviously, knowledge about principles related to projections is of vital concern to teachers and performers. To cover this subject adequately, this chapter is divided into three major divisions: (1) forces which affect flight, (2) angle and height of projection, and (3) the effects of impact on flight.

Forces which affect flight

When the body or an object is projected through space, three forces influence the course of flight:

1. The propelling force, which puts the object in flight
2. The force of gravity, which tends to pull the object downward
3. Air resistance, which retards the object's flight

The latter two forces work in opposition to the first force.

Propelling force

Muscular contraction is the source of the propelling force, whether the force is used in striking, kicking, throwing, or jumping. This idea has already been explained in detail in Chapter 13. But at this point, it should be reemphasized that for a force to exert its greatest influence, it must be applied at exactly the *right time*, in the *right place*, and in the *right direction*.

Point of application of propelling force. The propelling force produces certain effects depending upon its point and direction of application. If the appli-

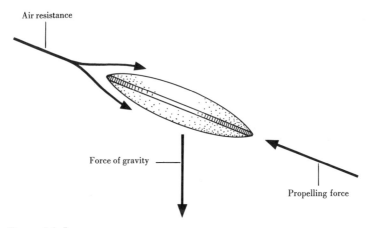

Figure 14–1.
There are three forces acting on an object in flight (discus). The flight pattern
is changed by altering any of the forces.

cation is directly through the projectile's center of gravity, only linear motion
results from the force. As the projecting force is moved farther from the center
of gravity, rotary motion of the object increases at the expense of linear motion.
If the force is below the object's center of gravity, backspin results. Forward spin
results when the force is above the center of gravity. When the force is off center
to the left, clockwise spin results, and when it is off center to the right, counterclockwise spin occurs.

Example A: A curve ball will travel slower than a straight ball (assume equal
magnitude of projecting force) because a portion of the projecting force is spent
in producing spin to cause the ball to curve, meaning that the force does not pass
directly through the ball's center of gravity. (Increased air friction on the spinning ball retards its speed even more.) *Example B:* If a golf club contacts a ball
below its center of gravity, the ball moves forward and upward from the point of
contact, and it has backspin. The greater the distance from the center of gravity
that contact is made, the higher will be the flight of the ball and the greater the
backspin.

Effects of spin on flight of an object.   An object propelled without spin
tends to waver because of air resistance against the object's irregular surface.
The amount of waver varies with the density of the object. A small amount of spin
on an object produces a stabilizing effect which tends to hold it on its line of
flight. Increased spin causes the object to curve in the same direction as the spin.
The amount that an object will curve in a given distance is determined primarily
by (1) the amount of spin and (2) the rate at which the object travels. Amount
and direction of wind and the shape and density of the object are also important
influences in some cases.

Example A: A volleyball served with slight spin follows a course of flight determined by the projecting force, but if the ball is contacted decidedly off center, the resulting increase in spin will produce a curve. If the ball is hit directly through its center of gravity, the ball receives no rotary motion, and it tends to waver. *Example B:* In baseball pitching, a knuckle ball (little spin) is thrown with the intention of causing a wavering action. In this case the amount of waver is related to the speed the object travels. The faster it moves, the more it will waver. *Example C:* A counterclockwise spin (golf hook, baseball outside curve, and volleyball or tennis serve where the ball is contacted on its right side) will cause a ball to curve to the left. A clockwise spin (golf slice, baseball inside curve, and volleyball or tennis serve where the ball is contacted on its left side) will cause a curve to the right. *Example D:* If a golf ball is hit with top spin, the distance it travels in flight will be reduced (parabolic curve will be increased), and it will tend to dive rather sharply to the surface. This action will be followed by a long roll, enhanced by the forward spin. If the ball is given backspin, it will tend to rise higher; therefore it will stay in flight longer. Upon landing, the length of its roll will be reduced by the backspin.

Force of gravity

Represented by the mass (weight) of the object, the force of gravity is ever present. As soon as contact is broken with a projected object, the force of gravity begins to diminish the vertical velocity of the object. Finally, gravity overcomes the effects of the vertical component of the projectile, and the object begins to descend. The factors that determine how soon gravity will cause the object to

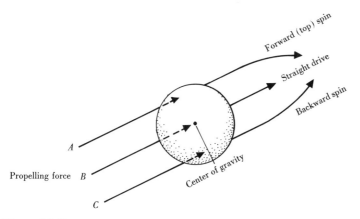

Figure 14–2.
The motion of a projected object is influenced by the exact point of application of the propelling force.

descend are (1) weight (mass) of the object, (2) amount of force driving it upward, and (3) the effects of air resistance on the object.

Effects of air resistance

As the speed of an object increases, air resistance plays a more significant role. Objects that are dense and streamlined are influenced less by air resistance, and the less surface an object presents, the less will be the effect of air resistance.

Example A: If a discus wobbles or an arrow quivers while moving through space, it causes a larger surface to be presented. This results in increased air resistance, thus reducing the distance of the flight. *Example B:* If a shuttlecock is hit with great force, its path will vary considerably from the usual path an object takes. Generally, the path of descent of a projectile is similar to the path of ascent, but in this case, the object will fall almost vertically from its peak, due to the light weight and odd shape of the "bird." It meets a great amount of air resistance relative to its weight. *Example C:* When an object such as a discus or javelin is hurled into a head wind, the object should present as little surface as possible, and its usual angle of flight should be reduced. If a tail wind is encountered, the angle of flight should be increased. In a tail wind, a discus would be thrown at an angle greater than 45°, with the nose pointed slightly upward.

Angle and height of projection

If the propelling force is constant, then the angle at which an object is projected determines the height it reaches. In turn, if the speed at which an object travels is constant, then the height that it reaches determines the distance it travels because the height determines how long the object remains in flight.

Angle of projection

When the beginning and ending points are on the same level, the optimum angle of projection with which to gain maximum distance is 45° from the surface. Since most projectiles are above the surface at the time of release, the angle of flight is usually reduced from 45° to compensate for this. If the angle is less than optimum, the projectile will not be in the air long enough to travel a maximum distance, and if the angle is greater than optimum, too much of the propelling force is wasted in vertical rather than horizontal flight.

Example A: A place-kick in football begins and ends at ground level, so for maximum distance the kick should be made at a 45° angle from the surface. *Example B:* When putting the shot or when long-jumping, the angle should be less than 45°, because the center of gravity of the projectile is lower at the com-

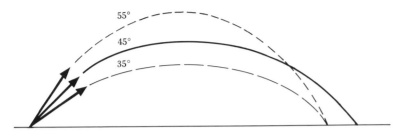

Figure 14–3.
The relative horizontal distance covered when a heavy object is projected at angles of 35, 45, and 55°. The propelling force is constant.

pletion than at the beginning of the flight. The shot is usually put at 38 to 41°, and the long jump should be executed at about 40°; however, the horizontal speed of the jumper makes this impossible. The usual angle of projection among long-jumpers is about 25°. *Example C:* When hitting a golf ball from a lower to a higher elevation, the golfer should select a club with a greater pitch (higher number) than he would if the terrain were level. In this case, the ending point is higher than the beginning point. *Example D:* In a baseball throw, the quickness of the ball's arrival to a teammate is almost always more important than maximum distance. With this objective in mind, the ball should be thrown as horizontally as possible within the limits of the force the thrower can muster. Obviously, if the thrower has insufficient force, he will be unable to obtain the needed distance unless he selects a high angle of projection.

Time in flight

The length of time an object remains in flight depends upon the height it attains. An object remains in flight only as long as it takes to move through the vertical plane. The horizontal component of force applied to an object is not related to the time of flight.

Example A: If a ball is projected at shoulder height in a perfectly horizontal path, it will strike the surface at exactly the same time as a similar ball simply dropped from the same height. If the ball is projected downward, it will strike the surface sooner than the dropped ball; if it is projected upward, it will strike the surface later than the dropped ball. The greater height the ball attains, the longer it remains in flight. *Example B:* If two identical objects are projected at different angles, causing the first object to reach a height of 100 feet and the second to reach a height of 50 feet, the first object will remain in flight almost twice as long as the second object. *Example C:* It sometimes takes less time to relay a baseball to the infield after a long hit than it would take for the retriever to throw the ball all the way to the infield because, in the latter case, the thrower must project the ball to a greater height in order to gain the needed distance.

Example D: A springboard diver must project himself high in the air in order to allow time to achieve the airborne movements (stunt) he desires. If his projection is chiefly horizontal, he has insufficient time to complete the maneuver in good form.

The effects of impact on flight

Objects receive impact when they are struck by various implements or when they contact stationary surfaces. In either case a rebound of the object from the surface results, provided resistance of the surface is greater than the momentum of the object. A rebound will occur if (1) the object moves, and the surface does not move, such as the basketball dribble or a handball shot; (2) the object does not move, but the stroking surface does move, as in the golf drive; and (3) the object and surface both move, as in striking a moving ball with an implement as in tennis or baseball. The angle and magnitude with which the object rebounds are influenced by several factors.

Angle of rebound

The angle at which an object will rebound from a surface may be predicted except for modifications which occur as the result of (1) irregular shapes of the two colliding surfaces, (2) the force resulting from elasticity of the object, and (3) spin of the object both prior to and after the contact. When these factors are discounted, the angle of incidence will equal the angle of reflection, meaning that the angle at which the object approaches a surface is equal to the angle at which it leaves that surface. If the object (a ball) is underinflated or the striking surface "gives" (such as a loosely hung canvas), part of the force is dissipated, and the rebound will be lower and shorter due to the loss of force.

Example A: A basketball shot at the backboard will rebound toward the basket at an angle similar to the angle at which it approached the board. *Example B:* If a handball player drives a ball into the front wall at an angle of 60°, the ball will reflect from the wall at an angle of 60° in the direction opposite the approach (assuming there is no spin on the ball). *Example C:* If a tennis ball strikes the court at an angle of 30°, it will rebound at the same angle, except when influenced by spin and elasticity.

Magnitude and direction of a rebound

The velocity of the object as it rebounds from a striking surface determines the distance it will travel. The rebounding velocity, in turn, depends upon the

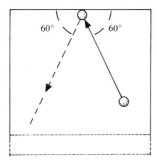

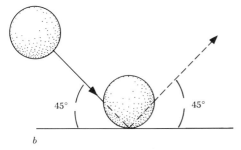

Figure 14-4.
(a) A handball approaching a wall at an angle
of 60° will rebound at 60°, unless spin influences the rebound. (b) A basketball bounced at
an angle of 45° will rebound at 45°.

momentum of both the object and the striking implement upon contact, the
physical characteristics of both, and especially the characteristic of elasticity
(restitution after compression).

A related concept discussed under Newton's third law of motion (counterforce)
implies that "give" in the striking surface results in a reduction of rebound force.
That law assumes that there is no quick restitution of the striking surface to its
normal shape. If, after being compressed, the striking surface tends to reassume
its shape quickly, it adds velocity to the object. This idea is demonstrated in the
case of a trampoline or a diving board. An air-filled pole-vaulting pit is an example
of a surface which does not reassume its shape quickly and, therefore, fails to
add velocity to the rebound.

Sufficient striking force.   The magnitude of the striking force must be
sufficient to overcome the inertia of the object being struck. The striking force is

determined by the momentum of the moving object or objects that are involved in the impact.

Example A: A football blocker may be unable to develop enough momentum to overcome the inertia of a heavier opponent. In such a case, the opponent (object) will not be caused to rebound from the striking surface. *Example B:* The striking force of a baseball bat on a ball is determined by the momentum of both the bat and the ball. A fast-moving ball will rebound with greater velocity than a slower ball, provided the bat has enough momentum to overcome sufficiently the inertia of the ball. *Example C:* A golf club with a heavy head will have greater momentum than one with a lighter head, if velocity is the same. Therefore, the heavier club will exert greater force on the surface of the ball.

Elasticity of the striking surfaces.   A highly elastic object will quickly spring back to its original shape after being compressed. Some substances compress easily but are not elastic enough to reassume shape quickly. Other substances are difficult to compress, but once compressed, their ability for restitution to original shape (elasticity) is great. Still other substances are neither highly compressible nor highly elastic. The greatest rebound occurs when the object is greatly compressed and possesses a high degree of elasticity.

Example A: Connection with the ball at the middle of a tennis racket produces a faster rebound of the ball because the strings are the most compressible at that point. The movement of the strings back to original position depends upon the quality of the strings and how tightly they are strung. *Example B:* A metal shot (shot put) lacks the ability to be compressed and is not elastic. Therefore, it rebounds very little upon landing on a hard surface. The same could be said of a rock. *Example C:* A softball is harder to compress and has less elasticity than a tennis ball; therefore, a softball has less rebound ability. *Example D:* Both a handball and a golf ball are highly elastic, but the golf ball is more difficult to compress. If the two balls were dropped from the same height (shoulder height) onto the same surface, the handball's rebound would exceed that of the golf ball. The reason is that the impact would be insufficient to produce enough compression of the golf ball to allow its elastic quality to function. When struck hard with a golf club, the golf ball compresses a considerable amount, thus allowing its elastic quality to function. As a result, the golf ball responds better than a handball to the impact of the club. *Example E:* A basketball with insufficient air will compress easily when bounced, but lack of air pressure within causes the ball to have little elasticity; therefore, its rebound ability is poor. When properly inflated, the ball is more difficult to compress, but it has increased elasticity and thus rebounds farther. *Example F:* To add to the elasticity of the strings, the tennis ball compresses upon contact with the racket. Then, due to its elasticity, it immediately rebounds from the racket. A "dead" tennis ball is one which has partially lost its elasticity.

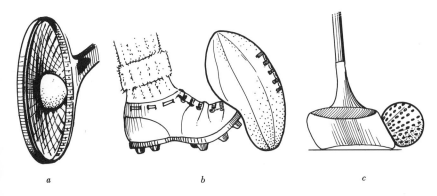

a   b   c

Figure 14–5.
The ability of an object to react to a force (rebound) depends on the object's compressibility and elasticity. (*a*) Both the tennis ball and racket face have a reasonable amount of compressibility and elasticity. (*b*) The football is more difficult to compress, but it has greater elasticity. (*c*) The golf ball is very difficult to compress, but it has great elasticity.

Rebound of two moving objects.   When both the object and the striking surface are moving, the momentum with which the object will rebound equals approximately the sum of the two momenta, minus the momentum retained by the striking surface. A slight additional loss of momentum will result from friction and heat. The direction of the rebound will be the same as the direction of the greater of the two momenta, provided they are moving exactly in opposite directions and the two centers of gravity pass through each other.

Example A: Assuming that the momentum of a softball bat exceeds the momentum of the ball, the faster the softball is pitched, the farther it may be hit. This is true because the momentum of the incoming ball is added to the momentum of the moving bat. *Example B:* It takes less striking force to return a fast-approaching tennis ball than a slow-moving one; however, the momentum of the striking racket must at least be sufficient to withstand the momentum of the approaching ball. *Example C:* To bunt a baseball effectively, a batter must be sure either to redirect or diminish the impact force, or else the ball will rebound too far. The faster the ball is delivered, the greater the batter's concern must be for this factor.

It should be obvious that maximum rebound is not always the greatest concern. In fact, reducing the rebound is sometimes the objective, as in the bunt. The basketball player attempts to control the speed of his approach when shooting a lay-up to prevent too much rebound from the backboard. Some baseball hitters sacrifice some momentum of their swing to achieve greater accuracy and/or more frequent contact. A well-placed shot in tennis, handball, volleyball, badminton, and other games is generally more effective than more forceful shots that are not well placed.

Effects of spin on angle and magnitude of rebound

Application of spin to an object may result from contact with either a moving surface (implement) or a stationary surface. Following are important facts relating to the effects of spin and how to achieve the desired amount of spin on an object.

Intentional spin resulting from striking.   To cause an object to spin in the desired direction, the striking implement should be drawn across the object in the direction of the desired spin. Forward (top) spin is caused by an implement striking forward-upward. Backspin is produced when the strike is made forward-downward. Right spin (clockwise) is generated by drawing the implement across the ball from right to left, and left spin is developed from contact of the implement in a left to right direction.

Example A: In tennis driving strokes, the ball should usually be hit with a forward-upward motion (the racket face tends to roll over the ball) in order to apply top spin to the ball. Top spin causes the ball to drop, producing a tendency for it to land within the opponent's court rather than to be too long. Also, top spin causes the ball to move faster on the rebound and to bounce at a lower angle. *Example B:* If the tennis stroke is forward-downward, a "cut" shot results, and the ball will backspin. A backspinning ball will "hang" in the air longer and rebound from the surface at a sharper angle, tending to rebound higher. *Example C:* If a golf club is drawn across the ball from right to left on contact, right spin (clockwise) will result. The ball will slice (right-handed golfer). The slicer also tends to "pull" his shots to the left when this "outside-in" swing contacts the ball dead-center. If the heel of the club leads the toe of the club at contact (face open), a slice results, even though the swing may be straight through. *Example D:* If a golf club is swung "inside-out" (club head contacts the ball from left to right), the right-handed golfer will create left spin (counterclockwise), which causes the ball to hook.

Spin resulting from contact with surface.   A moving object develops spin in the direction of its motion as a result of contact with a surface.

Example A: A bowling ball gains an increasing amount of forward spin as it progresses, due to friction between it and the surface. The additional spin reduces the friction against forward movement of the ball. If the ball is projected with backspin, it loses its velocity more rapidly. *Example B:* If a golf ball has forward (top) spin during flight, the spin will be increased as a result of contact with the surface. If the ball has backspin, the spin tends to be neutralized upon landing. If the backspin is excessive, its effects will supersede the effects of the landing.

Example C: Although a golf ball is struck directly through the center of gravity on a putt, it will still develop forward spin as a result of friction as it rolls along the green.

Effects of spin on a ball landing on a horizontal surface. A change may be expected in the rebound angle, in the distance of the bounce, and in the distance of the roll as a spinning ball contacts a horizontal surface:

1. *Top spin* causes a lower angle of rebound, a longer bounce, and more roll.
2. *Backspin* causes a higher angle of rebound, a shorter bounce, and less roll.
3. *Sidespin* causes the angle of bounce to change toward the direction of the spin (left spin-left bounce). The smaller the angle of the approach of the ball to the horizontal surface, the greater is the effect of sidespin. If the approach is perpendicular (90°), sidespin has no effect.

Example A: A basketball bounce pass may be given sidespin to change the rebound from the floor. If the ball is spinning to the right (clockwise), it will tend to bounce to the right on the rebound. The lower the pass (smaller angle to the floor) and the greater the spin, the greater the ball will deviate from its normal path of rebound. *Example B:* An opponent in tennis is often deceived by spin of the ball; for instance, the cut shot (backspin) results in a higher and shorter bounce than anticipated. *Example C:* The effect of a spin on a football is difficult to predict because of the shape of the ball; as a general rule, a longer roll can be expected when a ball turns end-over-end forward than when it rotates around its long axis (a spiral). Hence, the quick kick is usually more successful when projected low and end over end. Although with such a kick the ball travels less distance through the air, the long roll may result in more total distance, provided the ball is airborne beyond the deepest receiver (Figure 14–6).

Effects of spin on a ball striking a vertical surface. The vertical surface which a moving object strikes may be stationary (basketball backboard, billiard table rail, or handball front wall) or may be a moving implement (paddle, racket, bat, or hand). The following may be expected from contact with a vertical surface:

1. *Top spin* causes a higher rebound.
2. *Backspin* causes a lower rebound.
3. *Right spin* causes a rebound to the left.
4. *Left spin* causes a rebound to the right.

(It is interesting to note that an object with sidespin responds to a vertical surface in a direction opposite from its response to a horizontal surface.)

Example A: If a tennis opponent delivers a forehand drive with top spin on the ball, compensation in position of the racket face should be made to avoid a

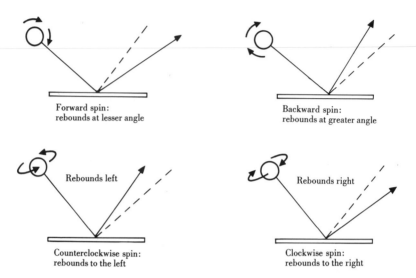

Forward spin:
rebounds at lesser angle

Backward spin:
rebounds at greater angle

Rebounds left

Rebounds right

Counterclockwise spin:
rebounds to the left

Clockwise spin:
rebounds to the right

Figure 14–6.
Influence of spin on angle of rebound from a horizontal surface.

return that is too high and too long. If a cut shot (backspin) is approaching, the performer should adjust his racket face to avoid the tendency of the ball to rebound downward into the net. *Example B:* A basketball backboard shot from the front will have a better chance to rebound into the basket if it has backspin, because it will rebound at a lower angle. *Example C:* A table tennis ball served with left spin (counterclockwise) will rebound from the receiver's paddle to the server's right (receiver's left). *Example D:* A baseball pitched with excessive backspin will tend to rebound downward upon contact with the bat. The batter would need to swing forward-upward if he wanted to hit a fly ball. *Example E:* The curve ball from a right-handed pitcher has a combination of left spin and top spin, which creates a tendency for the ball to be hit high and to the pitcher's right (left field line).

Reducing effects of spin by increasing striking force.   The more forceful the contact between an implement and an object, the less will be the effects of spin. The rebound path of the object will be dominated more by the path of the striking implement as its momentum increases. Spin produces greater effects as the force of impact becomes less.

Example A: The effects of spin produced by the baseball pitcher will be greater when the batter bunts than when he takes a full swing. *Example B:* Tennis players often err when they attempt to "baby" a critically placed shot, because they fail to realize that reducing the force of their stroke increases the effects of spin on the ball.

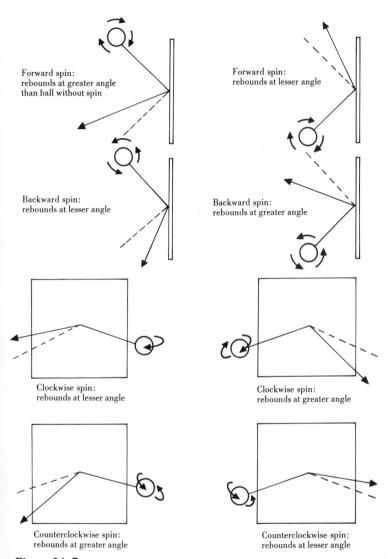

Forward spin:
rebounds at greater angle
than ball without spin

Forward spin:
rebounds at lesser angle

Backward spin:
rebounds at lesser angle

Backward spin:
rebounds at greater angle

Clockwise spin:
rebounds at lesser angle

Clockwise spin:
rebounds at greater angle

Counterclockwise spin:
rebounds at greater angle

Counterclockwise spin:
rebounds at lesser angle

Figure 14–7.
Influence of spin on angle of rebound from a vertical surface.

Recommended supplementary reading

Broer, Marion R.: "Efficiency of Human Movement," 2d ed., chap. 9, W. B. Saunders Company, Philadelphia, 1966.

Bunn, John W.: "Scientific Principles of Coaching," pp. 24–41, 61–71, 76–81, Prentice-Hall, Inc., Englewood Cliffs, N.J., 1955.

Cooper, John M., and Ruth B. Glassow: "Kinesiology," 2d ed., chap. 17, The C. V. Mosby Company, St. Louis, 1968.

15

Equilibrium

*W*hen the body is in equilibrium, an even adjustment exists between all opposing forces, and the body is in balance. The state of equilibrium may be secure or precarious. This chapter deals with important facts about equilibrium as it relates to performance. The chapter content is arranged under the following subheadings: (1) center of gravity, (2) balance and stability, and (3) posture.

Center of gravity

The center of gravity of the human body may be defined as (1) the point of exact center around which the body may rotate freely in all directions; (2) the point around which the weight is equal on all opposite sides; or (3) the point of intersection of the three primary body planes—sagittal, frontal, and transverse. The center of gravity in the body is normally located at a point along the mid-line, at about 55 percent of the person's height. However, its exact point varies from one individual to another, depending on body proportions. An analysis of the following factors is important to understanding center of gravity and its effects on performance.

Because of the differences in body structure between men and women, center of gravity is usually proportionately lower in women than in men. This gives women a structural advantage in stability, but it gives them a disadvantage when they are required to raise the center of gravity, as in high-jumping. On the average, center of gravity is proportionately higher in children than in adults as a result of the change in body proportions as one progresses from childhood to adulthood. The center of gravity is affected by amputations and other structural changes which cause the body to deviate from normal. In addition, the center of gravity is temporarily influenced by specific body positions; for instance, in diving, a person's center of gravity shifts forward as he moves from a layout to a pike or

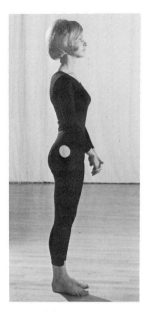

Figure 15–1.
Center of gravity in the human body.

tuck position, and it moves away from the midline of the body when he laterally flexes the trunk.

The human body rests on a base of support defined as the area of contact between the body and the supporting surface. If the base of support and other factors remain constant, then, as the center of gravity is lowered, the stability of the body is increased. This can be demonstrated by comparing two triangles with equal bases and different heights, one twice as tall as the other. The shorter triangle is considerably more stable than the taller one.

Balance and stability

When a body is in balance, an even adjustment exists between opposing forces. A balance center located in the inner ear, the kinesthetic sense, and the eyes all play a role in maintaining balance.

Principles of balance

For balance to be maintained in any stationary position, the center of gravity must remain over the base of support. Whenever the center of gravity passes out-

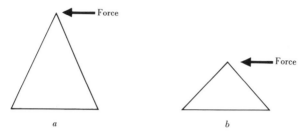

Figure 15–2.
The taller triangle (*a*) is less stable than the shorter (*b*).

side the base of support, the body is off-balance in that direction. This applies to all body positions, including upright, inverted (where the hands form the base of support), and three-, four-, or six-point positions. For balance to be maintained in a standing position, continuous forward body lean is necessary. This results in constant tension on the large calf muscles, and it places the center of weight approximately over the center of the feet.

To execute balance skills effectively, the performer must develop two primary qualities: (1) adequate strength to support the body in the given positions and (2) ability to shift the body weight quickly into the correct positions at the right time. The first quality (strength) is dependent on the three factors which compose it, namely, contractile force of the mover muscles, ability to coordinate all the muscles involved in the act, and mechanical ratio of the different levers. The second quality (shifting body weight) depends on several factors, namely, kinesthetic perception and visual perception (the awareness of the position of the body and its parts), function of the balance center of the inner ear, quick reactions, good neuromuscular coordination, agility, and flexibility.

Recovery of balance.   If the center of gravity moves outside the base of support, a quick adjustment must be made in order to regain balance. The base of support may be moved or enlarged, or a body part may be adjusted in order to return the center of gravity to a position over the base of support. After the adjustment is made, a lowering of the center of gravity makes the performer more stable; thus he is less susceptible to another loss of balance.

Example A: A loss of balance in the handstand may be regained if the performer handwalks (moves the base) in the direction of the overbalance until the base is again beneath the center of gravity. Overcompensations after the balance has been regained can sometimes be avoided by bending the arms (lowering of the center of gravity). *Example B:* In the head- and handstand, the area of the base can be enlarged by increasing the distances between the points of the triangle formed by the points of support, the head and the hands. Often the least stable performers place their hands alongside their ears (head and hands in a straight line), thus reducing the area of their base in the forward-backward direction. If these three points truly represent the area of the base, each must bear approximately equal weight. *Example C:* When the performer is working on a balance beam, the movement of a body segment can shift the center of gravity back over the base of support. While the movement of a segment may be effective immediately after a loss of balance, the same movement may be ineffective if the center of gravity has been allowed to move too far outside the base of support or if too much falling speed has developed. For this reason, very quick and correct reactions are essential for recovering balance.

Sensory receptor adjustments.   The reduction of unfamiliar sensations associated with balance receptors often reduces dizziness which may lead to a loss of balance. For instance, the eyes have been oriented to certain spatial relationships in an upright world, and deviations from the upright positions often affect sense of balance negatively. Also, fast-twirling head movements produce movement of fluids in the inner ear which give rise to the sensation of dizziness. These negative results can be partially controlled.

Example A: When bouncing on a trampoline, the performer should focus his eyes on a distant object which is relatively level with the usual upright head position, such as a point on a distant wall. This will reduce dizziness. *Example B:* When spinning rapidly in place during a dance or skating maneuver, the performer should select a fixed point upon which he keeps his eyes focused as long as possible during each turn. If he returns his concentration to this point as quickly as possible in each succeeding turn, he produces the least possible disturbance of the inner-ear fluids. *Example C:* Beginners often feel dizzy when performing gymnastic turning movements. Even simple stunts like a forward roll can produce this effect until the performer becomes accustomed to unfamiliar positions and movements of the head. Practice helps overcome this dizziness, because kinesthetic adjustments become keener as unfamiliar positions are repeated.

Carrying postures.   When external weight is applied to the body, as in lifts and carries, the body weight must be shifted in order to maintain balance around the line of gravity (a vertical line passing through the center of gravity to the surface).

Example A: If a 50-pound weight is held under the right arm, the line of gravity in the body must be shifted toward the left edge of the base of support in order to compensate for the change in the center of weight. *Example B:* If, when lifting a heavy object, the performer keeps the object close to his center of gravity, less adjustment will be needed and there will be less likelihood of a loss of balance.

Principles governing stability

Stability is firmness of balance. The stable body is less apt to be disturbed by any upsetting influences. The physical makeup of a person exerts strong influence

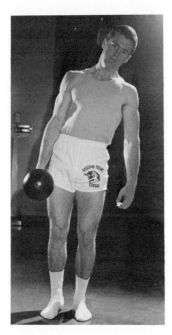

Figure 15–3.
External weight added to the body
calls for an adjustment in posture.
The body's center of gravity shifts
in a direction away from the external weight.

on his stability, but within the bounds of this limitation, one can purposely assume
positions which contribute to stability in any given situation.

Resisting undetermined forces.   If the direction of forces which tend to
destroy balance cannot be determined, the center of gravity of the body should be
placed over the center of the base of support, or as near to it as possible. This
applies to both foot-supported and arm-supported positions, as well as to three-
point, four-point, and six-point (hands, knees, feet) positions.

Example A: A gymnast performing a handstand is most stable when his center
of weight is directly over the center of the base of support, his hands. *Example B:*
A modern dancer in a half-crouched position or a wrestler in a standing position
is most stable when the center of weight is directly over the base of support,
which, in these cases, is determined by the exact positions of the feet.

Lowered center of gravity.   Stability may be increased by lowering the
center of gravity.

Example A: The wrestler, basketball player, football player, and modern dancer
all increase their stability at certain times by assuming a crouched position which

lowers the center of gravity. *Example B:* When in an unstable craft, such as a canoe, the chances of tipping become less as the center of gravity gets closer to the bottom.

Enlarged base of support.   Stability is enhanced by increasing the area of the base of support. As the base becomes larger, the center of gravity must be moved through a greater distance in order to disrupt the balance.*

Example A: The baseball batter broadens the base of support in the direction that he wishes to hit the ball. Similarly, when the golfer drives with greater force, he assumes a wider stance in order to increase stability. Basketball, tennis, badminton, and volleyball players all spread their feet apart to broaden the base of support, and dancers increase stability by properly positioning their feet. *Example B:* Football linemen increase stability by moving from a two- to a three-point stance. The four-point stance provides a still larger area of support.

Body size and proportions.   All else being equal, the greater the mass, the more stable the object is against external forces; in fact, the stability is proportional to the mass. Thus in performance where stability is important, weight becomes a consideration. Concentration of weight also influences stability. A larger proportion of body weight concentrated in the upper part of the body raises the center of gravity, which is a disadvantage in activities requiring balance and stability in an upright position, but is an advantage in arm support skills requiring balance.

---

* The principles relating both to lowering the center of gravity and to enlarging the base of support are subject to limitations and may be self-defeating. If the performer applies these principles beyond reason, he may produce undesirable angles of support and force weak muscular actions. It is generally true that beyond a certain point, an increase in stability reduces mobility; thus, if mobility is important, it may be desirable to sacrifice maximum stability.

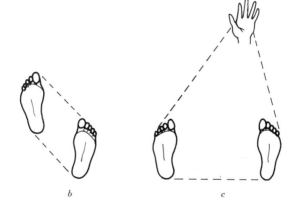

a   *b*   *c*

Figure 15–4.
As the base of support is enlarged, the object becomes more stable. (*a*) Unstable position; (*b*) more stable position; (*c*) very stable position.

Example A: A heavy basketball rebounder or post man, a heavy football player, or a heavy wrestler is more stable (harder to move) than a light one. *Example B:* A heavy concentration of weight in the upper portion of the body is a stability disadvantage for the skier, dancer, or skater, who may, however, compensate for it by other qualities. This same structure, though, would enhance performance in most gymnastic skills.

Friction. The greater the friction between the supporting surface and the body parts in contact with that surface, the greater the stability.

Example A: The use of gymnasium shoes on hard surfaces and the use of base-ball, football, and running spikes on their respective surfaces all increase sta-bility. *Example B:* When traction is insufficient, forces which are applied must have more of a vertical and less of a horizontal component. The performer runs more "up and down" on a slippery surface.

Stability against a known external force

Some of the principles included in the preceding section are not entirely useful when the direction of the force with which the performer must deal is known. **Moving the center of gravity toward the force.** If a known force is approaching, and the performer wishes to maintain his balance, his center of

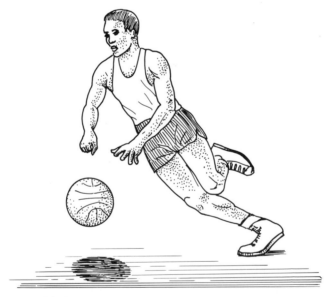

Figure 15–5.
Adequate foot-surface friction is necessary in certain perfor-mances.

gravity should be very near the edge of his base of support on the side nearest the oncoming force. He is most stable under these conditions because his center of gravity must be moved a maximum distance before it is outside its supporting base. He may further diminish the effects of the oncoming force by developing momentum of his own in a direction opposite that of the force.

Example A: The football lineman widens his base by stepping toward an oncoming blocker, and he moves his center of gravity in the same direction. (He also lowers the center of gravity.) If the blocker is to upset the lineman, he must move the lineman's center of gravity all the way through the increased distance of the base of support. *Example B:* The boxer or the wrestler usually carries his center of gravity forward of the base of support in order to be prepared for potential force from the opponent. The wrestler must be sure to not overdo the forward weight shift or else his opponent may pull him off-balance in the forward direction.

Destroying the stability of an opponent.   A person can be moved off-balance most easily by pushing or pulling him toward the nearest edge of the base of support or in the direction of the narrowest part of the base.

Example A: In wrestling, an opponent can be taken off balance most easily by pushing or pulling him in the direction at right angles to the line connecting his feet. *Example B:* In any two-point stance, as in football, an opponent will be least stable in one direction depending on his foot placement, because the measurement of his base in one direction can be only as great as the length of his feet.

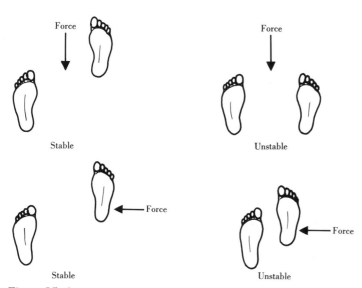

Figure 15–6.
The position of the feet should be determined by the direction in which stability is needed.

Tasks requiring instability

Some positions of readiness require instability rather than stability, because the shorter distance the center of gravity must move to clear the base of support, the more quickly the whole body can be put into motion in that direction.

Starts in a known direction.   If one wishes to start quickly in a given direction, he should move his center of gravity as close as possible to the edge of the base of support nearest the desired direction of movement.

Example A: The swimmer or runner desires to be almost off-balance in the direction of the start. *Example B:* Because a high center of gravity causes instability in the position of the track start, the position requires high hips to be most effective. However, the hips may be held *too high*, and when they are, the legs are too straight, thus reducing the leg force needed to propel the body. If the performer has his center of gravity near enough to the edge of the base, the shoulders will be slightly forward of the hands in the "set" position.

Compromise stances in the state of readiness.   The degree of stability desired in a state of readiness for any given performance is determined by the task to be accomplished.

Example A: Wrestlers, defensive basketball players, boxers, tennis, badminton, and volleyball players must be center balanced in order to move quickly in any direction. *Example B:* Four- and six-point football stances are highly desirable if the performer is going to move forward or attempt to hold his position. But, performers assuming such stances operate at a disadvantage when they are required to move laterally or backward. A compromise stance (3-point or very low 2-point) affords greater versatility.

Balance and stability while in motion

Many principles of balance in motion are the same as those applied to stationary postures. Important differences are (1) the base of support is constantly moving, (2) the base of support is often only as large as the one supporting foot, and (3) recovery movements must be especially quick and precise when the body is in motion.

Use of gravity.   Many locomotor activities depend upon a deliberate loss of balance to enable gravity to combine with muscular forces to move the body in the desired direction. The base of support is then moved beneath the moving body to support it for a brief period of time. This action is repeated rhythmically.

Example A: When a person leans forward to start walking or running, he shifts the center of gravity outside the base of support and then must step forward to regain balance, thus establishing a new base of support. The center of gravity, which is in motion, passes over the new base of support and continues its forward motion. Subsequently, the base of support is moved by stepping forward with the feet, and locomotion (walking) results. When walking, a person is supported simultaneously by both feet for a brief moment between steps, but when running, only one foot contacts the surface at a time. At any time during the run, the base of support is provided by only one supporting limb which demands intricate timing. *Example B:* When a swimmer or runner starts a race, he shifts the center of gravity forward of the base of support in order to utilize the force of gravity to help him move in that direction.

Increasing stability while in motion.   Stability can be gained while in motion by lowering the center of gravity and enlarging the base of support.

Example A: The ballcarrier in football has a low center of gravity and a wide base when running through a congested area. He adds lateral stability by widening his running stance. He may also run with short, choppy steps, which allow him to establish his base of support more often, and, thus he may change direction more quickly. This running technique results in a sacrifice of linear speed. When the runner clears the congested area, he should raise his center of gravity, narrow his stance, and take a longer stride to gain maximum speed. *Example B:* While walking on his hands, a person is most stable in a lateral direction when taking shorter and wider strides. Lowering the center of gravity also aids stability in this particular skill. *Example C:* Automobiles are more stable if they have large wheel bases and low centers of weight.

Control of momentum.   To stop quickly or change direction when in rapid motion, the performer should widen his base and lower his center of gravity. This principle is often neglected in teaching skills.

Example A: The basketball player on defense is better able to control momentum and to change direction quickly when his legs are reasonably well spread and his body is reasonably low. *Example B:* If the football pass receiver is to execute sharp and effective cuts, he must observe this principle. If he does not, he will be likely to round corners and be more easily covered by a defender. The greater his momentum, the more difficult it is to stop or change direction. *Example C:* The offensive basketball player is likely to lose balance and "travel" if he does not follow this principle. The skier, too, applies the principle when turning sharply, as in slalom racing.

Posture

Posture is both dynamic and static, and we must be concerned with both types. Static posture (standing, sitting, etc.) is the easier of the two types to study. It is relatively easy to establish guidelines for static posture, but it is very difficult to provide guidelines for dynamic posture (body positions during movement) because it takes many different forms. Many of the guidelines for static posture, however, can be applied effectively to dynamic posture.

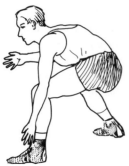

Figure 15–7.
The basketball defensive
player keeps a low center
of gravity and a wide base
of support for stability in
his position and readiness
to move quickly in any
direction. Similar "ready
positions" are employed in
tennis, badminton, wres-
tling, and other sports.

Correct posture is important because (1) it affects the functioning of the
organic systems; (2) it reduces strain on muscles, ligaments, and tendons; and
(3) it increases attractiveness of the individual. In addition to affecting one's
ability to function and his attractiveness, posture may influence a person's concept
of himself and how others view him. Therefore, posture has important psychological implications.

Evaluating posture

It is established that many of the traditional hard and fast rules of posture are
unjustified. Current thinking is that postural evaluation must be approached from
a highly individual and functional point of view. The judgment of how correct a
posture is must be based on corrections from the physiological, anatomical, and
aesthetic points of view.

Physiological correctness.   Posture is physiologically correct when it allows
the organic systems to function efficiently. Posture which restricts adequate circulation, respiration, digestion, and elimination is not correct; for instance, a rigid
(at attention) standing position restricts circulation. Research results indicate that
changes in posture influence heart rate in static positions and also influence the
required cardiac output during exercise.

Anatomical correctness.   Posture is anatomically correct when the body has good balance and alignment, the result of a minimum of muscle strain. In such positions the skeletal structure carries a maximum amount of weight, so posture demands minimum muscle effort. Poor posture means a body that is too rigid or too erect. Rasch (**61**) claims that the military attention position requires 20 percent more energy than an easy standing position and that an extremely relaxed standing position requires 10 percent less energy than the easy standing position. From the anatomical point of view, the best posture is a position where the bodily structure is vertically aligned and the muscles are as relaxed as possible.

Aesthetic correctness.   Posture is aesthetically correct when it contributes most to the attractiveness of the person. Aesthetically correct posture also tends to be anatomically and physiologically correct. Occasionally, however, the aesthetic point of view tends to lead people toward too much rigidity and too much precision in movement.

Guidelines for correct posture

Whether posture is evaluated from the physiological, anatomical, or aesthetic points of view, there are several guides that should be followed:

1. The weight-bearing segments should be correctly aligned, so that the line of gravity passes through them. This reduces unnecessary muscle strain and contributes to attractiveness.

2. The extension of the weight-bearing joints should be an easy extension not accompanied by strain, tension, or excessive rigidity.

3. The feet should be placed far enough apart to form a base of support over which the body can be balanced easily without excessive muscle use.

4. With respect to inward and outward rotation of the legs, the correct position is the patellae and feet pointed straightforward.

5. Excessive forward tilt of the pelvis should be avoided because it contributes to a swayed back and protruding abdomen.

6. The spinal column, when viewed laterally, will naturally exhibit three curves, a convex cervical curve, a concave thoracic curve, and a convex lumbar curve (see Figure 6–1). Efforts to eliminate these curves are undesirable, but it is important not to allow the curves to become excessive. When viewed from the rear, the spinal column should be straight.

7. The abdominal wall, which is composed mostly of muscle tissue, should be kept in good tone, and care should be taken to keep the wall straight and in proper support of internal organs.

8. Many people have a tendency to abduct and forward rotate the shoulder girdles. This position should not become part of habitual posture because the condition commonly known as sunken chest and rounded shoulders will result.

9. In good, erect posture, the neck should be held straight, but not rigid, and the head should be aligned with the spinal column so the neck muscles are not under unnecessary stress.

Relationship of posture to other factors

Postural characteristics may be inherited or developed, and they may relate to, and be derived from, other personal qualities. A parent with severe scoliosis will be likely to produce children with scoliosis, whereas a parent with round shoulders and a forward neck tilt will tend to produce children who are inclined the same way. Postural similarities between parents and children may result partly from heredity and partly from environment. Children inherit many qualities, but they tend to develop after the models that exist in their environments.

Nutrition affects body structure, and a person with poor nourishment may have neither the energy nor the muscular strength and tone to habitually hold the body parts in correct position. Inadequate nutrition may contribute to poor posture especially during the years of bodily growth when consistently poor temporary body positions gradually become part of habitual posture.

A person's height may influence his posture. Short people tend to extend their height by standing very straight, and extremely tall people tend to reduce their

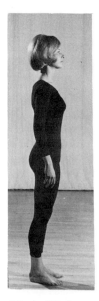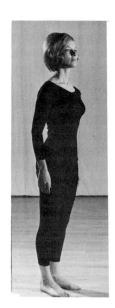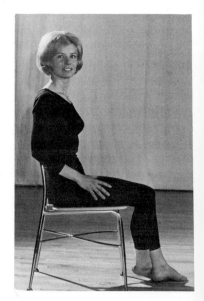

Figure 15–8.
Good posture: (*a*) standing, side view; (*b*) standing, diagonal view; (*c*) sitting.

height by settling at the joints and hunching at the upper back and neck. These people are trying to appear closer to medium height.

Training may have significant effects on posture. Dance, gymnastics, diving, and fencing all contribute to straight and slightly rigid postures and precision in body movements. Wrestling and boxing contribute to a slightly hunched posture. Long-distance running and swimming contribute to a relaxed and, often, slouchy posture. Other activities have specific effects on posture, although many activities are neutral as far as postural development is concerned.

Work conditions also affect posture. For instance, excessive study over a desk tends to develop round shoulders and forward head tilt. The same can be said of high-precision jobs requiring close hand-eye coordination and fine muscle movements, such as the work of a jeweler.

Posture has strong psychological implications. It tells much about one's personality. For example, withdrawn and shy persons often display a withdrawn-type posture, as if they are attempting to hide within themselves. The opposite-type personality (highly aggressive) often displays a very straight and outgoing posture, which makes him feel more obvious.

Correcting posture through muscle conditioning

Some cases of postural correction are more a task for psychiatrists than physical educators because the deviations grow out of psychological problems. But in most cases, the well-informed physical educator can help a student correct poor posture by (1) motivating him to want to correct his posture and (2) leading him through a program which will strengthen the muscles capable of correcting the particular deviation and add flexibility to the opposing muscles.

Experience shows that the following is the most successful postural corrective procedure:

1. Correctly identify the postural deviation and inform the individual of its nature and the importance of correcting it.
2. Attempt to identify the basic causes of the deviation, and control the causes.
3. Motivate the individual to want to correct the deviation. (In the absence of such motivation, postural corrective exercises will probably fail.)
4. Prescribe an exercise program designed to correct the condition.
5. Periodically evaluate the effects of the program.

After studying muscular actions in the earlier chapters, you should be able to select exercises to suit your needs in postural correction. You should be able to tell which muscles must be strengthened and which ones must have increased flexibility in order to bring about the desired postural changes. With this information you will be able to select exercises which will add the desired strength and flexibility, thereby favorably influencing posture.

Recommended supplementary reading

BROER, MARION R.: "Efficiency of Human Movement," 2d ed., chap. 4, W. B. Saunders Company, Philadelphia, 1966.

BUNN, JOHN W.: "Scientific Principles of Coaching," pp. 13–21, 193–194, Prentice-Hall, Inc., Englewood Cliffs, N.J., 1955.

COOPER, JOHN M., and RUTH B. GLASSOW: "Kinesiology," 2d ed., chaps. 12 and 13, The C. V. Mosby Company, St. Louis, 1968.

WELLS, KATHERINE: "Kinesiology," 4th ed., pp. 30–39, 390–406, W. B. Saunders Company, Philadelphia, 1966.

16

Mechanical analysis of a specific skill

*T*he golfer is told, "Keep your eye on the ball" and "Keep your left elbow straight" (right-handed golfer). But neither of these coaching tips is necessary for an effective golf shot; they are merely devices to help the performer assume a swing arc which will assure correct contact with the ball. The important factor is the *contact,* and not whether or not the left elbow is straight and the eye is on the ball. These factors do not affect the efficiency of the motion. The stroke will be less effective, however, if the back foot is not securely in contact with the surface upon impact or if the force of the club head does not pass through the center of gravity of the ball. In these cases basic laws of motion and force are violated, thus reducing the propelling force. Such laws are the basis for mechanical analysis of a performance, serving as the foundation upon which correct technique is determined.

The value to the student in doing a mechanical analysis is apparent. As he proceeds, he will find support for many teaching tips and will find that some commonly used tips have no basis for support. Also, he will understand better the reasoning behind established techniques of performance and why pieces of equipment are constructed and used as they are. A mechanical analysis of one skill has great carryover value in understanding other skills which involve some of the same laws and principles.

After the skill to be analyzed is selected, the logical procedure is to refer to each law, principle, or concept presented in the preceding four chapters and decide whether it is applicable. If the principle does apply to the particular skill, it should be stated and then discussed in light of that skill. Finally, the most important aspects of successful performance of the skill should be summarized.

Mechanical analysis of the golf drive (right-handed)

The golf drive was selected because its success depends upon adherence to a wide variety of principles. The purpose of the golf drive is to achieve maximum distance and accuracy. The technique may be varied to meet different conditions, especially by a performer of advanced skill, but the purpose remains essentially the same for all golfers. The skill includes (1) the development of a maximum and accurate striking force, (2) control of balance by the performer during the swing, and (3) factors involved in the behavior of the projectile. Essentially, the desired qualities of the swing are (1) maximum club-head momentum at impact, (2) correct position and direction of motion of the club head at impact, and (3) contact of the ball directly through its center of gravity. All the techniques employed should produce these desired results.

Principles of motion

The following principles of motion are evident in the golf drive:

PRINCIPLE—Combining translatory and rotary motions. Successful performance often calls for effectively combining translatory and rotary motions.

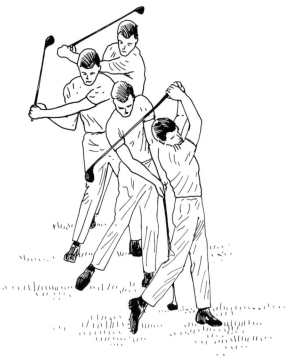

Figure 16–1.
Sequence of the golf drive.

Application. Angular (rotary) motion is the only kind that a body lever can experience. The golf drive requires successive actions of several body levers, and the arc of the club head undergoes angular motion as a result of the lever actions. The whole body experiences a limited amount of linear motion from the shift of weight from the back to the front foot. This shift tends to flatten the arc of the club head at the bottom of the swing, thus increasing the length of time that the club head can contact the ball directly through its center of gravity. If this "flattening" did not occur, chances would be greater that the strike would be made on either the downswing or the upswing, because the club head would move from the downswing to the upswing more quickly. In addition, the weight shift contributes to the striking force. The timing and the extent of the weight shift are extremely critical. It starts just prior to the downswing, and in so doing, it helps place the mover muscles on stretch for the swing to provide a more forceful contraction. If the weight shift is completed too soon or too late, its beneficial effects are lost because it is not integrated into the continuous flow of forces. Also, if the shift occurs too soon, the swinging action will lag too much, and a "push" or possibly a slice will result because the club face will still be open when the ball is contacted. The same result occurs if the body is too far forward of the ball at the time of address. If the shift occurs too late or in insufficient amount, the opposite results. Furthermore, the performer with too much weight on his back foot at contact will tend to lift, cutting the swing short and increasing chances of "topping" the ball by contacting it decidedly on the upswing. From such observations, coaching tips such as "keep the head directly over the ball" and "keep your eye on the ball" were evolved.

In addition to the body experiencing linear and rotary motions, the ball undergoes both kinds of motions. When struck, the ball undergoes curvilinear motion which becomes increasingly curvilinear as air resistance reduces its velocity. At the same time, the ball usually encounters rotary motion (spin), applied either purposely or inadvertently. The amount and direction of the spin may influence the flight of the ball a significant amount.

PRINCIPLE—Continuity of motion. When performing activities in which two or more consecutive motions contribute toward movement in the same direction, the performer should not pause between motions.

Application. Each successive motion of body parts should occur so that the club head undergoes constant acceleration. The appearance of a swing which develops in this manner is smooth and flowing; the smooth swing will produce a greater final momentum than the jerky swing because inertia against the action is less. Also, energy is conserved when the forces are smooth and consistent in intensity.

PRINCIPLE—Effects of momentum. When a moving object strikes another object, the greater its momentum at impact, the greater will be its force.

Application. Because momentum is the product of velocity and mass, the increase in either of these factors results in increased momentum. In the golf swing it would appear that a heavier or longer club would produce greater momentum, and thus a greater impact. This is true provided velocity is not sacrificed; however, the key factor here is whether the performer has adequate strength to handle the heavier or longer club so that the same final velocity results as would with the lighter or shorter club. Theoretically, as a person increases in strength, he is able to handle a heavier club at the same velocity; therefore, the momentum of his drive is increased. It should be noted that the momentum developed in the backswing must be overcome before the downswing can begin, which explains the reason for a slow backswing, especially with a heavy club. It is obvious, then, that additional strength in the correct muscles is one key to more distance off the tee.

Control is another aspect of momentum. The club movements may destroy the balance of the performer or may alter the swing arc, causing inaccuracies in the contact. A greater club momentum tends to magnify these tendencies. A golfer who swings harder (faster) or who uses a heavier club becomes more susceptible to such inaccuracies. He will be able to cope better with these conditions if the muscles controlling the club and body balance are stronger.

In conclusion, the performer needs adequate strength in muscles that produce striking forces and in muscles that maintain balance. Usually, he will need additional strength in these muscles if he wishes to increase the distance of his drive either by swinging harder or by using a heavier or longer club.

PRINCIPLE—Transfer of momentum. Momentum developed in a body segment is transferred to the rest of the body only while the body is still in contact with the supporting surface.

Application. The momentum of the club and the movements of the body in the direction of the swing will tend to pull the body off-balance in that direction. Maintaining of balance is discussed more fully in Chapter 15.

PRINCIPLE—Maximum acceleration and efficiency of motion. All available forces should be applied sequentially with proper timing, and as directly in the intended line of motion as possible. Body movements extraneous to the desired motion should be reduced to a minimum.

Application. The major forces of the golf swing in proper sequence follow:

1. Inward rotation of the front hip (a reversal of customary muscle function—the pelvis rotates on the fixed leg)
2. Left rotation of the thoracic spine
3. Abduction and outward rotation of the left shoulder (this may vary some from true abduction), coupled with scapular adduction to the left side and extension of the right elbow.

4. Ulnar flexion (adduction) of the left wrist and flexion of the right wrist (the right wrist may also tend somewhat toward ulnar flexion)

These forces are in addition to the total body weight shift which has already been discussed. Each of the forces makes a particular contribution to maintaining the accuracy of the swing. If too much or too little motion results from any one force, inaccuracies result. If the timing of any force is too early or too late in the sequence, the result will be inaccuracy, reduction of momentum, or both.

Few extraneous movements are seen in golf swings, but a common one is too long a backswing, which tends to pull the golfer off-balance. Another common undesired motion is extension of the trunk, which pulls the golfer away from the ball just prior to contact, causing him to top, slice, or completely miss the ball. Overeagerness to watch the flight of the ball also contributes to this mistake.

It appears that extra force would become available for generating momentum if the left elbow were flexed in the backswing and extended just prior to contact. But this movement has not been advocated; in fact, golfers are cautioned to keep the left elbow straight throughout the swing. In a way, this can be compared to punting a football without using the extension of the knee. The reasoning behind this restriction is twofold: (1) the timing between forces 2, 3, and 4 above is so precise that the inclusion of another force would be impossible to control consistently and (2) if the elbow did not return to complete extension prior to contact, the length of the lever would be shortened, and a complete miss could result. It appears prudent to sacrifice some possible additional momentum for consistency and accuracy.

PRINCIPLE—Rotational speed. If a constant force causes a body to rotate, then as changes in the radius of rotation occur, variations in the speed of rotation (the term angular and rotational speed can be interchanged) will result. As the radius is lengthened, the body rotates more slowly; as the radius is shortened the body rotates more rapidly.

Application. We can assume the available muscular force is constant and the distance from the shoulders to the club head represents the radius of rotation. The point of grip on the handle can be varied slightly to alter the radius of rotation. It will take less force to achieve a given angular velocity if the grip is farther down the club; however, unless there is considerable increase in angular velocity, the performer can expect less club head momentum at contact because of the shorter radius of swing. The shorter grip will probably aid accuracy at the expense of speed of the club head.

PRINCIPLE—Counterforces in striking activities. The amount of force a striking implement imparts to an object depends upon the combined momentum of the implement and the object at the moment of impact. Any "give" in the implement at impact reduces the propulsive force.

Application. Obviously, strong contractions of the agonist and stabilizing muscles are essential for reducing loss of force due to "give" at the moment of impact. Foot contact with the surface must be secure, and the grip must be firm. Instructions to relax in the swing refer to antagonist muscles and muscles not directly involved in the action or support of the action.

PRINCIPLE—Direction of the counterforce. The counterforce is directly opposite and equal to the applied force.

Application. The applied forces in the golf drive are the push with the right (back) leg, the strong body rotation to the left, and the arm actions in the downswing. The first force requires firm footing to avoid the tendency of the feet to slip backward, and the second force requires firm footing against the tendency of both feet to turn to the right in reaction to the striking force to the left. Cleats of golf shoes are designed to hold the feet firmly in place; without proper footwear, it is likely that reduction in the force of impact will occur, due to slippage (give). A slippery surface exaggerates this effect.

A stance with the feet wider than shoulder width increases the tendency to slip, because forces are directed further away from a line perpendicular to the surface and the body weight is less concentrated directly over the two points of support (the feet).

PRINCIPLE—Temporarily stored counterforce. If a surface, implement, or object used in a performance has elasticity, then an applied force produces bend or compression, which represents stored energy.

Application. The shafts of golf clubs vary in flexibility; a more flexible shaft bends with the forces of the downswing, only to snap back to original shape at impact. This energy adds to the striking force, but at the same time, it makes accuracy more difficult. Some golfers prefer a stiffer shaft rather than contend with the possible loss of accuracy.

PRINCIPLE—Leverage. By changing the amount or type of leverage, either speed (and distance) or force can be gained at the sacrifice of the other.

Application. Practically all the body levers used in the golf drive are in the third class. This type provides speed and range of motion (distance) at the expense of force. Class three levers are especially effective in producing a fast striking force with a relatively light object. These levers require great amounts of muscular force to accumulate momentum because of their short effort arms, but this problem is rectified by the successive application and precise timing of the numerous separate levers, each adding to the same motion. To obtain the optimum effect, the total range of motion must be great enough to allow time for each lever to make its fullest contribution.

Principles of force

Because of the direct relationship between force and motion, some of the principles of force have been touched upon under the previous section, "Principles of Motion." Those principles of force not yet identified are:

PRINCIPLE—Total force. The final velocity (or force) is the sum of the velocities of all contributing movements, if the movements are applied in a single direction, in the proper sequence, with proper timing.

Application. At the moment of contact, the club head has a velocity approximately equal to the sum of the velocities of the contributing levers. In order to accumulate the greatest velocity, a particular movement in the sequence of movements should be applied at the peak velocity of the prior movement. Because so many levers operate in such a short time in the golf swing, the importance of timing becomes apparent. Much practice is needed to develop correct timing, and conscious attempts to intensify forces without regard to timing in the swing ("pressing the swing") are often disastrous. This principle explains why the strongest individual may not necessarily hit the ball the farthest if his ability to correctly time the individual forces is inadequate.

PRINCIPLE—Duration of force application. If a constant force is applied to a body, the body develops greater acceleration as the duration (distance) over which the force is applied increases.

Application. For maximum duration of force application, the backswing should be as long as possible without destroying the swing arc or pulling the body off-balance. It should be understood that the backswing is only to gain correct position for an effective downswing and to place on stretch those muscles used in the downswing. If optimum back swing and optimum total body shift are used, then the optimum duration of force will result.

PRINCIPLE—Follow-through. Emphasis on a correct follow-through eliminates a tendency to decelerate the striking action prior to contact.

Application. Adequate follow-through is vital to a forceful and complete swing. Lack of follow-through contributes to a "chopping" or "punching" action. Also, an adequate follow-through allows the golfer to select a "point of aim" on the ball and to drive with full force toward that point. The coaching tip is "throw the club head toward the target." Concentration on the follow-through may also help to control the consistency of muscular contractions during the downswing.

PRINCIPLE—Effects of spin on the ball. The flight of an object is influenced by the direction and amount of its spin.

Application. We know that a spinning ball curves from an accumulation of air resistance on the forward spinning side of the ball and from a reduction of air resistance on the opposite side. The curve is magnified if the ball remains in flight for a longer time as a result of a slowing of the ball which allows a greater effect of the spin. Therefore, inaccuracies in the club-ball contact (causing spin) are of greater concern when the driver is used because it produces great linear velocity which results in long flight. The ball will slice, hook, rise, or drop to a greater extent for a given amount of spin if it is driven farther.

PRINCIPLE—Centrifugal force. Centrifugal force creates the tendency for an object to continue momentum in a straight line instead of in a curved path.

Application. During the swing, the golfer feels the results of the force attempting to pull the club head away from the desired arc. Applying the precise amount of opposing force to counteract this effect is extremely difficult, and it is one of the keys to accuracy of the swing. If the grip is not secure, the club may fly from the hands. If the golfer pulls back too far, he will miss the ball or top it. The need to contend with this force also illustrates the importance of assuming an address stance which is relatively close to the ball (no need for reaching), which is rather upright (reduces tendency to straighten up), and which distributes weight over the whole foot (reduces tendency to shift weight forward or backward during swing).

The greater the momentum of the club, the greater the centrifugal force. This again points to the driver as a difficult club to master, and it illustrates that the relatively unskilled golfer will experience more accuracy if he does not attempt to drive too hard. Some professionals advocate hitting with all available force, but this appears to be good advice only for certain exceptionally skilled golfers.

Principles of balance and stability

The principles of balance and stability which relate to the golf drive have influenced the adoption of techniques which provide a relatively stable base of support.

PRINCIPLE—Enlarged base of support. Balance and stability are enhanced by increasing the body's base of support.

Application. Because the total body shift is from right to left and the momentum of the swing is basically in the same direction, the stance must be broadened in the lateral direction. This keeps the center of gravity over the base throughout the swing. Care must be taken to avoid developing so much momentum on the backswing that balance is adversely affected. Also, the feet must not be spread too far apart because hip rotation (a powerful force) will be restricted.

From the standpoint of balance, the least room for error is in the forward-backward direction, because the size of the base in this direction is only as great as the length of the feet. For this reason, it is very important for the golfer to place his center of gravity as near the middle of the base as possible. Consequently, the weight should be distributed evenly over the feet rather than on the balls of the feet, as recommended for many other activities. For this stance, the coaching tips given are "keep the weight on your heels" or "pretend you're sitting on a high stool."

The back foot must be perpendicular to the line of drive for purposes of adequate support. The front foot may deviate slightly from the direction of the back foot, but any significant deviation will affect hip rotation adversely.

It is recommended that a slightly closed stance be used; that is, the left (front) foot should be slightly forward of the right foot. The ball should be placed well forward, directly outward from the inside edge of the left foot. This lengthens the swing prior to contact. The swing should move slightly from the inside (close to the body) at the backswing to the outside at the point of contact.

The obvious check to determine whether poor shots are caused by loss of balance is to see that the shot is completed in a balanced position and that the feet have not moved to correct loss of balance.

PRINCIPLE—Lower center of gravity. Stability is increased by lowering the center of gravity.

Application. The correct address position includes slight flexion at the ankles, knees, and hips. This flexion lowers the center of gravity and increases stability. It would appear that an advantage could be gained by bending the knees even more, but such is *not* the case. The correct address position establishes exactly the right relationship for club-ball contact. If any additional flexion of body joints occurs during the swing (bending of the knees is a common error), this correct relationship is lost. It is important to maintain the same stance throughout the address and the swing.

Principles of projection

Some of the important principles of projection apply to the golf drive. They are as follows:

PRINCIPLE—Angle of projection. When the beginning and ending points are on the same plane, the optimum angle of projection to gain maximum distance in flight is 45° from the surface.

Application. When only the distance in flight is considered, the 45° angle is the optimum angle of projection. But in the golf drive, there are two factors which change this condition and cause the optimum angle to be less than 45°. First, the great air resistance encountered by the ball moving at high velocity favors a lower angle of projection. Second, the total distance of the drive is a combination of the flight and the roll, and an angle of considerably less than 45° will produce a longer total distance (flight plus roll), providing the terrain is suited to a long roll as fairways usually are. Also, the amount and direction of wind must be considered in selecting the most desirable angle.

PRINCIPLE—Force causing the projection. The force causing the projection produces varying effects depending upon its point of application.

Application. Off-center contact produces rotation. If this contact is below the ball's center of gravity, backspin results; if it is above the center of gravity, the ball gains top spin. If the ball is struck on the right side, it curves to the left; if struck on the left side, it curves to the right. Except under specific conditions, these spins are unwanted because they detract from the linear direction the ball will travel. Obviously, force in the desired direction is greatest when the club face is square to the ball and the line of swing is directly through the ball's center of gravity. The angle of the face of the club head, then, determines the angle of flight, and it also determines how much of the force contributes to the linear motion of the ball.

Summary statements

This example of a mechanical analysis is rather detailed; however, much detail was omitted that could have been included. For instance, the chapter on projections contains much additional material that could be applied in special situations. Such principles as time in flight, magnitude of the rebound, elasticity of the striking surfaces, intentional spins, and the effects of spin, present fertile ground for a more detailed analysis. Also, the analysis could have included points specific to the golf drive, such as a comparison of popular gripping methods and their effects. Recall that the only reference to the grip in this analysis was in relation to firmness throughout the swing and extra firmness upon impact.

Additional material could have been brought into the analysis from popular articles which stress certain styles or techniques. Do their contents stand up to a thorough mechanical analysis?

Another approach is to question popular coaching tips, such as "keep the left heel on the ground," which is obviously violated by almost all professionals. Why is it still found in the literature? Another approach is to select a common error, investigate the causes, and suggest the possible corrections.

In the present analysis, the movements producing the major forces were identified, and their correct sequence and timing were emphasized. The contributions of the swing technique and the maintenance of balance to the production of force and accuracy were stressed. Other important factors related to equipment, flight, and special effects and conditions were observed.

Some words of caution seem to be in order. (1) Just because the teacher is aware of the factors necessary for successful performance, it does not necessarily follow that the performers should be bombarded with a multitude of instructional points. It is pathetic for a performer to try to concentrate on a multitude of individual aspects of a skill when the skill requires one fluid motion. The mechanics of the total motion must be gradually improved by improving specific points, one at a time. (2) Balance principles are easily recognized in a skill whose primary objective is balance, but often the principles are unrecognized and unheeded in throwing, striking, jumping, or locomotor activities, even where balance may be of vital importance. Correct balance is basic to almost all athletic performances, and it is very important in the golf drive.

Student project

Select a specific skill of interest to you and perform a thorough mechanical analysis of it. Let the contents of this chapter serve as your guide. Draw heavily from the material in Chapters 12 to 15, but do not necessarily limit yourself to those chapters or to this book.

Part 4

Application of kinesiology to basic patterns of performance

In Part 4 physical education performances are conveniently grouped into five general patterns of performance. One chapter is devoted to each performance pattern. In each of the chapters the more important facts are identified relative to (1) the general nature of the performance pattern, (2) the major actions and muscle groups involved, (3) the application of natural laws and principles, and (4) generally how to improve performances included in that group. This part is the practical application of kinesiology to performances in general.

Chapter 17 deals with the most basic and frequently used skills, locomotion. Chapter 18 is the application of kinesiology to throwing, putting, and striking-type skills (projecting objects). Chapter 19 has to do with performance involving jumping, leaping, and hopping (projecting the body). Chapter 20 deals with arm-supported skills. Chapter 21 covers skills performed in the water, and Chapter 22 is a summary of the important considerations involved in improving performance.

17
Locomotion

*A*ny self-produced movement that transports the body from place to place is locomotive. Some locomotive skills are discussed in other sections of the text (i.e., body projections, arm-supported skills, and locomotion in water). The most common forms of locomotion, walking and running, are discussed in this chapter along with other forms, including skating and skiing.

Walking

If a person walked at the rate of 120 steps per minute for eight hours, he would execute 57,600 steps. If he weighed 200 pounds, the bottoms of his feet and his muscles would bear 11,520,000 pounds in the eight-hour period. In walking at 120 steps per minute with a three-foot stride, one moves at a rate of 4.1 miles per hour. Many individuals may walk inefficiently, but regardless of the level of efficiency for each of us, walking is probably our best learned skill. It has been practiced since infancy, and, consequently, neural pathways used in walking are deeply ingrained.

Walking results from successive losses of balance of the two alternating feet. Each balance loss is followed by a newly established base of support and a regaining of balance. Forward progress in walking results from a combination of three forces: (1) muscular force causing pressure of the foot against the surface, (2) force of gravity which tends to pull the body forward and downward once it is off-balance, and (3) force of momentum which tends to keep the body moving in the same direction and at a constant speed. Limited additional force may result from the transfer of momentum from the arm swing, which is performed primarily to aid balance.

In walking, the leg movements (stride) occur in three phases: (1) *propulsion*, (2) *swing*, and (3) *catch and support*. The propulsion phase starts with the push-off leg in a flexed position. The joint actions during propulsion are simply

275

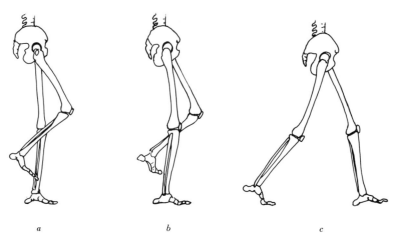

a   *b*   *c*

Figure 17–1.
The three phases of the walking stride (right leg). (*a*) Swinging phase, (*b*) support phase, (*c*) propelling phase.

extension at the hip, knee, and ankle (plantar flexion), and flexion of the toes. The main muscles involved in this phase of the stride are the hip extensors, knee extensors, ankle plantar flexors, and toe flexors. These muscles must be well conditioned if extensive walking is done. Hip rotation inward (medial) accompanies the propulsive phase of the stride.

During the swinging phase, the hip, knee, and ankle of the swinging leg flex to allow clearance for the foot to swing forward. The hip flexion movement is especially ballistic in nature, and the other flexion movements are also ballistic, but to a lesser extent. This means that the initial movement is caused by muscle contractions and that the remainder of the movement results from momentum of the moving segment. Hip rotation outward (lateral) accompanies the swinging phase to keep the toes pointing in the line of progress. Hip rotation results in the pelvis twisting in the direction of the stride. The outward hip rotator muscles cause the movement, but as the femur rotates to a point near the correct line of direction, the inward rotators contract to hold the leg in line. The longer the stride, the greater is the amount of outward hip rotation.

The catch and support phase of the walk begins by dissipating the force of the landing. The ankle, knee, and hip joints absorb the shock by gradually flexing, but the force for flexion is provided by the body's momentum and the force of gravity. As a result, the extensor muscles of these joints contract eccentrically to reduce the forces slowly; the muscles "apply the brakes." When the forces are sufficiently reduced, flexion is halted, and there is a momentary isometric contraction of the leg extensors, during which no apparent changes in the positions of the joints are noted. This does not mean the body is motionless, as it still maintains its horizontal momentum. The support phase smoothly flows into the propulsion phase, and the cycle is completed.

Besides the three phases of the stride, *other body movements* are important in walking. With each stride, the pelvis twists toward the lead leg to the point diagonal to the line of progress. If the right leg is providing the force (trail leg), the left hip leads and the right hip trails. This pelvic twist contributes significantly to the length of stride and to smoothness of the gait. Rotation occurs at both hip joints to keep the feet and legs pointing straight ahead. The back hip rotates medially while the lead hip rotates laterally. Actually, the pelvis rotates on the support leg, and the lead leg rotates on the pelvis. Therefore, the hip rotator muscles are important contributors to walking.

As the pelvis turns, the upper trunk turns in the opposite direction to keep the upper body on line with the forward movement. Therefore, the trunk rotator muscles are important contributors. The rotation of the upper trunk occurs primarily in the thoracic region of the spine.

In both walking and running, the arms swing diagonally forward and inward. Diagonal movement should not be so excessive that the arm swing appears awkward. The arm movements are opposite the leg movements, thus aiding the upper portion of the trunk to rotate counter to the rotation of the pelvis.

Speed of walking

Walking speed is determined by the combination of the *length* and *frequency* of the strides. As length of stride increases, the lead leg flexes more. This puts the leg in better position for application of force, allows propulsion in a more horizontal direction, and thus permits a longer stride. As frequency of stride increases, the period of double support decreases slightly; as the frequency con-

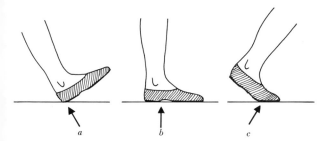

Figure 17–2.
Foot contact pattern during walking. The body weight rolls from the heel across the sole of the foot and onto the toes. The arrows *a, b,* and *c* indicate the direction in which the force is applied during each phase of foot contact.

tinues to increase, the double-support phase disappears, and the walk becomes a run. With the reduction of double support, there is a corresponding proportionate increase in the swing phase of the stride.

For adult males the optimum walking speed in terms of energy cost is 3.0 to 3.5 miles per hour (2.5 to 3.0 miles per hour for females). When the pace exceeds 4.0 miles per hour for males, the walk becomes more fatiguing.

Incorrect mechanics of walking

Many people walk with the feet in a slightly "toed-out" position, which results from outward rotation at the hip joints. This walking style is very undesirable. Toeing-out results in a diagonally directed propulsive force, and it almost eliminates the use of the four small toes. In addition, the length of the foot as a lever is reduced, and the stride is shortened.

Some people walk with the feet "toed-in" (pigeon-toed). This practice does not reduce efficiency a great amount unless the toes turn in excessively. Usually the main concern about this deviation is its awkward appearance. Both toed-in and toed-out deviations can be corrected to some extent by the individual if he concentrates on keeping the feet pointed straightforward during walking, standing, and sitting.

Excessive accumulations of fat on the thighs force the walker to assume an undesirable spread of the feet to avoid friction. Knock-knees require a similar adjustment. Such a foot position results in misdirected forces resulting in a swaying or a ducklike "waddle." Infants tend to walk in this manner to aid lateral balance.

Tight hamstring muscles restrain both walking and running and increase the probability of injury while running. Often, older individuals suffer from this affliction unless a special effort is made to maintain the flexibility of this muscle group.

Ascending and descending

Adjustments must be made for walking on inclines. If the walker wishes to locate his center of gravity properly for an uphill grade, he leans farther forward than usual. Such leaning places the body in a position where applied force will propel the body forward, helping to bring the powerful gluteus maximus muscle into hip extension (not ordinarily effective in the last $15°$ of extension). However, this forward lean has some detrimental effects. It reduces the length of the stride and increases the work of the back extensor muscles which support the trunk in a forward-leaning position. The adjustment in forward lean is made primarily at the ankle and hip joints. A flat-footed landing is most efficient when walking upstairs, because rest is provided for the calf (plantar flexor) muscles when the heel is supported.

In walking down an incline, a backward lean from the lumbar area of the spine and from the ankle joints causes the center of gravity to align over the supporting base (foot). Gravity provides all the necessary force for the descent, and the walker's efforts are mainly limited to controlling the effects of gravity. The knee extensor muscles (front of thigh) are used the most and usually tire from walking downhill. The hip extensors are also important contributors.

Running

Running is not only an athletic event itself (track events), but it is also a very important part of other sports. Running and maneuverability are very important in almost all court and field games. Running and walking are very similar except the *actions are greatly accentuated in running*. Two other apparent differences are:

1. In running, there is a brief period during which there is no contact with the surface (body totally suspended).
2. In running, there is no period in which both feet are in contact with the surface at the same time.

In running, the support phase is a much smaller proportion of the total cycle than in walking, and the propulsion phase can begin almost immediately after the foot contacts the surface because the center of gravity is moving forward rapidly. Because the body is moving at a fast rate, the propelling force must be perfectly timed, and it must develop quickly. This means the hip, knee, and ankle extensor muscles and the toe flexors must be able to contract rapidly and with great force.

The direction of the driving force is more horizontal in running than in walking, and the push-off leg inclines much farther forward before surface contact is broken. In a sense, this is another way of saying the stride is much longer in running (about 6 to 7 feet for the adult male). It should be emphasized that overstriding increases the resistance provided by the lead leg upon contact; thus overstriding is mechanically inefficient. On the other hand, chopping the stride too much is inefficient because it prevents each stride from making its optimum contribution.

Generally, in running, the body has a greater forward incline than in walking, the rotary actions in the spine and pelvic regions are greatly increased, and the arm actions are higher and much more vigorous.

Running speed

Speed is determined by the *length of stride* and *frequency (speed) of stride*. For increased running speed, one or both of these factors must be increased.

Length of stride is dependent primarily upon leg length and the power of the stride. Leg speed (frequency) is mostly dependent upon speed of muscle contractions and neuromuscular coordination (skill) in running.

Running mechanics vary from one individual to another, and they vary in the same individual running at different speeds. More specifically, running mechanics change with speed in the following ways:

1. Amount and type of foot contact with the surface
2. Amount of joint flexion and extension
3. Amount of body inclination

At a slow running speed, complete foot contact is used. The foot-surface contact with each stride goes from the ball of the foot to the heel and back to the ball (restful to calf muscles). As running rate increases, the amount of foot contact becomes less, until finally at full speed only the forward part of the foot contacts the surface. The sprinter "runs on the toes."

At a slow running speed, a relatively small amount of action occurs in the joints throughout the body, and the runner tends to run with the arms low. As speed is increased, more flexion and extension occur in the arm and leg joints, and other joint actions increase accordingly. Also, the arm action is higher.

At slower speeds, runners tend to run more erectly, whereas at full speed, the typical sprinter leans forward at about 20° from the perpendicular. Forward lean usually comes naturally with the increased propulsive forces, and conscious attempts to increase lean are not usually necessary. However, on occasion it is necessary to teach a runner to increase forward lean.

Sprinting.   Sprinting is essentially a power performance. It depends on one's ability to project the body forcefully and rapidly from alternate feet. Developed relatively early in life, about age twenty for men and about fifteen for women, running speed is a quality that can be improved a limited amount. The best possibilities for increasing speed are (1) to increase the power (force × velocity) of the leg extensor muscles, thus causing more powerful propelling forces, and (2) to practice running at top speeds, which should improve sprinting technique and the specific coordinations involved in sprinting. In certain instances, errors in the mechanics of sprinting may be corrected, which may improve speed.

Middle-distance running.   Middle distances are run at a fast pace and with a style that is somewhat more relaxed than the sprinting style. Of course, the speed and running form varies with the length of the particular race. But, generally speaking, when compared to sprinting, middle-distance running requires less joint action, less forward inclination, and more complete foot-surface contact. Pace is very important, and physiologists generally agree that an even pace over the entire distance is the most economical. In middle distance races, success is determined by the correct combination of (1) running speed, (2) running effi-

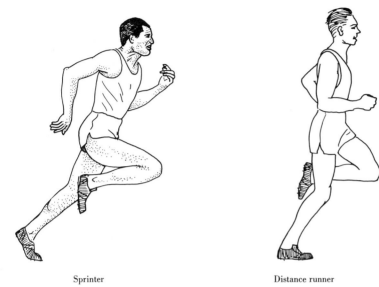

Sprinter   Distance runner

Figure 17–3.
Differences in running styles at different speeds. When compared to the
sprinter, the distance runner typically runs with low strides, less vigorous- and
lower-arm actions, a more upright body position, and more foot-surface contact.

ciency, and (3) running endurance. Circulorespiratory endurance exerts the greatest influence in middle distances where a relatively long distance must be covered
at a rapid rate.

Long-distance running. Long distances are run at a slower pace, with great
emphasis placed on a relaxed and easy running style, which conserves energy.
As compared to middle-distance running, the long distances require still less joint
action, less forward lean, and maximum foot-surface contact. Here again, an even
pace over the entire distance is recommended. Whereas endurance (especially of
the circulorespiratory system) has limited influence on sprinting, it becomes
increasingly important up to middle distances and then subsides. In long distances
the prime factors are (1) total body endurance and (2) ability to conserve
energy. Of course, a reasonable amount of running speed is always beneficial.

Running in sports other than track. Field and court games like football,
basketball, and baseball often require changes in direction, changes of pace,
stability from lateral forces, and other changes which demand agility-type movements while running. These maneuvers are always made at a sacrifice to straight-
ahead speed. Under such conditions, the location and movement of the center of
gravity need to be more precisely controlled. The length of stride is often reduced
so foot-surface contact will be more frequent, making possible quick changes in

direction. Also, more lateral spread of the feet is often desirable. The trunk is usually carried with less forward incline than in sprinting. The typical even cadence of the running strides may be interrupted as adjustments are made in speed and direction.

Incorrect mechanics of running

Even some champions run incorrectly, and if their running styles could be corrected, some of them would run faster. If running mechanics deviate from the following important guides, then incorrect mechanics are used, resulting in some loss of running efficiency:

1.   The knees and toes should point straight in the line of progress. Deviation from this in either direction results in loss of power.
2.   The inner sole of each footprint should be directly under the middle of the body. Any lateral deviation from this results in loss of power and a weaving action of the total body.
3.   The total body should incline forward at about 20° from perpendicular at top running speed. The amount of incline will gradually reduce as running rate is reduced. If the incline is too far forward, the propelling forces will be too horizontal. Too little incline will cause the forces to be too vertical. If, when viewed from the side, a runner's head moves up and down excessively with each stride, misdirected propelling forces are indicated.
4.   The arm swing should be close to the body, and the hands should swing forward to a point in front of the chest. Almost all arm action should occur at the shoulder joint. There should be only slight movement at the elbows.
5.   Rotary movements in the spine and at the hip joints should be reasonably free, because these movements can greatly enhance the length of stride. In a way, the rotation of the pelvis substitutes for the limited amount of hyperextension available at the hips (restricted by the strong anterior capsular ligaments). Any excessive spinal curvatures (lordosis, kyphosis, scoliosis) restrict the amount of spinal (pelvic) rotation because the bone structure will not allow it.

Controlling momentum—stops, reverses, and changes of direction

The process of *stopping* involves an absorption of momentum. Resistive forces are gradually applied over several short steps, and the center of gravity is carried farther backward and lower. The main muscular actions involved are eccentric contractions of the hip, knee, and ankle extensors. The ability of these muscles to resist force (their strength) is very important to stopping quickly.

A *reverse* is a stop with an immediate reversal of momentum. After the momentum has been dissipated as described above, the body is immediately turned, led by upper body rotation, and put into motion in the opposite direction. The body should already be inclined in the new direction of movement; however, some additional lean may be needed at the moment the reversal occurs. The same muscles (hip, knee, and ankle extensors) that contracted eccentrically to stop the body now contract concentrically to put it into motion in the new direction. The toe flexors are also important contributors. Both reversing and sharply *changing direction* with a jab-type step while running involve essentially the same actions. The force for direction change is always applied at about right angles to the length of the foot. For a 90° turn, the planted foot continues to point along the initial line of direction. If a 45° turn is desired, the foot is toed-out about 45°. If more than 90° is desired, the foot is toed-in a corresponding amount.

In football, for example, a ballcarrier is in constant danger from outside forces and may require sudden, unexpected direction changes. There is an obvious inability to change direction when unsupported, so the more often the foot contact occurs, the more prepared the performer is to change direction. He must sacrifice speed to achieve short, choppy steps, a small amount of lean, and a wide lateral base. Most of his cuts (turns) will be made forward between 25 to 90° from the initial direction. Crossover steps cannot provide sharp cuts with direction changes, but they are sometimes advantageously used for other reasons.

Overcoming inertia from stationary positions (starting)

Starting from a standing position is basically the same as reversing direction after momentum has been overcome. The body is inclined in the anticipated direction of movement so the center of gravity may be quickly shifted off-balance in that direction. The signal to start must be anticipated mentally in order to respond quickly. In some instances, rolling the center of gravity in the direction of movement will increase one's ability to move quickly once the signal is given. However, in racing starts, such action is illegal. In other activities, such as baseball, tennis, football, and basketball, this procedure often makes the difference between success and failure. However, occasionally it results in error when a quick adjustment in the anticipated direction of movement must be made, and the body is already off-balance in the anticipated direction.

The positions of the crouch, track, and football starts were discussed in the chapter on equilibrium, but the process of gaining acceleration following the start has not been discussed. The short and powerful strides used in accelerating are energy-consuming; however, they are necessary to accelerate rapidly. One reason for the short strides is that the base must be reestablished often because of the excessive amount of forward body lean. A second reason for short strides is that the leg joints experience optimum mechanical advantage through only a small range of motion, and it is this range that is used in short and powerful strides. It should be emphasized that the short stride is the result of contacting the surface quickly with the lead leg and *not* a lack of full extension in the propelling leg.

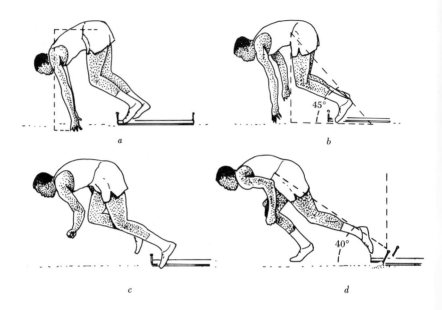

Figure 17–4.
A sprinter must design his starting technique so the forces are correctly directed. The above illustrations show world record-holder Bob Hayes at the start. Illustration *a* shows him in a high hip position with his shoulders 3 or 4 inches beyond his hands. Illustrations *b* and *c* show his low body position (body at a 45° angle, back parallel to the track). Illustration *d* shows the extreme horizontal components of his initial drive. Illustrations *e* and *f* show him a few yards from the blocks.

Hip rotation is restricted when the hips are flexed; therefore, the typical twisting action of the pelvis is limited during acceleration. As the runner assumes the erect running position, hip flexion is reduced gradually, and hip rotation then fully contributes its part to a long running stride.

Hard driving actions with the arms are very important to acceleration. The arm actions should be more directly forward (less diagonal) during the acceleration phase of a sprint. For most sprinters, a full running stride is achieved at about 20 yards from the start. According to experiments by Bunn [11], top speed is achieved after 15 to 20 yards of running.

Locomotion on skis

In downhill skiing the propelling force is provided by the force of gravity. Skis are especially designed to provide a minimum amount of friction against the snow, and waxing the skis may reduce the friction even more. The various body

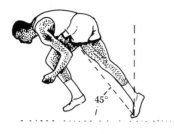
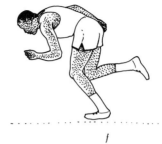

e   f

segments are used only to support and balance the body and to execute maneuvers.

Skis enlarge one's base of support in the forward-backward direction, thus making greater lean possible, either forward or backward, without loss of balance. The base of support in the lateral direction is determined by the width at which the skis are placed from each other. Beginning skiers tend to keep the base wide in the lateral direction so they can maintain balance. Expert skiers narrow the base as much as possible, because this aids them in maneuvering.

The typical body position of the skier is (1) skis parallel and close together, (2) partial flexion at the ankles, knees, and hips, (3) elbows close to sides and bent to about 110° angle, and (4) the whole body leaning forward of the line perpendicular to the skis so the center of gravity is over the balls of the feet. Generally, the steeper the slope, the more forward the center of gravity should be and the more flexion there should be in the lower extremities. The flexion of the legs provides the skier with several advantages: (1) it lowers the center of gravity, and this aids in balance; (2) it places the skier in a position of readiness so he can make quick adjustments in body position; and (3) it provides him the opportunity to cushion over rough spots.

As the skier extends the legs, he temporarily unweights (lifts his weight from) his skis, which allow them to move faster over the snow. Flexing the legs has an opposite effect on speed because it weights the skis. The muscles used mainly in supporting body weight on skis are the hip, knee, and ankle extensors. These

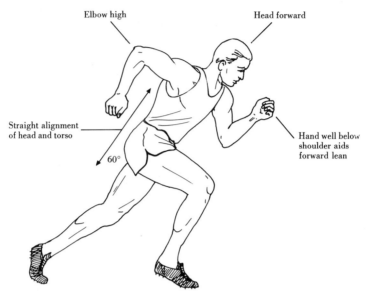

Elbow high

Head forward

Straight alignment
of head and torso

60°

Hand well below
shoulder aids
forward lean

Figure 17–5.
Correct body position greatly enhances acceleration.

are also the muscles used in weighting and unweighting the skis. In weighting (leg flexion), the extensor muscles contract eccentrically; in unweighting (leg extension), the extensor muscles contract concentrically. Other muscles of great importance to skiing are the hip and spinal rotators.

The forces used to effect a change in direction (turns) are (1) deflecting force—resistance against the side of the ski, which is caused by the snow and results from the correct edging of the skis during a turn; (2) turning force—moving one ski at an angle to the direction of descent and using a transfer of body weight to that ski thus causing the turn, as in snowplow and stem turns; (3) turning power of the body—counterrotation of the body to cause the skis to turn, as in the short swing and the wedeln techniques.

Locomotion on skates

Skating action is much like walking action. The support phase of the walk becomes the skating glide. During the glide, the skate blades are placed approximately in the line of progress because this position presents minimum resistance against forward movement. The propelling foot must have the toes turned outward at the time of the push (outward rotation at the hip) in order to utilize the sharp edge of the blade and to present as much of the blade edge as possible to the ice. This foot position is necessary to gain sufficient friction between the blade and the ice, but it results in glides that, of necessity, must be somewhat oblique to the line of direction. Sharp blades add a great deal to propulsion. Forward momentum is greatly aided by forward lean at the hips and long sweeping arm actions with the arms fairly straight. Diagonal movement of the arms is emphasized.

Training for locomotive skills

Locomotive skills vary so much in their nature that it is necessary to analyze each skill separately to determine what should be included in the training program. However, a few generalizations should be made. (1) In most locomotive skills, leg power is of prime importance, so in training for such skills, *increasing leg power* should receive serious consideration. (2) Each method of locomotion requires specific skill patterns, and development of the skill patterns requires extensive practice of the correct technique. Therefore, *extensive practice of the particular locomotive skill* is an important part of any training program. (3) Certain locomotive events require much endurance of the total body, with emphasis on circulorespiratory endurance. The training programs for these events must concentrate on *increasing endurance*. The most effective means known for developing such endurance is interval (repetition) training with emphasis on underdis-

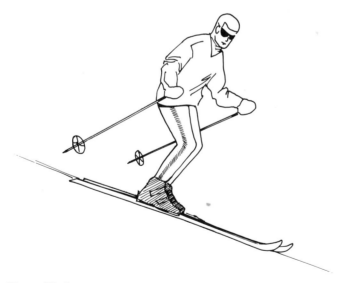

Figure 17–6.
Side view of a good straight-run skiing position. Joint flexion and forward body lean are essential.

tance and fast speed (distances shorter than the competitive distance at speeds faster than the competitive speed). The ideal number of repetitions for a practice session is not established; this number can be greatly influenced by the length of each repeated distance, the speed at which it is performed, and the condition of the performer. For additional information on interval training, refer to Chapter 8.

Recommended supplementary reading

BROER, MARION R.: "Efficiency of Human Movement," 2d ed., chaps. 11–13, W. B. Saunders Company, Philadelphia, 1966.

COOPER, JOHN M., and RUTH B. GLASSOW: "Kinesiology," 2d ed., chap. 15, The C. V. Mosby Company, St. Louis, 1968.

RASCH, PHILLIP J., and ROGER K. BURKE: "Kinesiology and Applied Anatomy," 3d ed., chap. 19, Lea and Febiger, Philadelphia, 1967.

WELLS, KATHERINE F.: "Kinesiology," 4th ed., pp. 407–427, W. B. Saunders Company, Philadelphia, 1966.

18

Jumping, leaping, and hopping skills

*J*umps are defined as body projections characterized by landing simultaneously on both feet. Takeoffs for jumps can be from either one foot or both feet. *Leaps* and *hops* occur only with takeoffs from one foot and landing on one foot. The leap differs from the hop in that in the leap the landing foot is not the same as the takeoff foot, whereas in the hop the same foot is used for takeoff and landing.

Several mechanical principles are common to all jumps, leaps, and hops. (1) They all depend upon the counterforce available from the supporting surface. All factors which reduce maximum counterforce, such as insufficient friction between the performer and the surface or "give" in the supporting surface and/or any of the performer's joints, are detrimental to a maximum projection. (2) They all involve similar patterns of sequential muscular actions. In each case the main propulsive force comes from the supporting leg (or legs), beginning with hip extension, followed by knee extension, ankle and foot extension (plantar flexion), and toe flexion. (3) In each case the "transfer of momentum" principle is applied when nonsupporting body parts (arms, shoulders, and often the free leg) are thrust in the direction of projection; these motions are initiated prior to the application of the propulsive force. The transfer of momentum (thrust of body parts) exerts its maximum influence only if the body segments are moving rapidly in the direction of the projection when the performer leaves the surface. If deviations from this ideal timing occur, the effectiveness of the thrust is reduced.

In addition to the mechanical factors already mentioned, the following influence body projections:

1. Individuals possessing high centers of gravity enjoy an advantage when the purpose is to project their bodies vertically over barriers, such as high-jumping, pole-vaulting, or hurdling, or when reaching height is important, such as basketball rebounding or the basketball lay-up shot. These individuals also have an advantage, though less obvious, in horizontal projections for distance, such as barrel-jumping

289

on ice skates, long-jumping, and triple-jumping. When the center of gravity begins at a point higher above the surface, less vertical force needs to be applied by the performer, to remain airborne for a given length of time, which makes more horizontal force possible. This advantage results from application of the principle that a body remains in flight only as long as it takes to move through its vertical plane of flight, regardless of the horizontal distance the body covers. A lower center of gravity is one reason why women cannot equal men in body projection performances. On the average, women are shorter, and their centers of gravity are proportionately lower than men's. However, there are other more important factors involved.

2. Another advantageous anatomical feature is longer levers. If bones are longer, more linear velocity can be developed at their ends, provided angular velocity remains constant. The long-geared performers enjoy this advantage if they have sufficient strength to achieve comparable angular velocity.

Physiological factors which contribute significantly to body projections are *strength* and *speed of movement*. Projections performed for maximum distance are tests of power. Power is a combination of force (strength) and velocity (speed of movement). Therefore, the force and speed with which the mover muscles contract will greatly influence projections. Antagonist muscles must relax to reduce resistance to the development of power.

Excessive weight, especially due to fat which does not contribute to performance, hinders projections of the body. Weight due to additional muscle also adds resistance, but its contribution to the action may exceed its detrimental effects. Small dumbbells held in the hands have been shown to improve long-jumping performances significantly. Such devices are outlawed in the rules of competition but do demonstrate the important contribution of the transfer of momentum.

Inflexibility at certain joints may restrict the needed range of motion for a maximum projection. By analyzing the mechanics of a performance, the body regions which need unusual flexibility can be identified, and specific exercises can be used to develop the flexibility necessary for maximum performance.

Stationary takeoffs

Projection of the body from a stationary position depends almost entirely upon two factors: (1) explosive power from leg and trunk extension and (2) ability to transfer momentum from other body parts. The momentum of the swinging body parts (arms and shoulders) overcomes part of the body's inertia, and this action aids in shifting the center of gravity to a position where the forces from the legs can be directed through it. The leg extension action must encounter the center of gravity when it is located in the best position for optimum results.

If the objective is to project the body forward for a maximum horizontal distance, then leg extension must occur when the center of gravity is well forward of the feet, and the arm and upper body thrust must be directed partly toward the horizontal. If, at the time of leg extension, a line were drawn from the feet through the center of gravity, that line would create nearly a 45° angle with the surface. The pressure of the feet on the surface is both downward and backward.

If the objective is to project the body vertically, thrust is made upward, and leg extension occurs when the center of gravity is directly above the base of support. If the movement is to be made in a backward direction, the center of gravity must be behind the base of support at the time of the leg extension.

Double-leg stationary projections

The use of both legs in stationary takeoffs affords two advantages over single-leg projections: (1) the projecting force is increased about twofold and (2) the larger supporting base enhances balance. The feet should be spread about the width of the shoulders in order to aid balance and ensure that the forces will be properly directed. The two legs must contribute about equally. If one leg generates more force than the other, or if the two legs do not extend simultaneously, the projection will not be in the intended direction. Similarly, the two arms must produce momentum of about equal amounts simultaneously. Check points in leg and foot positions include feet below the shoulders, toes pointing in the intended line of flight, and knees directly above and pointing in the same direction as the toes.

The optimum amount the legs should flex to develop maximum force depends upon the strength of the extensor muscles. If the crouch is deeper, force can be applied over a greater distance to develop more acceleration. Conversely, the greater depth of crouch signifies that more work must be done to lift the body, and as the joint angles become less, the muscles must "pull around corners" at the joints. Strong muscles are more effective when joint flexion is slightly less than 90° (deep crouch); weak muscles contribute best with lesser amounts of flexion (shallow crouch).

Greater muscle forces are developed when the stretch reflex adds nerve impulses to those impulses voluntarily provided. Recall, the stretch reflex is initiated by sudden stretching of the agonist muscles, provided the stretch is followed immediately by contraction of those muscles. (Refer to discussion of stretch reflex in Chapter 10.) Basically, this means that a slight, sharp dipping action (sudden crouch) should immediately precede and flow into the leg extension action. If a pause occurs at the bottom of the dip, the effects of the stretch reflex are lost. If the dip is extensive, too much downward momentum develops, which wastes contractile force in the reversing of such momentum.

Standing long jump.   Studies have shown that at takeoff inferior jumpers do not have their centers of gravity as far forward as better jumpers. Upon landing, the feet of the inferior performers are usually not as far forward of their centers of gravity as the feet of superior performers. When a jump is correctly executed, the angle of projection with the surface is slightly less than 45°, because the center of gravity is at a lower level upon landing than it was at takeoff.

The driving force is initiated with an arm swing directed forward and upward, which is combined with thrusting actions of the shoulder girdle and trunk. Momentum from these movements is transferred to the total body during the jump—this momentum can add greatly to the distance of the jump. However, the primary driving force comes from hip, knee, and ankle extension and toe flexion. The center of gravity should be well ahead of the feet at the time of leg extension in order that the force from the legs be correctly directed.

During flight, leg joints must quickly be flexed so the lower body can swing through rapidly, resulting in the feet reaching as far forward as possible upon landing. Care must be taken not to reach too far with the feet because loss of balance backward may result from insufficient momentum to carry the center of gravity forward to a position above the base of support.

The main muscles contributing to the projection are the shoulder flexors, shoulder girdle elevators, back extensors, hip, knee, and ankle extensors, and toe flexors. Note that the gluteus maximus, the strongest hip extensor muscle, contributes only when the hip is flexed beyond 15°; therefore, deep flexion at the hip is important. During flight, the abdominal muscles must contract strongly to stabilize the pelvis, which enables the hip flexors to lift the thighs during the flight.

Common errors in this skill are (1) incorrect angle of projection, (2) lack of precise coordination of the swinging parts with leg extension, and (3) loss of

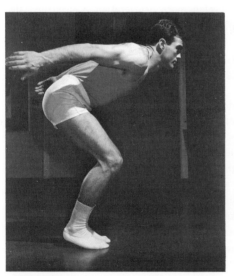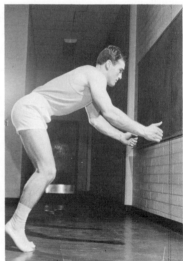

Figure 18–1.
Source and direction of the projecting forces in the standing long jump.

distance resulting from improper positioning of the feet upon landing. The landing errors occur when the feet fail to reach forward enough or when too low a projection does not permit sufficient time in flight to achieve a correct landing position.

Racing dive.   This skill is different from the standing long jump in only three ways: (1) The center of gravity shifts much farther forward before leg and trunk extension occurs, in fact, so far forward that the projection is almost horizontal. (2) The toes curl around the pool's edge so that the last push may be perpendicular to the resisting surface (the pool's vertical edge). If this situation did not exist, the lack of friction between the two slippery surfaces would detract a great deal from the projection. (3) Projected into a prone position, the body is as straight and slender as possible in order to reduce water resistance against forward motion upon entry into the water. Upon landing, the body should be at an angle of only 5 to 10° below the horizontal.

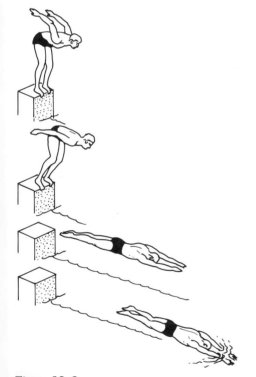

Figure 18–2.
The ability to project the body horizontally is very important in the racing dive. The angle of projection and angle of entry must be correct to get maximum horizontal distance.

Vertical jump.   The vertical jump for height is highly dependent upon leg power, and it is highly correlated with the standing broad jump. The widest use of the vertical jump is in basketball, volleyball, and dance activities, but it is also used in many other performances. The basic technique is similar to that of the standing long jump, except the forces are directed upward and the projection takes place with the center of gravity directly over the base of support. Some individuals achieve better results when they assume a stance with one foot slightly forward of the other. This position provides improved stability in the forward-backward direction; however, it should not be overdone so that less advantageous joint angles appear.

After initiation of the upward movements of the arms and shoulders, the movements that follow in close sequence are hip, knee, and ankle extension and toe flexion. The combined forces from these movements determine how high the body will be projected.

Trampoline bounce.   The trampoline bounce is a unique kind of vertical bounce performed on an elastic mat. The important body actions necessary to create and utilize the energy stored in the mat are discussed in Chapter 12, under Newton's law of counterforce. The arms and shoulders are used to transfer momentum, as in the vertical jump, but they have an additional use when great heights are attained. They maintain balance while the body is in flight, and they serve this purpose best when abducted to the horizontal position. When the arms are in the abducted position, their weight is farther from the body, thus the movements of the arms are more effective in controlling balance. The tightrope walker uses this effect when he selects a long balance pole. Balance during flight is essential because if the base of support is not directly under the center

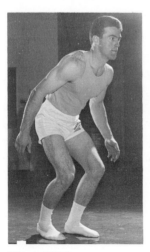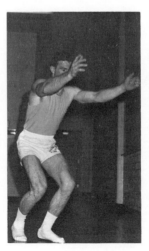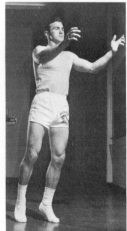

Figure 18–3.
Source and direction of projecting forces in the vertical jump.

of gravity in the landing, little can be done to control the direction of the subsequent bounce.

The technique of landing following each bounce has great influence on the subsequent bounce. The performer should contact the mat with the legs straight and rigid, which causes maximum depression of the trampoline mat, allowing the mat to store more energy. Near the bottom of the bounce (mat almost fully depressed), the arms and shoulders should be thrust downward to add a final bit of downward momentum, and the legs should assume slight flexion. As the mat responds (releasing its stored energy), the arms and shoulders are thrust upward, and the legs are extended. These body movements must be correctly timed to the response of the trampoline mat. It is important to land near the center of the mat to get maximum benefit from its elasticity, and thus avoid being thrown off-balance by its response.

Back dive.   Various back dives and some backward projections in tumbling begin from stationary stances and depend upon double-leg projections. Most of the same principles apply to these projections as apply to projections in a forward direction. Exceptions are (1) the transfer of arm and shoulder momentum is more upward and backward, (2) the center of gravity is shifted behind the base of support, and (3) the projecting force is reduced somewhat because a major force (ankle plantar flexion) is partly eliminated in backward projections.

Rotations.   Some projections require rotation of the body in either a forward or backward direction (diving and trampoline stunts). It should be understood that the force for the rotation is created at takeoff and only accelerated or decelerated by body positions in flight. For example, if one wished to perform a backward somersault from a diving board, the amount of rotation produced would depend on the timing of the leg extension in relation to the position of the body's center of gravity. If the line of force is directly through the center of gravity, no rotation occurs; however, if the center of gravity is off center from the line of force, the body will tend to rotate in the direction in which the center of gravity is displaced. For the performer to accomplish a forward somersault, his center of gravity must be slightly forward of the line of force. A backward somersault requires that the center of gravity is slightly behind the line of force. After a given rotating force has been applied, the speed with which the body rotates depends upon its weight and the position of its segments. The less it weighs and the closer its segments are to its center, the faster it will rotate. This is the reason a diver rotates relatively slowly in a layout position, faster in a pike position, and still faster in a tuck position.

Single-leg stationary projections

Single-leg projections from stationary positions are not often used. A few movements may qualify as single-leg projections, but they appear more as exaggerated weight shifts. Among these movements are dodging actions from stationary positions and standing leaps in dance. In any case, such activities are limited in use, and the principles involved do not differ from the principles already discussed.

Moving takeoffs

The principles discussed in the previous section, stationary takeoffs, also pertain to skills found in this section. The primary difference between projections involving a stationary takeoff and those involving a moving takeoff is that the latter includes an approach used to develop horizontal momentum of the whole body. In a projection involving an approach, the key to success is to add a correct vertical component of force to the horizontal momentum. This involves correct positioning of the center of gravity in relation to the line of the projecting force, as was the case with stationary takeoffs. But with the running approach, the skill becomes more intricate and the timing more precise. In moving takeoffs, the center of gravity moves at a greater velocity, balance is harder to control, the muscles must act with greater speed and more refined timing, and the projecting forces must act in concert with the momentum of the approach; these actions, along with power, project the body a maximum distance at the desired angle.

Double-leg moving projections

Few double-leg projections are used in combination with a moving takeoff because the double-leg takeoff requires that forward momentum be reduced in order to assume the double-leg takeoff position.

Tumbling, gymnastic, and diving skills.   Double-leg moving takeoffs are used in various gymnastic performances on the long horse and in such tumbling performances as the forward roll and dive and roll. In these performances, considerable horizontal momentum is necessary to carry the body through the performance. At the same time, it is necessary to project the body straightforward in a position square with the direction of movement, a position which can be accomplished only by using moving double-leg takeoffs. Following the run, a short and rather high hurdle step is taken. The hurdle step checks the horizontal speed and converts some of it to vertical momentum. Also, the hurdle step allows the performer time to position the body for a double-leg landing. Upon landing on both feet simultaneously, the performer assumes a position very similar to that at the beginning of the standing long jump, and the subsequent movements are practically the same as those discussed earlier in the standing long jump. The body is moving forward rapidly; therefore, the projecting movements must be precisely timed.

In springboard diving, the approach is terminated with a hurdle step. The main objective of the approach is to gain height and correct body position during the hurdle. The more height the performer gains, the more downward force he can apply to depress the board. The farther the board is depressed, the more energy it stores, and the stronger will be its reaction. The body actions during the double-leg projection in diving are almost identical to those in the vertical jump. In the dive, the body actions must be perfectly timed with the rebound of the board. Placement of the feet in relation to the end of the board is very important to the responsiveness of the board. For best results, the toes should be near the end (within 1 or 2 inches), but not extended beyond the end. The objective of the spring is to gain as much height as possible to allow time to execute the desired dive. *Remember,* a body remains in flight only as long as it takes to move through its vertical plane of flight.

Barrel jump on ice skates.   The objective is to jump horizontally over barrels as far as possible. Great horizontal momentum, combined with a strong upward projection at the correct angle, is necessary. Most of the movements of the standing long jump are also required in this performance. The main differences are in the barrel jump (1) the body is in rapid horizontal motion and (2) most of the thrusting force from the two legs must be directed upward because the lack of friction between the ice and skates will permit very little horizontal thrust from the legs.

Ski jump.   The development of momentum for the ski jump is provided by a push-off at the top of the runway followed by acceleration due to gravity. The skier can develop even greater momentum if he can reduce friction and air resistance as he moves down the runway. The technique of the takeoff is about the same as for the barrel jump, except the skier is less concerned with powerful extension and more concerned with balance and perfect timing. Because of the excessive speed of the jumper, excessive forward lean is necessary.

The airborne phase requires the use of some principles of aerodynamics as the jumper utilizes air resistance to prolong his flight by correctly positioning his body and skis. The ski tips are angled slightly upward to catch the wind, and the total body is angled forward and upward for several reasons, one of which is to increase upward lift. The arms are held close to the sides with the hands slightly back of the hips. Air resistance has unusual potential in this event because of the long period of time the jumper is airborne and the great velocity he attains during the approach. The jumper must maintain balance and good form upon landing (he is judged on this); he does so by (1) increasing the forward-backward base of support by placing one ski slightly forward of the other, (2) absorbing the landing shock with controlled flexion at several joints (eccentric contraction of extensor muscles), (3) maintaining the center of gravity over the base of support, and (4) spreading the arms sideward to aid lateral balance (the skis should be spread very little).

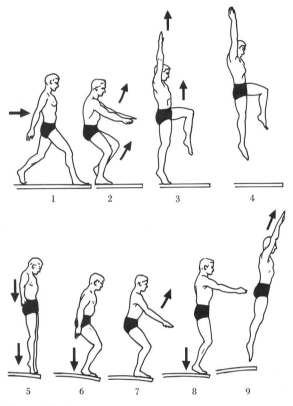

Figure 18–4.
Body actions during the *hurdle* and *takeoff* in springboard diving. The body thrust must be perfectly timed with the response of the board. The transfer of momentum by the arms and swinging leg is very important to the height of the hurdle; transfer of momentum downward from arm and shoulder action to depress the board is equally important.

Single-leg moving projections

Single-leg projections with a running approach provide the greatest amount of momentum (except for the ski jump); consequently, they are used when maximum height or distance is the objective. In these performances, the free leg, arms, and shoulders are thrust vigorously to contribute to the development of momentum in the desired direction. The momentum of the run, the thrust of the free leg, arms, and shoulders, and the projecting force from the push-off leg must all be perfectly coordinated and timed to provide maximum momentum in the desired direction.

Running long jump (broad jump.)   The long jump can be conveniently divided into the *approach, gather, takeoff, flight,* and *landing.* The approach need be no longer than it takes the performer to attain maximum running velocity. A longer approach than necessary is commonly used because most performers prefer to begin slowly and gradually achieve full speed. Because success in the long jump is highly dependent upon running speed, sprinters are usually good long jumpers. In addition to speed, the other important feature of the approach is the achievement of a consistent running stride so that a step pattern can be developed which will cause the performer to jump consistently from the takeoff board.

The positioning of the center of gravity and slight flexion of several joints (sinking action) in preparation for the jump are referred to as the gather, and they result in the loss of some forward momentum. This loss of momentum is desirable in one respect, because it allows a little more time for the takeoff leg to provide the vertical component of force. The gathering action results in flat-footed contact with the board, followed by a rolling action to the ball of the foot. This practice requires that the takeoff heel be afforded special protection from heel bruises.

The takeoff itself results from the combination of three forces: (1) forward momentum from the run; (2) push-off from the leg; and (3) thrusting actions with the swinging leg, arms, and shoulders. Each of these forces must make its maximum contribution, and the three forces must be perfectly timed. The major muscle groups involved in the takeoff are the hip, knee, and ankle extensors of the takeoff leg, the hip flexors of the swinging leg, shoulder flexors, and shoulder girdle elevators.

Optimum angle of projection at takeoff varies slightly with individuals depending upon their jumping styles. Even though the optimum angle would seem to be about 40°, the rapid horizontal speed from the run makes it impractical to project the body at an angle greater than about 25° from the surface. Most inexperienced performers tend *not* to jump high enough. The takeoff and flight utilize most of the principles of projections discussed in Chapter 14.

The "run in air," or hitch kick, flight is the most widely used. Actions while in flight are used to aid balance and to assume a good body position with which to land. The movements also help to rotate the upper body backward so the legs can reach out front upon landing. Airborne movements do *not* change the angle of flight or prolong the flight.

The correct landing technique is very important to success of the jump, for the feet must reach forward as far as possible and still allow the center of gravity to move forward over the base of support. The jumper lands in a pike (jack-knife) position with the feet spread apart so the buttocks can pass between them. He cushions the landing by bending the knees. Momentum carries the body past the points of support (feet).

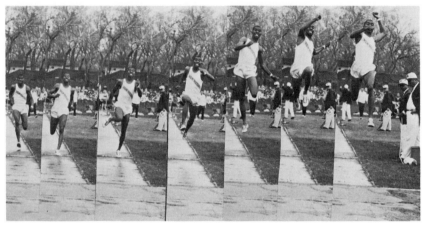

Figure 18–5.
Illustration of good technique in the running long jump. (*Athletic J., February, 1966.*)

Running high jump.   The tall, long-legged individual has a definite structural advantage in the high jump. The center of gravity must be raised above the crossbar, and if it is already located in a relatively high position, it need move a lesser distance upward in order to clear the bar. Consider the following example:

Location of the center of gravity generally varies between 55 and 56 percent of total body height in adult males. If a person 6 feet tall has long legs in comparison to his height, his center of gravity could be located about 42 inches above the surface in normal standing position. This means that if he projected the center of gravity vertically an additional 42 inches, he could reach a height of 7 feet. A person whose center of gravity is 4 inches lower (38 inches) in standing position would have to project the body an additional four inches to achieve the same height of 7 feet.

For purposes of analysis, the high jump can be conveniently divided into the *approach,* the *lift, crossing the bar,* and *landing.*

The approach is designed to serve two purposes: (1) to develop horizontal momentum which can be converted to momentum in a vertical direction and (2) to place body parts in position to contribute best to the vertical thrust at takeoff. There is disagreement among both coaches and performers about the angle and velocity of the approach. A relatively slow approach at a 45° angle has been commonly recommended in the past. But several of today's better jumpers approach more head-on and with greater velocity. Standardization of approach techniques may be inadvisable because of individual differences, but it is important to consider the effects of variations in approach angle and velocity.

The high-jumper wants to devote as much momentum as possible to raising his

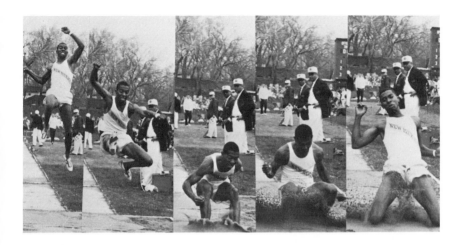

body vertically. Yet some horizontal momentum must be applied to move the body across the bar. A faster, more head-on approach is capable of producing more horizontal momentum to carry the jumper across the bar, and the faster approach also permits development of more rotary momentum, which is needed to cause the rolling action over the bar. This indicates that individuals with problems of trail-leg clearance should emphasize a faster, more head-on approach. The faster approach makes the timing of the vertical lift more critical and, in that sense, is disadvantageous. The more direct approach does not allow as much clearance for the swing of the free leg, which is a disadvantage because the performer must either shorten the length of that lever, thus limiting the momentum it can produce, or take off farther from the bar. If he chooses the latter, he is forced to direct less momentum in a vertical direction. Also, there seems to be less time to adjust for error in the more head-on approach.

Other important conditions of the approach follow: (1) A step pattern must be developed to make the point of takeoff and the velocity at takeoff consistent. (2) The last stride should be longer, placing the center of gravity well behind the planted foot. This enhances backward lean and the gather for the jump. (3) The toe and knee of the takeoff leg should point in the intended direction of flight. (4) The free leg should remain slightly bent during its swing, but then should extend fully as it passes over the bar.

At the completion of the approach, the body must be gathered for the lift. The lift must begin when the center of gravity is almost over (but slightly behind) the takeoff foot; the center of gravity must be slightly forward of the vertical at its completion. The lift involves coordinated and precisely timed upward thrusts with the swinging leg, the push-off leg, the arms, and the shoulders. Each of these movements makes an important contribution to the vertical rise. The forward-upward drive of the swinging leg, combined with the backward tilt of the trunk, are the primary movements in converting momentum from the horizontal to the vertical. The arm and shoulder thrusts occur simultaneously with the leg swing, and extension of the takeoff leg follows slightly behind. The lift is by far the most vigorous action of the jump, and from the standpoint of muscular involvement, it is dependent primarily upon the hip, knee, and ankle extensors of the takeoff leg, the hip flexors of the swinging leg, the shoulder flexors, and the shoulder girdle elevators. The abdominal muscles are important stabilizers of the pelvis.

The action over the bar is basically the same for practically all jumpers, but emphasis on certain movements varies among performers. The body rotates around its long axis as it moves horizontally across the bar. As soon as one part of the body crosses the bar, that part should be lowered to cause elevation of other body parts. The body crosses over in segments so that the whole body need not be above the bar at any time. Following are various popular tips which help to bring body parts down after they have crossed the bar: "Look down and back under the bar;" "Throw the lead shoulder down;" "Outward rotate the hip of the trail leg." These hints contribute to rotation of the body and practically assure that the landing will be on the back. If an adequate jumping pit is provided, the landing action does not require special attention.

The foregoing discussion refers to the straddle or bellyroll style which is used almost exclusively today. Obviously, the most efficient style should be used, because all other popular styles require a greater lift of the center of gravity to clear an identical height of the bar.

Triple jump (hop, step, and jump).   When performing three body projections successively after a running approach, as this skill requires, it is essential for the performer to place great emphasis on preserving horizontal momentum. Excessive loss of momentum during any part of the performance reduces total distance, which means the hop must be rather low, the step (leap) somewhat higher, and the jump the highest of the three. Some of the possible distance from the first two phases (hop and step) is sacrificed in order to conserve horizontal momentum for the third phase (jump).

The landing after each of the first two phases results in precarious balance, and complex coordination and timing are required to maintain good balance for the next phase. Both the hop and step are one-footed landings with the center of gravity moving at a high velocity. Such landing, along with a subsequent projection, requires very powerful hip, knee, and ankle extensor muscles. As these landings occur, the extensors of the leg must contract eccentrically to cushion the shock and produce joint flexion in preparation for the next projection. Almost immediately, the muscle contractions change to concentric contractions, thus causing the leg to extend. Arm, shoulder, and free leg movements must be perfectly timed and coordinated with extension of the push-off leg. The muscle actions of the total body in the triple jump are essentially the same as in the long jump. Very powerful leg extensors and a good deal of specific skill are required for success in this event.

Hurdling. Hurdling action is classified as a leap, which in turn can be thought of simply as an exaggerated running stride. Hurdling was analyzed in detail in Chapter 9; therefore, it does not receive detailed attention here. But a few additional points of information should be established at this time.

The efficient hurdler attempts (1) to raise the center of gravity as little as possible and yet provide clearance, (2) to remain in the air as short a time as possible, and (3) to land in good balance and in a position conducive to continuing the drive to the next barrier. To keep the center of gravity low when passing over the hurdle, the performer must develop great flexibility of the hip region. The hip adductor muscles of the trail leg and the extensors of the lead leg must be especially flexible.

A person with a high center of gravity has an advantage in hurdling, for the same reason explained in the high jump. Individuals who have this advantage show little change in the vertical position of the center of gravity when leaping a hurdle. Other important attributes of a hurdler are the same as those for a sprinter—a top hurdler must be a good sprinter. For the specific movements and the muscular actions involved in hurdling, refer to Chapter 9.

The leap in dance. In order to retain correct form or to create an illusion, in some skills the performer must sacrifice maximal projection. The leap in dance is one such skill. The meaning expressed by a certain posture during a leap may be vital to good form, and certain joint alignments aid the illusion of "hanging." Though maximum height and/or distance is usually desirable, it is of secondary importance. Transfer of momentum principles (involving the free leg and arms) sometimes must be disregarded to accomplish the more important objectives of the particular leap.

Kick turns. Essentially, kick turns are hops with varying degrees of twist. Various types of kick turns are widely used in dance and figure skating. In skating they are called axles. Even though kick turns vary from one another in appearance, the basic actions and principles governing them are the same. The takeoff is initiated by a dipping action of the trunk and takeoff leg, followed by the usual trunk and leg extension actions. To supplement the force from the takeoff leg, momentum is transferred to the body at takeoff by actions from the free leg and the arms. Usually this takeoff is preceded by horizontal momentum of the total body, so an important problem becomes one of correctly converting horizontal motion to a more vertical direction. The projection should be high enough to allow time for the necessary movements in the air.

For a turn to the left (left leg takeoff), the takeoff involves two major twisting actions around the body's vertical axis before the takeoff foot leaves the surface: (1) inward rotation at the left hip (the pelvis rotates on the fixed takeoff leg) and (2) left rotation of the thoracic spine (torso rotation), which results in

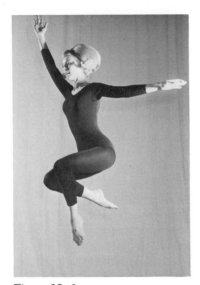 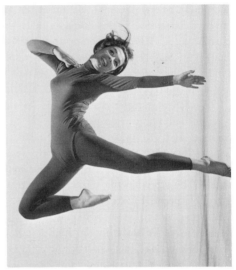

Figure 18–6.
Body position is important in the dance leap in order to create the desired visual impression.

upper body rotation to the left. The direction of motion of the swinging leg and the arms may also favor the left to add to the twist. The amount of twist that occurs is dependent upon (1) how much twisting force is developed and (2) how well it is conserved. Conservation of the twisting force is greatly influenced by the position of body parts. For example, extending the arms away from the body reduces the amount of turn, but drawing them near the body (closer to the axis of rotation) results in faster and more turns.

The landing usually is performed on the same leg as the takeoff, which classifies the skill as a hop. Greater vertical and lesser horizontal momentum in the flight permits better control upon landing. A more vertical flight also results in gaining greater height and, consequently, more time for the completion of movements in the air. But the amount of horizontal momentum that should be retained is influenced a great deal by the subsequent movement to be performed.

Hurdle step.   The diver or tumbler uses a hurdle step in preparation for a double-leg takeoff from the board or the mat. The primary purpose of the hurdle is to convert horizontal momentum to vertical momentum, as exemplified by the basketball player executing a lay-up shot. He uses a modified hurdle step just prior to the lay-up to reduce his horizontal momentum and to increase his vertical momentum. If the diver executes too flat a hurdle, he tends to project out too far from the board and does not get enough height.

A hurdle step movement is characterized by a slight backward lean of the trunk, a sharp upward motion of the swinging leg in the bent position, a spring from the takeoff leg, and a vertical thrust with the arms and shoulders. The arm and shoulder thrust and the lifting action of the swinging leg greatly aid the development of vertical momentum. The leg bent at the knee results in a faster leg action and more direct vertical lift.

Improvement of jumping, leaping, and hopping skills

These skills, when performed for maximum distance, are power events. They depend on one's ability to project the body through space. Therefore, the factors that can influence them are (1) improved coordination through the particular skill patterns, (2) increased power of the muscles used in the projection, and (3) reduced resistance to the projection (less weight). The less experienced performer should devote more time to development of the specific skill (coordinations), because it offers him the greatest opportunity for improvement. It is very important that he practice the correct technique. The more experienced performer should have already developed a high level of skill, so he should place greater emphasis on increasing power of the particular muscles involved. But the advanced performer must not forget that sharpening skills as often as possible is still vital to him. The physiological changes resulting from training may call for frequent reestablishment of timing in the skill pattern.

Upper body exercises may be beneficial, but are of less direct concern. In projections, the hip flexor muscles act with great velocity but not against great resistance, so the development of power in the hip flexors is of limited concern. The prime concern is with the hip, knee, and ankle extensors (plantar flexors) and the abdominal muscles which stabilize the pelvis. Training exercises should include leg presses, squats, step-ups, jumps for height, body curls, sit-ups, leg lifts, and other similar exercises. It should be remembered that the objective is not strength alone, but power; therefore, the exercise should be performed with great speed against reasonably heavy resistance. Exercises performed against constant resistance must be done with increased velocity in order to ensure power overload. Isometrics may serve as a weak substitute, but their limitations involving speed of contraction should be obvious. Some athletes claim to benefit a great deal from functional overload activities. Weighted vests, belts, and/or anklets are most commonly used. Many coaches and athletes think that functional overload interferes with correct timing and coordination.

In performances where a running approach is used, such as the long jump, running speed, endurance, and consistency of stride are important; so training programs should be designed to improve these factors. For example, endurance is of little importance to a long-jumper because he jumps few times during a contest, and with a reasonable level of endurance, he will adequately recover between jumps. However, a lack of endurance will hamper him in practice sessions. He will be unable to perform enough repetition of the skill to improve it. The importance of speed and consistency of stride is apparent.

A reasonable amount of flexibility, especially of the hip extensor muscles, is important. Lack of such flexibility may restrict the desired range of motion and contribute to injury. Flexibility can be increased best by repeatedly placing the muscles on steady stretch for short periods of time.

Recommended supplementary reading

BROER, MARION R.: "Efficiency of Human Movement," 2d ed., chap. 13, W. B. Saunders Company, Philadelphia, 1966.
WELLS, KATHERINE F.: "Kinesiology," W. B. Saunders Company, Philadelphia, 1966.

19

Throwing, striking, and pushing objects

hrowing and pushing receive more attention in this chapter than striking, because Chapter 15 provides a detailed mechanical analysis of a striking activity, the golf swing. The reader should refer to that analysis for principles which apply to striking activities. The analysis is also partially applicable to throwing, for the movements which develop striking momentum are similar to those that contribute to velocity of the hand in throwing, and objects in flight behave similarly, whether thrown, struck, or pushed.

Throwing, striking, and pushing objects all result in projection of the objects. And success in these activities is dependent primarily upon the *velocity* (momentum in striking) or *accuracy*, depending on the objective of the particular performance. The acceleration and control of the projected object are produced by muscle contractions, which must cause body movements in correct sequence. These kinds of performances are usually initiated by foot pressure against the supporting surface, followed by sequential movements progressing upward through the body, and finally terminating in the object to be projected. Each body segment receives the velocity produced by the preceding movements. A buildup of velocity occurs as each successive body movement adds to the sum of the velocities of the previous contributing movements. For example, in throwing a ball, the velocity of the ball at the moment of release is equal to the sum of the velocities of all contributing body movements, provided the movements are performed in correct sequence and each new movement is timed to add to the peak velocity of the movement which preceded it.

In the case of striking, *momentum* rather than velocity is of prime importance. When a baseball is struck with a bat, the velocity combined with the mass ($v \times m$ = momentum) of the bat determines the amount of impetus given to the ball. The lighter the bat, the greater velocity it must have in order to give an equal amount of impetus.

Several points are common to skills in which external objects are projected, regardless of the method used to set the objects in motion:

1. Lack of firm footing reduces the velocity of body segments necessary to gain maximum final velocity of the projected object. For example, a football jump pass is less forceful than one made from a set position where the feet are in firm contact.
2. As the length of the preparatory phase of the movement (backswing or windup) increases, ability to gain velocity in the action phase increases because the levers move through a greater range of motion and the muscles contract with greater initial force when placed on stretch. But an increased preparatory phase introduces greater chance for errors in accuracy.
3. Conscious attempts to speed up the action in a sequential movement pattern are often destructive to the sequence and timing, which may result in an unsatisfactory performance.
4. Distance magnifies errors in accuracy. More specifically, a longer backswing will increase the effects of errors in movements, and the farther the object is projected, the more apparent inaccuracies in direction of flight become.
5. Denser objects are influenced less by air resistance and air movements than less dense objects.

Throwing

Arm motion at the shoulder joint makes possible these convenient classifications of throwing actions:

1. Underarm—shoulder flexion
2. Sidearm—shoulder horizontal flexion
3. Overarm—shoulder inward rotation and horizontal flexion
4. Overhead—shoulder extension

Some throws can be performed either with one or both arms; some are executed from a stationary position (usually initiated by a shift of body weight), and others utilize forward progress of the total body in an approach run. An approach puts the object in motion in the desired direction before the throw actually begins.

The weight of the object may determine the throwing pattern used; heavier objects are usually projected with the underarm or pushing pattern. But for most people, the overarm and sidearm patterns produce the greatest speed and accuracy. The purpose of the throw and its place in game strategy normally determine the throwing pattern used and the type of preparatory action for the throw.

L

Underarm patterns

The underarm pattern is characterized by shoulder flexion. Perhaps the most forceful underhand pattern is the softball pitch. Other similar actions are the badminton underarm shot, handball and paddleball underarm shots, horseshoe pitch, bowling, and deck and ring tennis shots. Most underarm patterns progress with the following sequence of actions—and these actions indicate the muscles involved. In general, the movements flow from the ground upward through the body and out the arm.

1. Initiation of total body weight shift
2. Left hip inward rotation (right-handed pitch)
3. Left rotation of the trunk (spine)
4. Scapular abduction
5. Shoulder joint flexion and outward rotation
6. Elbow flexion (slight)
7. Lower arm rotation outward (in some cases only)
8. Wrist flexion

Though the relative importance of each movement varies with different performances, in many cases they are all important contributors to the velocity of the projected object.

Cooper and Glassow (**18**) found that in underarm patterns, shoulder flexion consistently makes the greatest contribution. For example, they found that in the underarm pitch, the relative contributions of the different joints are shoulder flexion 45 percent, wrist flexion 32 percent, hip rotation 15 percent, and trunk rotation 8 percent.

Underarm pitch. A very powerful underarm action, the underarm pitch requires that all contributing body segments make their maximum contribution. This demand calls for an extensive windup (preparatory action) to allow greater time for acceleration. As explained earlier, extensive windup is conducive to inaccuracy; therefore, the correct combination of velocity and accuracy is of prime concern to the softball pitcher. Major muscle groups which contribute to left-right accuracy are the shoulder joint adductors and abductors in concert with the left rotators of the trunk. Very fine coordination of these muscles is required. Of greater concern to accuracy, though, is high-low errors, which result from improper timing of the ball's release. The ball should be released at the lowest point of the arc; if it is held too long, the flight is high, and if released too early, the trajectory is low. Although the bottom of the arc is passed almost immediately in a fast pitch, its time can be extended by emphasizing two other body actions. The shoulder girdle moves forward because of scapular abduction, and the whole body moves forward because of the stride (shift of body weight) into the pitch.

Extending these actions keeps the ball at its lowest point for a longer period of time (flattens the bottom of the arc), permitting a greater tolerance for errors in the time of release.

If the underarm pattern includes both arms, as does the underhand free throw in basketball, the hip and trunk rotatory movements and the shift of total body weight are eliminated. Leg extension substitutes for the shift of body weight. Fewer joint movements are used, and the force is sacrificed for accuracy and control.

Sidearm patterns

In sidearm throwing, greater reliance is placed upon the hip and spinal rotator muscles, and less emphasis on muscles of the arm and shoulder. Basically, the arm becomes a long lever, lying horizontally, rather than a series of short levers. This arm position lengthens the levers which act in hip and spinal rotation. The primary movements for a right-handed pitcher are:

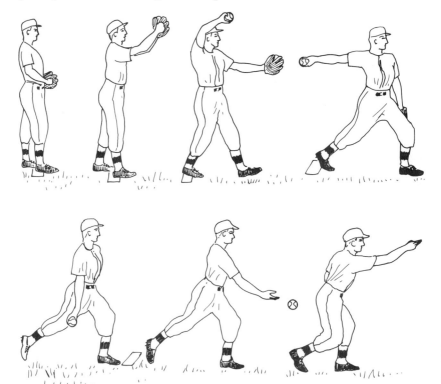

Figure 19–1.
Body actions in the underarm softball pitch.

1. Initiation of total body weight shift
2. Left hip inward rotation
3. Left rotation of the trunk (spine)
4. Scapular abduction
5. Shoulder horizontal flexion and slight medial rotation
6. Wrist flexion

Sidearm pitch.   In this method of throwing, the high-low accuracy becomes less of a problem, but errors to the left or right become more prevalent. Here the left-right inaccuracies are caused mostly by errors in the timing of the release. The arc of the hand movement can be somewhat flattened in the sidearm throw by the same techniques as described in the underarm throw. In the sidearm throw, flattening of the arc helps to control left-right errors.

If a baseball pitcher delivers a sidearm throw, the point of release is not from the center of the field, but from a point nearer the third base line (right-handed pitch). If such a ball is thrown to a right-handed batter (discounting any appreciable spin), the angle of delivery causes the ball to move at an angle away from the batter. This reduces the power with which the batter can meet the ball, and it reduces the area of playing field (left field) to which he may hit with maximum power. The right fielder can play especially shallow if the pitcher is effective with the sidearm throw.

The sidearm throw is used by ballplayers other than the pitcher when the situation requires quick release and a fast throw for a short distance. This pattern involves less arm action than the overarm pattern, so a sidearm pitcher is less apt to develop arm trouble. The sidearm pattern is often used when larger and heavier objects are hurled and the arm is to be protected from strain. This pattern ordinarily supplies more speed than the underarm pattern, but less speed than the overarm pattern.

Discus throw.   Difficulty in gripping the discus explains, in one sense, why the sidearm delivery is used. But even if its shape were more appropriate for grasping, its weight might still be great enough to force a sidearm delivery for protection of the arm. Since accuracy is of little concern in discus-throwing, it is advantageous to utilize a full range of shoulder motion as well as maximum hip and torso rotations.

The discus is put into motion by a total body spin. As the performer spins, he moves forward across the ring in the direction of the throw. Then he adds the final thrust (throw) to these movements. The velocity of the discus results from the combination of the three types of movements, namely, (1) total body rotation, (2) forward progress of the body, and (3) actions involved in throwing. An increase in force from any of these movements will increase the velocity of the discus at release.

Experienced performers attain approximately 20 to 25 percent additional distance from the spin as compared to a stationary throw. When a very rapid spin is used, the event becomes a real test of body balance, and many mediocre performances are caused by loss of balance during the spin. It is presently common to use 1½ turns in the spin. Conceivably, future record breaking will be the result of an additional fraction of a turn.

One common problem resulting from the turn is the centrifugal force pulling on the discus during the spin. This tends to draw the arm away from the fully cocked position, thus reducing the length of the action at the shoulder joint when it becomes time to deliver. Another common problem of discus-throwing is releasing the missile with its leading edge too high in relation to its trailing edge. This occurs when forearm rotation is not properly controlled, causing a "thumb-up" delivery. In this position, pronation of the forearm is insufficient, for the best flight is obtained when the palm of the hand is down and the leading edge of the discus is pointed at the angle of flight. The air pressure then provides aerodynamic lift similar to that of an airplane wing. Still another frequent problem is falling away from the throw. Usually, this problem is the manifestation of balance loss. Almost invariably, if the performer is off-balance at the release, it is in the backward direction. Because discus-throwing is a very complex skill, it requires many hours of practice and unusual neuromuscular coordination.

The muscles which contribute the most during the spin are the hip rotators and the hip, knee, and ankle extensors. During the throw the key muscles are the ankle, knee, and hip extensors of the back leg, hip and trunk rotators (to the left), the shoulder horizontal flexors of the right (throwing) arm, and the horizontal extensors of the left (opposite) arm. Because the discus throw is a power event, muscle-conditioning programs should be designed to increase muscle power.

There are a limited number of two-handed sidearm patterns; the most common one is the hammer throw.

Overarm patterns

We commonly identify the baseball throw as the standard overarm throw; although it does serve as a good standard, some other overarm throws deviate from it slightly. The overarm pattern is distinctive in that the performer often has an incorrect mental image of the mechanics of his arm actions. Many visualize the major arm force resulting from a downward and backward movement (extension) of the humerus beginning from the vertical. In truth, the major force results from inward rotation of the humerus, and the humerus is not vertical; it is usually almost horizontal and parallel with the surface. Even at times when the point of the elbow is higher than the shoulder, the relationship of the humerus to the trunk is changed very little because the higher elbow results mostly from lateral flexion of the spine.

The sequence of movements which are involved in the whiplike action of the overarm throw include (right-handed thrower):

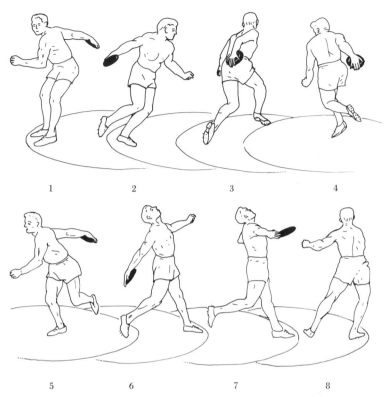

Figure 19–2.
Body actions in the discus throw.

1. Initiation of the total body weight shift
2. Inward rotation at the forward hip (the pelvis rotates on the fixed leg)
3. Left lateral flexion, and strong left rotation of the trunk
4. Strong inward rotation and horizontal flexion at the shoulder joint
5. Elbow extension, combined with lower arm rotation, to give correct direction to the throw
6. Strong wrist action, the direction of which depends on the purpose of the throw (Straight flexion is the dominant wrist action, but ulnar flexion is often used.)

Overarm pitch.   Among expert throwers, about one-half the force is derived from the movement of the legs and trunk and one-half from the arm actions. (This ratio may be influenced considerably by the size and shape of the object being thrown.) This demonstrates the importance of total body action. The overarm method is the one method which allows the greatest opportunity to utilize all available levers through their greatest range of motion. Therefore, with

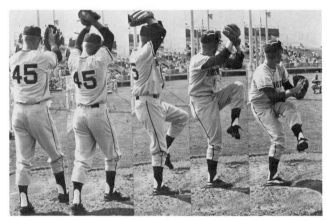

Figure 19–3.
Body actions in the overarm baseball throw. (*Athletic J.*, pp. 56–57, January, 1968.)

relatively light objects, this is the throwing method with which the greatest speed can be developed. Cooper and Glassow (**18**) found that in the baseball throw, wrist flexion was the greatest contributing action. Hip rotation, spinal rotation, and medial rotation at the shoulder (humerus) were also very important.

Most errors in accuracy in this pattern are high-low errors. The overarm throw generally produces more left-right errors than the underarm, but fewer than the sidearm throw.

Incorrect technique resulting in loss of force in the overarm throw is most commonly observed in young girls, although such errors are not exclusive of others. The most serious error occurs when the wrong foot is placed forward; the wrong foot, in this case, is the one on the side of the throwing arm. This action eliminates almost all contributions of trunk rotation, and the shoulder actions begin too soon in the sequence, causing their contributions to be almost fully spent before they can add acceleration to the ball.

Accuracy in the overhand throw appears to develop at the speed at which it is practiced. An individual may be fairly accurate at one speed but much less accurate at another speed. In consequence, practicing throws at slow speed appears to be of limited value if the performance must be at fast speed. Repetition in practice is needed at all the velocities to be used.

It has been said that throwing without the use of the fingers is like taking a flat-footed jump. Failure to use these levers limits the opportunity to develop maximum velocity. In order to use the fingers effectively, the performer must hold the ball by the fingers, not in the palm of the hand. If these levers are lengthened by moving the ball closer to the finger tips, effectiveness is increased,

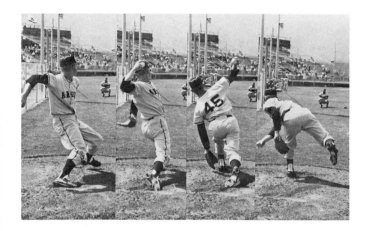

but the ball must not be so far toward the finger tips that the force does not pass through the ball's center of gravity. If the object is heavy, finger and wrist flexor muscles may be unable to contend with it when the weight is placed too far toward the finger tips.

The muscles which contribute most to the overarm pitch are the ankle, knee, and hip extensors of the back leg, hip and trunk rotators to the left, shoulder horizontal flexors and medial rotators, elbow extensors, and wrist and finger flexors.

Curve ball. Throwing a curve ball differs from throwing a fast ball in movements of the elbow, wrist, and fingers. The elbow extends in either case, but while the forearm is pronated for a fastball delivery, it is supinated with a "snap" for a curve-ball delivery. The wrist moves sharply through ulnar flexion for the curve, but the fast ball requires straight wrist flexion. At least two fingers are behind the ball in the fast-ball delivery; whereas, for the curve ball, the thumb remains behind the ball, and the ball is released by rolling it forward over the index finger. For more information about the grip and release of curve balls, refer to the chapter on projections.

Football pass. The football pass is nearly the same as the overarm baseball throw already described. The forearm position is between that of the fast-ball and that of the curve-ball throws. The wrist action is mostly ulnar flexion. A sharp downward movement at the wrist and the inward rotation at the shoulder produce the spiral flight of the ball. Large hands are an aid to better control.

Compared with the baseball pitch, the football pass involves less action at almost all joints, especially at the hip, and it results in more of a push and less of a whip action, because the football is harder to grip and control and must be released in such a way that it will travel in a spiral. The football throw may be preceded by several sideward shuffle steps, and right lateral flexion of the trunk

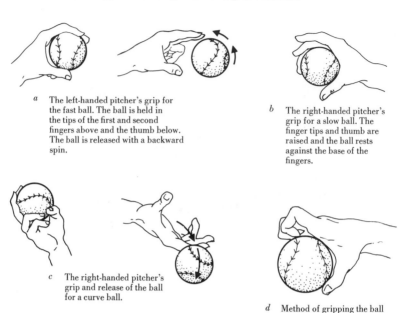

a   The left-handed pitcher's grip for the fast ball. The ball is held in the tips of the first and second fingers above and the thumb below. The ball is released with a backward spin.

b   The right-handed pitcher's grip for a slow ball. The finger tips and thumb are raised and the ball rests against the base of the fingers.

c   The right-handed pitcher's grip and release of the ball for a curve ball.

d   Method of gripping the ball for pitching the knuckle ball.

Figure 19–4.
Grips used to cause different effects on the flight of a ball. (*After Daniel E. Jessee, "Baseball," A. S. Barnes and Co., Inc., New York, 1939.*)

is used in preparation when more distance is needed. The follow-through actions are less extensive than in the baseball pitch because the football throw involves less action at all joints and less velocity. Another factor influencing follow-through is that the baseball pitcher assumes a position of readiness for fielding after the throw, but the football passer wants to protect himself from contact. The same major muscle groups are involved in the football pass as in the baseball pitch.

Javelin throw.   The javelin delivery is somewhat similar to the football pass, except for the following: (1) A running approach serves the dual purpose of putting the javelin in motion and the body in throwing position. The most effective approach yet developed involves a run followed by crossover steps with the back leg crossing in front of the lead leg. The cross steps put the performer's side to the direction of the throw without appreciably reducing his momentum. With each crossover, the toe of the crossing leg points more to the side. (2) The forearm begins in a fully supinated position and progresses toward pronation during the arm action. (3) The throw starts with the arm fully extended. (4) There is more movement in the shoulder and less flexion and extension at the elbow, resulting in a more straight arm delivery. These movements are such that the hand (and javelin) pass directly above the shoulder, at nearly full arm length.

Correct position of the javelin during the approach is very important. It should be held at an angle approximately equal to the angle of projection, and the point must not be allowed to drift upward and/or away during the approach (should stay close to the thrower's ear). If it drifts away from the ear, misdirection will result when the throwing forces are applied.

The balance of the javelin must be in accord with the ability of the thrower. For throwers whose distance will probably be short, more weight is located in the javelin's point, whereas for throwers of longer length, less weight is needed in the point for maximum flight. Only throwers of long distance can afford this luxury because when the javelin is in flight for a longer period, it requires less weight in the point to pull the point down in time for a correct (point first) landing.

Expert throwers also concern themselves with the position of the forward leg just before the release. They recognize the importance of the long lever extending from the toe to the lead leg to the javelin; the longer this lever is, the more it will contribute to the speed of the javelin, and the higher the javelin will be at release. Both these factors are favorable to greater distance, and consequently, the experts throw "against" a *straight* lead leg and attempt to rise to the toes and reach high with the hand at release.

The same major muscle groups are involved in the javelin throw as in the baseball throw, and the objective of a conditioning program is also the same— to increase muscle power.

Double-arm overarm patterns.   Examples of this type of throw are the overhead toss in soccer and the overhead two-handed pass or shot in basketball. In these skills, as in other throwing skills, total body action is essential. This involves precisely coordinated extension at various joints of the legs, trunk, and arms, which may be accompanied by a jump from both feet or a forward step to add force to the throw. The hands should be held on opposite sides of and partially behind the ball. The hands act as clamps. The elbows should be out front and above the shoulders. If the elbows are too far apart, forward force is sacrificed. During the action, there is slight extension at the shoulders, elbow extension, wrist flexion, ulnar flexion, and finger flexion. When accuracy is desired, the finger and wrist movements are very important because they put the "final touch" on the ball.

Single-arm circular overhead actions

Few activities can be classified within this category. The most common are the basketball hook shot and hook pass. Accuracy of this technique is less than that

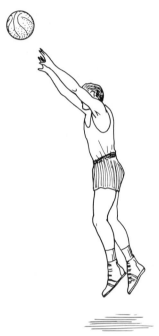

Figure 19–5.
Basketball two-handed overhead throw at release.

of other overarm throwing techniques, mainly because it is not suited for good
hand-eye coordination. However, some players become reasonably proficient in
shooting basketball hook shots when they shoot from known spots on the floor.
The action is most often preceded by a hurdle step approach which gains height
and makes it difficult for an opponent to interfere with the shot. Often a smaller
man finds the hook to be the best shot to avoid blocking by a larger opponent.
Large hands are obviously advantageous in controlling a hook pass or shot. Most
errors in accuracy result from too high a projection, which indicates inadequate
control of the ball.

Pushing actions

As compared with overarm throwing, pushing patterns involve less arm action
and leverage that is less favorable to producing great speed against light
resistance. But pushing patterns involve very powerful movements, movements in

which the leverage is highly favorable to application of force against heavy resistance. In pushing, the more powerful muscle groups are used, especially in the arm and shoulder movements. Also pushing patterns are conducive to great accuracy in certain performances because the hand moves linearly in the line of flight, which makes timing of the release less critical than in throwing.

Single-arm pushes

The most common single-arm pushing actions are shot-putting and the one-handed push shot in basketball. In the first case, the primary consideration is distance, and in the second, accuracy is of prime importance.

When *maximum velocity* of the missile is desired, as in shot-putting, actions of the legs and trunk are greatly emphasized. (They are similar to those of the overarm throw.) When *accuracy* is wanted, as in the basketball push shot, body and leg actions are limited to correspond with the objective of the skill.

Shot put. The shot is put (pushed) and not thrown. The prime objective is distance, and assuming the angle of projection is correct, the distance is dependent upon the velocity at which the shot is moving at release. One's ability to develop velocity of the shot is dependent upon his power, which is a combination of strength and speed. The shot-putter, then, is essentially concerned with increasing his power and perfecting the specific skill of shot-putting. Because of the importance of power, the shot-putter spends much of his training time attempting to increase strength and speed of movement against heavy resistance. He must also give adequate attention to the development of shot-putting skill, because the mechanics of movement and the sequential timing of the movements are of tremendous importance.

Shot-putting combines three kinds of body movements: (1) linear movement of the total body across the 7-foot ring, (2) rotation of the total body through about 180°, and (3) the pushing actions of the various body segments. Each type of movement must be correctly timed and fully utilized in order to make its maximum contribution. To illustrate the importance of each kind of movement, consider the "O'Brien style," which has revolutionized shot-putting. Its unique feature is that the performer starts the put with the back, rather than the side, toward the direction of flight. This position allows an additional one-quarter turn of the total body, thus increasing the time over which the body rotational forces can be applied.

After movement across the ring and just before the final thrusting movement, all body segments should be in correct position, the same position as if a stationary put were being made. In consequence, at the completion of movement across the ring, the legs and spine should be sufficiently flexed to provide for optimum effects from extension at those joints. The most effective depth of flexion in preparation is directly related to the strength of the extensor muscles.

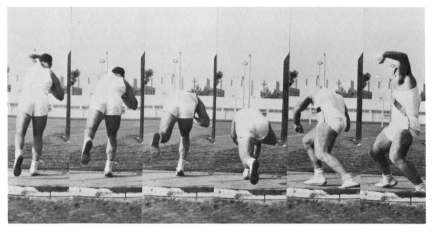

Figure 19–6.
A good technique in shot-putting. (*Athletic J.*)

Certainly the muscles contribute little if the joints are nearly extended after the glide across the ring and before the thrust.

The major force of the thrusting action in shot-putting results from the following body movements: extension at the various leg joints, with emphasis on the back leg; rotation at the hips and trunk; horizontal flexion at the shoulder; elbow extension; and wrist and finger flexion. As in the overhand throw, the movements generally flow from the legs upward. One very important movement often not recognized is horizontal extension of the opposite arm. This vigorous movement can add greatly to the speed of hip and trunk rotation.

The idea of maintaining contact with the surface is especially important in this event because if foot-surface contact is broken too early, the driving forces of the body are greatly reduced. Holding the shot high on the fingers can provide extra leverage, provided the fingers are strong enough to overcome the resisting force of the shot. If the fingers lack sufficient strength, then placing the shot too high on them will be self-defeating. The reversal (follow-through) at the completion of the putting action is important because it allows the performer to continue his thrusting movements longer, while it places the body in better position to maintain balance.

Basketball one-handed push shot.   The most widely used basketball shot today is the one-handed push shot performed with a jump (jump shot). In this performance, accuracy, and not force, is of prime importance.

The jump is usually initiated from a double-leg takeoff which is essentially directed upward, though some performers jump somewhat forward; on occasion, the backward "falling away" jump shot is useful. The main reason for the jump is to provide height to gain clearance over an opponent. In addition to the

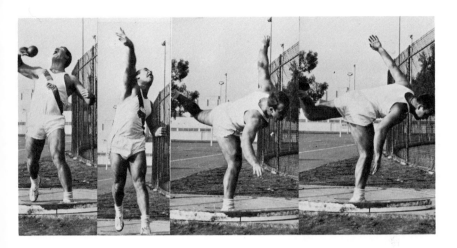

increased height, two other factors have contributed to the popularity of this technique: (1) the unexpectedness of the time and direction of the takeoff and (2) the delay of the shot, which makes it difficult to anticipate when to block. These factors have led some coaches to label the shot as indefensible. It should be noted that the delay, especially if it extends until the shooter begins his descent, eliminates the contribution of the legs and trunk to the force of the projection. As the shot becomes longer, shooting earlier in the jump becomes more necessary, and power in the hand, arm, and shoulder muscles becomes more essential.

Aside from the jump, almost all the actions in this shooting technique occur in the shooting arm. They are shoulder flexion, elbow extension, and wrist and finger flexion. Wrist and finger flexion are the final movements, and they are very important because they put the correct "touch" on the ball. For accuracy it is important that the ball be controlled with the fingers; when the ball is held high over the head, less action occurs in the shoulder and elbow, and more reliance is placed on the wrist and finger actions. Some performers shoot with the elbow in front of the shoulder; some shoot with the elbow almost directly to the side; and others have the elbow at some intermediate point between the front and side. There is no evidence that any of these styles is superior in accuracy.

The one-handed free throw shot or the one-handed set shot follows about the same pattern as the jump shot, except the leg and trunk actions are used more to contribute to the force.

Double-arm pushes

A few skills involve double-arm pushes. The most common ones are the basketball chest pass and the medicine ball pass. In these performances, the initial

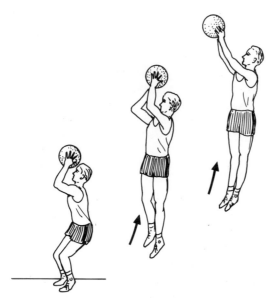

Figure 19–7.
Illustration of body actions during the basketball jump
shot.

force come from forward movement of the total body as a step forward is taken. The other important movements are shoulder flexion, elbow extension, wrist flexion, ulnar flexion, and finger flexion. As in other thrusting actions, the movements flow from the ground upward.

Striking activities (including kicking)

Most of the principles which apply to throwing and pushing also apply to striking, and the arm movement patterns used in throwing are very similar to those used in striking. The one essential difference between throwing and striking is that the emphasis in striking is upon the *momentum* of the striking implement rather than the *velocity* of the throwing hand.

Arm striking patterns

Examples of *underarm striking patterns* are the volleyball serve, badminton serve, tennis pickup shot, and the badminton underarm clear shot. Examples of *sidearm patterns* are batting a baseball and tennis forehand and backhand drives.

Overarm patterns include the tennis serve, tennis smash, badminton overarm clear shot, badminton smash, and the volleyball spike. A *circular arm pattern* is illustrated by the left hook of the boxer. Boxing also incorporates pushing patterns which produce striking forces. Examples are the jab and cross.

In striking, as in throwing and pushing, the movements flow from the feet upward, and the final motion is that of the striking implement. If all the contributing body motions occur in correct sequence with correct timing, then the velocity of the implement will represent the sum of the velocities of all contributing levers. The actual magnitude of the striking force is determined by the velocity and weight (momentum) of the implement.

In arm striking patterns, most of the force is provided by the following actions: total body weight shift (stepping into the strike), hip rotation, trunk rotation, horizontal flexion at the back shoulder, and horizontal extension at the front shoulder. In certain striking actions, elbow extension and wrist flexion, or ulnar flexion, are also important movements.

In Chapter 15 a mechanical analysis of a striking activity (golf drive) was presented. Many ideas relating to the mechanics of striking actions can be gleaned from that chapter. Following are interesting points about striking that were not discussed:

1. An oblique striking surface, off-center contact, and/or glancing blows produce spin on the object at the expense of force. The spin may significantly influence the flight of the object in different ways, depending on the direction of the spin.

2. If the object (ball) is moving toward the striking implement, and the momentum of the implement is greater than that of the object, the momentum of the object adds to that of the implement. This means that the faster a ball approaches, the farther it can be hit, as long as the implement's momentum exceeds that of the ball.

3. Maximum distance or force is not always desired, and often accuracy and quickness of movement can be gained by sacrificing maximum force. This concept is especially useful in baseball batting and tennis, where placement of the ball is very important.

4. The length of levers may be altered to suit the strength of the performer. The weaker man must sometimes shorten levers so he can maintain the desired speed of movement. He "chokes up" on the baseball bat or tennis racket in order to be sure he will overcome momentum of the ball and still not sacrifice accuracy. If he were strong enough to lengthen the lever, he would achieve a longer arc of swing and thereby gain the advantage of a more powerful swing. In the case of the tennis serve, the longer lever would give the ball a better approach angle to the net. When a very heavy implement is used, the performer may have to shorten the levers to achieve any degree of success.

5. In bunting a baseball, either the sacrifice or the drag bunt usually requires that the bat move away from the ball at contact and/or a loose grip is used to absorb the striking forces, thus reducing the distance of the rebound. Accuracy in directing the ball downward is also important to reducing rebound distance.

6. If great force is desired, it follows that the grip must be very firm, especially at contact. If the hands are spread in the grip, speed of movement of the implement is sacrificed for accuracy. The closer the hands are to each other, the more they act as a single unit.

Kicking patterns

In sports performances, kicking is most commonly used in American football and soccer. The investigation of kicking reveals that a backward inclination of the trunk almost always precedes a kick in which force or distance is the objective. This backward inclination contributes to the "stretch" of the rectus femoris muscle, a major contributor to the kicking action. The stretch stimulates the stretch reflex and removes slack in the muscle, enabling its contraction to have immediate and strong effect on knee extension. The backward inclination is most obvious in football and soccer punts. In place-kicking it is less obvious but still exists. Another result of backward inclination is that it starts the forward-upward motion of the thigh prior to the time hip flexion begins. This movement contributes to the force of hip flexion which follows. The action of the kick is best described as "whiplike," with the backward swing of the trunk as the initial motion, followed by the lashing action of the leg.

The placement of the supporting foot is very important to the place-kick. If the foot is placed too far forward, sufficient time is not available to build momentum before contact is made with the ball. If it is placed too far back of the ball, the peak force of the kick will be spent before contact is made. For the greatest force and best control, contact should be made at the bottom of the kick arc. The arc is flattened by the forward movement of the whole body and by a slight bending of the knee of the supporting leg. This provides greater tolerance for error.

The instep soccer kick has recently gained popularity for football place-kicking. It is difficult to assess the potential of each kicking technique in terms of force. The instep kick makes use of one long lever (from the hip) in an adducting movement. The adductor muscles are very powerful, and the lever is long. On the other hand, the toe kick utilizes two levers (lower and upper leg), which probably allow a greater development of momentum over a longer range of motion.

For accuracy the area of contact on the inside of the foot appears to be superior to the toe. Not only is a broader area of contact available, but the concave foot fits well with the convex ball. The square-toed kicking shoe partially alleviates this disadvantage of toe kicking.

In summary, it seems that greater force is available with use of the toe kick, and greater accuracy is possible with the instep kick. Accuracy may develop more slowly with the instep kick, however, because the line of sight is not along the line of movement as it is in the toe kick.

Improvement of throwing, pushing, and striking activities

Most of these activities are power events of a ballistic nature. Therefore, the components of fitness that should dominate the time available for training are (1) muscular strength, (2) speed of muscle contraction, and (3) flexibility in certain body regions. Of course, practice of the correct mechanics and specific coordinations necessary to the performance must not be neglected.

The natural amount of body power is usually insufficient for maximum performance in throwing, striking, and pushing activities. Therefore, each skill should be evaluated in terms of the requirements of power for its success. Then artificial overload (weight training, isometrics, or functional overloads) should be used to provide the needed power-building stimuli. For power, exercises should be performed explosively to improve both strength and speed of contraction. Although increasing power in the upper body should be emphasized, the trunk and lower extremities cannot be neglected, because these areas provide much of the force for throwing, pushing, and striking. Special exercises should be selected to increase flexibility in the areas where muscle tightness restricts the desired range of movement.

It seems to be rarely profitable to break these skills down into parts for practice, because they are so dependent upon correct timing and sequence. Also it is of little value to substitute similar skills, for these tend to disturb the timing of ballistic movements. For improved coordination of a particular pattern, the skill as a whole should be practiced extensively.

Recommended supplementary reading

BROER, MARION R.: "Efficiency of Human Movement," 2d ed., chaps. 18 and 19, W. B. Saunders Company, Philadelphia, 1966.

COOPER, JOHN M., and RUTH B. GLASSOW: "Kinesiology," 2d ed., chaps. 7–11, The C. V. Mosby Company, St. Louis, 1968.

20

Arm support and suspension skills

*T*his category of skills is dominated by gymnastic activities. Arm support, however, is also used in several starting stances, and arm suspension is used in the rope climb and pole vault. A great deal of strength and muscular endurance in the upper body are prerequisites to the successful performance of these skills, and precise control of muscular contractions is of utmost importance. Here, precision of the muscular contractions is highly dependent upon incoming information from the kinesthetic sense. In essence, the basic aspects of these skills are (1) sufficient strength to support the body in the desired positions and (2) effective manipulation and control of the center of gravity to maintain balance. In most arm-supported and suspension skills there is little room for error.

When the body is in arm-supported positions, the elbow extensor muscles contract strongly to resist the pull of gravity. Other joints of the upper extremities may either be in movement or be stabilized; therefore, few muscles in the upper body can relax. Unlike that of the lower body, the upper body bone structure is not well suited for weight bearing, and deficiencies in structure must be compensated for by extensive muscular use.

Inverted balances

All the principles of stability discussed earlier are applicable to inverted balance skills. In addition, factors pertaining to the base of support apply to these skills. For instance, in the inverted position, it is important to keep the center of gravity of the body over the base and to keep the center of gravity as low as possible within the confines of desirable form. If the performer's weight is proportionately greater in his upper body than in his legs, then his center of gravity is lower in the inverted position, and he gains an advantage in balance and stability. Of course, any position which lowers the body toward the surface aids in stability.

Once a balanced position is accomplished, the subsequent problems involve muscular strength-endurance and ability to make adjustments necessary to regain balance when deviations occur. Some necessary, though often undesirable, adjustments to preserve balance include (1) flexion of the elbows (to lower the center of gravity), (2) movement of the legs (to the side opposite the balance loss), and (3) reestablishment of the base of support to keep it underneath the center of gravity.

Handstands on the *floor* involve a base of support which is narrow in the front-back directions. Because of this narrow base, great strength is required in the muscles surrounding the wrist to oppose body sway. Effective stabilization of certain joints (elbows, shoulders, thoracic and lumbar spine, hips, knees, and ankles) may relieve tension on wrist muscles by reducing the amount of body sway. Also, correct movements in those joints will help to maintain control.

A handstand on the *parallel bars* is easier than on the floor, because the wrists are in stronger positions, due to the fact that (1) forward and backward

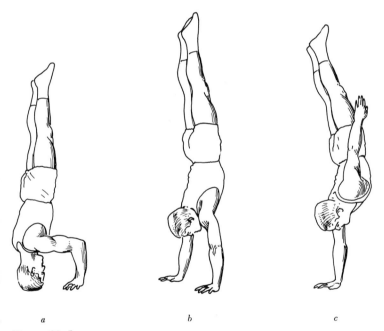

a   b   c

Figure 20–1.
As a performer progresses from the headstand to a two-handed stand, to a one-handed stand, he must demonstrate an increased sense of balance and greater strength, in order to compensate for the smaller base of support and fewer supporting limbs.

deviations are now controlled by the wrist adductors and abductors instead of the flexors and extensors and that (2) the grip on the bars provides a firmer base of support. The same circumstances are true to a lesser extent on the *rings*. During a handstand on the *horizontal bar*, the wrist flexors and extensors are in control, and the base of support is extremely narrow (diameter of the bar), making this a very difficult balance skill.

One-handed stands are still more difficult, because the supporting muscles carry a double load, and the base of support is reduced to the size of the one-handed contact with the surface. The center of gravity must be held over that small base. As additional body parts come in contact with the surface, the base of support is enlarged. Examples are the shoulder stand on the parallel bars and the head-and-handstand on the floor. In the head-and-handstand, an additional stability advantage is gained because the center of gravity is lowered from the bending of the arms. Also, the head-and-handstand affords the opportunity to widen the base of support in the forward-backward direction, as well as in the lateral direction.

Arm-supported travels

Skills like the handspring, cartwheel, handwalk, and progressing forward on the parallel bars are examples of traveling while being supported by the arms. The first two constitute linear movement accomplished by rotary motion of the entire body, and the last two result from linear movement by a progression of balance losses, each followed by successive reestablishment of the base of support.

Travels by rotary motion of the entire body

These skills depend upon an approach run to build sufficient forward momentum, followed by a takeoff of sufficient force and in the correct direction to provide enough rotary momentum to complete the skill. Examples of these skills are the forward roll and the handspring. The primary function of the supporting arms in such skills is to provide a stable base at the correct time. If the skill is done well, the joints of the upper extremities bend very little, and therefore, they provide limited force to aid the rotation.

Travels by a succession of alternate supports

These skills involve the same principles as the upright walk. The center of gravity is pitched forward of the base of support as one support is advanced to produce a new base beneath the displaced center of gravity. The propulsion of the body occurs mainly as a result of thoracic spinal rotation and backward-downward pressure by the trailing arm. These skills are done best with an optimum length of stride and continuous linear motion. If the performer has adequate strength and endurance in the upper body, then the main difficulty lies in the ability to maintain balance while advancing. This calls for each new base of support to be established while the body advances smoothly and steadily.

Stationary positions involving arm support

The exact stance used in any position of readiness is determined by the task to be accomplished. *Track and football starting stances* are established for the purpose of moving quickly in a predetermined direction. The stance of the dash man in track is obviously designed to initiate motion in the forward direction as quickly as possible. For this reason, the center of gravity is placed as far forward as possible without sacrificing balance which results in considerable weight on the arms and the base of support defined by the positions of the hands and feet. The football stance with the center of gravity well forward is desirable only if movement is to be in a forward direction. If the player must be ready to move in any direction, then the center of weight should be located near the center of the base. This is a stance of compromise which is not highly suited to movement in any particular direction, but well suited to quick adjustment in direction.

In a *front-leaning rest position* on the floor, the arms carry most of the weight. This position is used in exercises like the push-up or the squat thrust, and it may also be used during floor exercise routines in gymnastics. Its effective execution depends largely upon muscular strength and endurance of the shoulder girdle abductors, shoulder flexors, elbow extensors, and wrist flexors. The abdominal muscles bear the special burden of opposing a tendency for the pelvis to sag as a result of the pull of gravity.

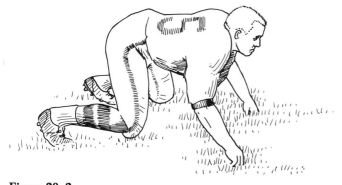

Figure 20–2.
The football 4-point stance combines two important factors: (1) great stability and (2) ability to move quickly and forcefully in the forward direction.

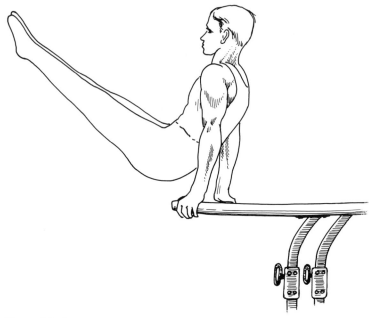

Figure 20–3.
Maneuvering in the arm support position on parallel bars (or similar apparatus) requires great arm and shoulder strength.

An *upright rest (support) position* varies with the gymnastic apparatus on
which it is performed. On the horizontal bar or the side horse, the performer
need only produce arm support against gravity, because balance is very easy
if he leans forward onto the apparatus and maintains body rigidity. In the support position on the parallel bars and still rings, the shoulder flexors and extensors must actively oppose each other to prevent the center of gravity from
swinging forward or backward beyond the supporting hands. The still rings pose
an additional problem because of their tendency to spread laterally. This calls
for strong contractions of the shoulder adductors. The upright rest position on
the flying rings becomes even more difficult because the supporting muscles must
also contend with a center of gravity which is in motion from the swinging action
of the rings.

Mounts and vaults

A good number of mounts and vaults are very much alike during the initial
phases. They involve a leg spring combined with a downward-backward thrust by
the arms. It is very important that the arm and leg actions are precisely timed

so they complement each other. As the center of gravity rises and the arms assume support of the body weight, it is important that the arms are completely straight to achieve the highest possible point of elevation. At this point the mount and the vault differ. The vault requires the momentum of the original thrust to continue in order to provide clearance of the apparatus by the body; whereas, the mount requires the performer to control the momentum in order to assume (usually) a resting support position. This dissipation of momentum can be aided partially by a slightly different direction of thrust (more upward) than that of the vault, but, mostly, it requires controlled absorption of the force of the thrust. This absorption calls for muscle contractions which gradually bring the body to a stop in the desired rest position.

Skills while suspended from the arms

Suspending the body from the arms tends to separate the joints, especially in the arms and shoulders. Therefore, the muscles must partially contract to protect the connective tissues at the joints; and a strong and enduring handgrip is necessary.

Grasps

Effect grasps depend primarily upon the strength-endurance of the finger and thumb flexor muscles. Grasps are more secure, especially during swinging or

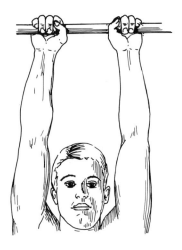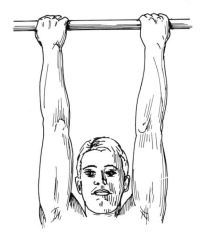

a   *b*

Figure 20–4.
Grips. (*a*) Forward; (*b*) reverse.

circling movements, if the thumbs encircle the apparatus opposite the fingers. During swinging or circling, it must be decided whether a forward or reverse grip is best. The decision mainly depends upon the direction of the action. The guide which applies is that the greatest amount of centrifugal force in the movement should be directed toward the palm, rather than toward the opening between the thumb and fingers. For instance, in the giant swing, where the body circles the bar in a forward direction, the forward grip (palms forward) is preferred. If the giant swing were done in the opposite (backward) direction, then the reverse grip would be used.

Hangs

Hanging by the hands taxes the muscles very little—except for the handgrip muscles. In fact, such a position can be very relaxing to all parts of the body except the hands, and it can be used to increase muscle flexibility in various portions of the body if the muscles are purposely relaxed during the hang.

A special kind of hang, the *iron cross on the rings*, can only be accomplished with very strong and sustained contractions of the muscles of the arms and

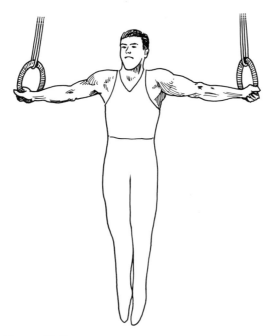

Figure 20–5.
The iron cross hang illustrates poor mechanical ratio
and the need for very strong muscle contractions.

shoulders. The performer starts in an upright support position and slowly spreads the rings sideward until his arms are abducted to the horizontal position. He then holds this position. The performer counteracts the pull of gravity by strongly contracting the shoulder girdle adductor (retractor) and depressor muscles, the adductors of the shoulders, the extensors of the elbows, and the wrist and finger flexors. The skill requires extreme strength because of very poor leverage in this position. The resistance arms of the main levers (from each hand to the shoulder joints) are very long in proportion to the length of the effort arms. The resistance arms can be shortened slightly by edging the rings closer to the wrists, thus placing them near the heels of the hands, and by flexing the elbows very slightly. Stronger muscles of the arm and shoulder regions may be brought into action by rotating the arms and shoulders forward.

Swings and circles

In vigorous swings, especially the giant swing on the high bar, an unusual amount of strength is required in the handgrip muscles. Other muscles of the arms and shoulders also must be very strong. Several mechanical factors apply to this category of skills; the most important are concerned with initiating and conserving angular momentum and contending with centrifugal force. In swinging, the body acts as a pendulum which swings as a result of certain muscles contracting and relaxing, causing the body to move toward the bar, then away from the bar at the right times. (In gymnastics these actions are restricted to certain joints, determined by acceptable form.) Gravity provides the force for gaining momentum, and consequently, the body length must be shortened on the upswing when gravity tends to decelerate the movement. Full body length is assumed on the downswing when gravity acts to accelerate the movement. This same principle is applied in all swinging actions, even in the case of playground swings. In working up on a playground swing, the performer crouches down during each downswing to move the weight farther away from the point of rotation, thus utilizing the force of gravity to gain momentum. During the upswing, he stands straight to move the body weight closer to the point of rotation, thus conserving momentum.

A circle in gymnastics is simply a swinging movement that continues through the full angular motion of the 360°. The skill on the horizontal bar known as the giant swing is actually a series of successive giant circles (see Figure 12–5).

Initiation of the swing. Swings are initiated by using muscular actions to place the center of gravity away from the point directly below the support so that gravity can initiate pendulum action. In some activities, such as the pole vault and certain gymnastic mounts, the force for starting the swing is the result of momentum developed in the approach. In gymnastics, if the performer begins from an arm suspension or arm support position on the apparatus, the starting action is called an upstart or a cast-off. Muscular actions project the center of gravity from its normal suspended position. Once this occurs, the force of gravity contributes to momentum of the swing. To begin a swing on the high bar from a hang, for example, the performer pulls upward and forward to move his center of gravity in that direction. At this point he extends his body to lengthen the radius of rotation. The extension enables gravity to exert its greatest force toward the pendulum action of the body.

If the performer is to do a back hip circle on the high bar, he begins from a front support position. The center of gravity is projected backward and slightly upward away from the bar. This movement provides linear momentum as the hips return to the bar. This momentum is converted to angular momentum as the hips meet the bar at a slightly lower point than the level of the starting position. The hips are then flexed to conserve the angular momentum during the time that the lower portion of the body is moving forward and upward against gravity. This same principle is applied on the parallel bars when the forward cast is used in swinging up to a handstand position. In this case, the forward-upward movement of the lower body from the support position leads to the position from which gravity can act on the body to produce momentum for the swing.

Kip.   The kip is a movement from a swing (suspension) in which the center of gravity is raised to a point that enables the performer to pull himself to a support position in a single thrust. It may be done on the rings, parallel bars, or horizontal bar. The principles are essentially the same, regardless of the apparatus on which it is performed. Its success is highly dependent upon precise timing.

At the end of the forward swing, forceful shoulder extension, trunk flexion, and hip flexion elevate the center of gravity to a level comparable to that in the support position. As the backswing begins, trunk and hip extension are quickly and powerfully applied when the body's center of gravity passes below the bar. This is the critical time. The hip extension at the bottom of the backward swing shortens the radius of the angular motion (brings the center of gravity close to the handgrip). The force of hip extension produces angular motion of the total

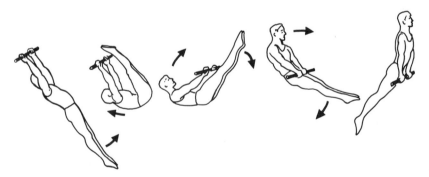

Figure 20–6.
Kip on the high bar illustrates importance of quick and correctly timed weight shifts.

body at the time when the handgrip and the center of gravity are at about the same height. The hips are kept close to the handgrip, and if the force of momentum is great enough, the arms can shift from suspension to support so the performance will be successful.

Regrasps and dismounts while swinging.   At either end of a swing, velocity is zero; at about the middle of the swing arc, velocity is maximum. It is obvious, then, that all regrasping (adjusting or changing the grip) and most dismounting maneuvers are easier at either end of the swing where there is no need to contend with momentum. If the grip release is inappropriately timed and too much momentum from the swing is retained, maintaining balance upon landing is difficult, if not impossible.

Travels while suspended

Traveling in an arm-suspended position may be in a horizontal direction, as in hand travel on an overhead horizontal ladder, or in a vertical direction, as in the rope climb. Progression in a horizontal direction is accomplished by trunk rotation to the left as the right hand reaches forward and the left hand maintains the grip. The lower body naturally turns in the opposite direction (Newton's third law of motion), becoming a preparatory movement for the development of momentum for the succeeding reach. The succeeding reach brings a reversal of the actions of the previous reach. The longer the reach, the greater is the momentum resulting from the swing. Within reason, then, longer strides are more efficient. Shorter strides may be advantageous to a weak individual because of the shorter period of time needed to support himself with one arm during each swing. However, the slower progress results in additional taxing of the muscles.

Most of the same points apply to vertical travels (climbing) as apply to horizontal travels. A high reach is advantageous provided the elbow does not fully extend. A fully extended elbow places the flexors of that joint under a severe mechanical disadvantage. The reaching action should come primarily from shoulder joint flexion, shoulder girdle elevation, spinal rotation (to the side opposite the reaching arm), and a slight lateral pendulum action of the body, which adds to the vertical momentum. The major propelling force should be provided by the large back muscles (especially the latissimus dorsi), which contribute to shoulder joint extension, adduction, and inward rotation. Shoulder girdle depression and elbow flexion are also very important. Hip flexion of the leg opposite the pulling arm results in a transfer of momentum which contributes to the upward body lift. Much skill is needed for efficiency in the rope climb, and the more skillful climbers require less strength. If the legs are used in contact with the rope, they wrap around the rope and push.

Either of these travels (horizontal or vertical) is accomplished with greater ease if the actions are continuous because then the loss of momentum is not permitted before the application of the next force. If momentum is lost, each stroke encounters greater inertia (Newton's second law of motion).

Principles of muscular involvement

Some muscular actions in arm-supported and arm-suspended skills are deceptive and obscure. A few generalizations may be helpful to the student attempting to analyze muscular actions.

Stabilization

Stabilization in arm support positions almost invariably requires contractions of opposing muscle groups in nearly all planes of movement, chiefly because the bone structure of the upper extremities is not designed to bear heavy weight. For example, in the upright arm support position on the parallel bars, the shoulder joint flexor and extensor muscles actively oppose each other, but no apparent movement takes place. The abductors and adductors and medial and lateral rotators also act in similar fashion.

Shoulder girdle muscles

It is often difficult to comprehend which muscles acting on the shoulder girdle are bearing the body weight because the muscular actions are often opposite what they appear to be. To illustrate, during a hang from an overhead support, the shoulder girdle is elevated, but the elevators are not contracting. Rather, the depressors contract to hold the scapulae from being pulled completely out of position; these muscles oppose the pull of gravity on the body.

If the performer is in an arm-supported position with the body upright and vertical (support positions on various types of gymnastic apparatus), then the depressors are again active. If the body is vertical but inverted (handstand), the shoulder girdle elevators are contracted. In front support positions (push-ups and various starting stances), the scapular abductors become very active regardless of the specific scapular position.

In all the foregoing instances, the contractions are isometric (static) although the muscles may be either at resting length, elongated, or shortened, depending on the stabilized position of the shoulder girdle.

If we keep in mind the concept of the movable girdle, the nonmoving arms, and the pull of gravity on the body, then muscular actions in the various positions become more clear. When analyzing an arm support position, it is helpful to think of the body weight being transferred directly through the supporting arms to push the shoulder girdle in that direction.

Contractions causing little or no apparent movement

Although no movement is observed at a particular joint, it is still important to assess the muscular actions present. A case in point is the action of the elbow flexors during the rope climb. It was pointed out earlier that little flexion or extension of this joint is noticed during skillful climbing. This does not suggest an absence of muscular activity in the elbow. During the time that the weight is supported, the flexors of the bent elbow are highly active to prevent the pull of gravity from forcing the elbow to extend. A similar illustration is the use of the shoulder girdle elevators in the hand walk.

The role of kinesthesis in arm-support balance skills

As a result of the kinesthetic sense and other senses associated with balance activities, such as a handstand, a constant flow of sensory information makes the performer aware of adjustments in muscular contractions that are needed to maintain the balanced position. The result of such information is the addition of nervous impulses to the proper muscles, at the proper time, and of proper intensity to correct the body position and keep the body in equilibrium. If a person has a strong kinesthetic sense, he is acutely aware of the exact positions of body parts, and he knows of deviations from the desired positions. This awareness makes it possible for him to initiate quickly correct adjustments in body position. The muscle contractions which maintain balance are constantly varying for several reasons, the most significant of which is fatigue of active motor units and their replacement by other motor units. This explains loss of balance from expending muscular endurance. The switch must be made from the fatigued motor units to fresh ones, which temporarily changes the kinesthetic information. Eventually, an insufficient number of rested motor units are available, and balance is threatened due to fatigue.

Improving arm-supported and arm-suspended skills

For effective performance of arm-supported and arm-suspended skills, two primary qualities are essential. They are (1) *adequate strength and endurance* to support the body in the necessary positions and (2) *ability to shift the body weight quickly* into the correct positions at the right time. The first quality (strength) is dependent upon the three factors which compose it, namely, contractile forces of the mover muscles, ability to coordinate all the muscles involved in the movement, and the mechanical ratios involved. If the person lacks adequate arm and shoulder strength to support the body with ease, it is impossible for him to effectively perform skills in arm support positions. Therefore, additional strength may be the key to improving performance—up to a certain point. If the skill calls for prolonged or successive contractions, then muscle endurance, in addition to strength, becomes important.

The second primary quality, ability to shift the body into correct positions at exactly the right time, depends on the following several specific factors: (1) *Insight into the task to be accomplished.* This requires a vision of the specific movements that must occur and their correct sequence. (2) *Adequate kinesthetic perception.* This is demonstrated by the degree to which one remains aware of the exact position of the body and its parts in space. (3) *Agility.* This is very important because it is the ability to change direction of the body and its parts rapidly. (4) *Fast reactions.* Fast reactions contribute to agility, and the two factors combined contribute greatly to one's ability to make fast adjustments in body position in order to maintain balance and perform desired movements with precision. (5) *Coordination.* Specific neuromuscular coordinations are essential; they may be improved from repeated practice of the specific skill. (6) *Precision and timing.* In arm-supported skills, the specific movements of body segments must be executed with great precision and timing. Any movement made out of sequence or with insufficient quickness and precision will detract from a successful performance.

A training program for improving these kinds of skills should include the following: (1) Exercises to increase strength and endurance of the muscles which carry the heavy loads during the performances and exercises to increase flexibility, especially in the hip, back, and shoulder regions. (2) When the skill is very complex, it should be broken into parts so that each part may be studied and practiced; then the skill should be put together in total sequence. (It is important not to segment a skill too much, because good performance usually requires a smooth flow of movements throughout the performance.) (3) The skill as a whole should be practiced extensively in order to improve coordination, timing, and form throughout the performance.

Recommended supplementary reading

Bunn, John W.: "Scientific Principles of Coaching," chap. 13, Prentice-Hall, Inc., Englewood Cliffs, N.J., 1955.

Cooper, John M., and Ruth B. Glassow: "Kinesiology," 2d ed., chap. 14, The C. V. Mosby Company, St. Louis, 1968.

21

Performance in water

hen a person moves from a solid surface into water, he experiences different problems involving performance. Correct solution to these problems requires special knowledge about such matters as buoyancy, propulsive forces in water, resistive forces in water, and correct mechanics of various swimming strokes.

Buoyancy

According to Archimedes' principle, "a body emersed in fluid is buoyed up with a force equal to the weight of the displaced fluid." This means that if a body displaces water weighing more than itself, the body will float. A rock displaces water weighing less than its weight, therefore the rock sinks. A cork displaces water weighing more than it weighs, therefore a cork floats.

When a body displaces water weighing exactly the same as it weighs, it has a specific gravity of 1. In other words, its density is identical to the density of water. When expressed in a formula:

$$\text{Specific gravity} = \frac{\text{weight of the body}}{\text{weight of an equal volume of water}}$$

If a human body has a specific gravity of less than 1, it will float. If its specific gravity is 1, the body will sink barely below the surface. The farther the specific gravity is above 1, the deeper the body will sink.

Specific gravity of most human beings is slightly less than 1 (with lungs filled with air), meaning that people are generally buoyant. However, a few people are not buoyant. With lungs filled, nearly all adults will float; with lungs empty, almost all adults will sink.

The factor that most influences density of the body, and therefore its buoyancy, is percentage of weight composed of bone and muscle. Bone and muscle tissues are more dense than other body tissues. On the average, men have a higher percentage of bone and muscle than women; therefore, women are more buoyant. For this reason, children are more buoyant than adults, and fat people are more buoyant than skinny people.

Floats

The best test for buoyancy is either the tuck (jellyfish) or pike float. In these positions, a portion of the upper back protrudes above the water's surface if the body is buoyant. A person who is buoyant in one of these positions can learn to float in either a vertical or supine position with the face out of the water. Whether a person floats in a vertical or a supine position depends on his body build, which determines the position of the body's center of gravity. Women's centers of gravity are proportionately lower than men's; therefore, women float in nearly a supine position. Men typically float in nearly a vertical position.

Locomotion in water

Several different strokes and kicks are effectively used to propel the body through water. But regardless of the particular swimming technique used, certain basic facts apply.

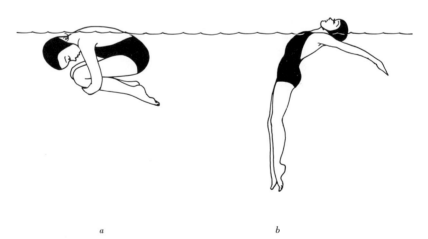

a   *b*

Figure 21–1.
Floating positions. (*a*) Tuck float; (*b*) vertical float.

In swimming there are propelling forces and resistive forces. The propelling forces result from the stroke and kick. Resistive forces result from (1) skin resistance (friction), (2) wave-making resistance, and (3) eddy resistance. Skin resistance is by far the most important factor in most cases. In attempting to improve swimming skill, the general objective should be to bring about changes which increase the propelling forces and decrease resistive forces. This can be accomplished by assuming correct body positions and by correctly executing the strokes and kicks with sufficient force.

Resisting force.   Body position in the water has great influence on resistance to forward progress. The body should be kept near parallel to the water's surface and should present as little body area as possible in the direction of progress. Available evidence from research indicates: (1) The prone position offers less resistance than either the back or side swimming positions. (2) As body rolling action is increased, water resistance increases. (3) At very slow swimming speeds (2 feet per second), resistance is greater than at faster speeds (5 feet per second), primarily bcause at the slower speed correct (horizontal) position is not maintained. As speed increases beyond 5 feet per second, resistance increases rapidly. (4) Tight-fitting suits made of lightweight silk or nylon cause no measurable resistance. The same, however, is not true of cotton and wool suits, although the fit of the suit is more significant than the fabric; loose-fitting suits offer considerably more resistance.

Incorrect techniques of recovery of the stroke and kick can add greatly to resistance. Recovery should be designed to present as little surface of the arms and legs as possible in the direction of progress. Up-and-down movements of the body increase the wave-making forces, which add to resistance. Therefore, vertical motion of the body should be held to a minimum; in other words, the body should move smoothly in a straight line. The force of inertia can be another source of added resistance if a steady pace is not maintained. Changes in speed result in greatly increased resistance during the acceleration.

Another important source of resistance, although not water resistance, is internal muscle resistance resulting from inability to use a "relaxed" swimming style. Because of the tenseness of some swimmers, the antagonist muscles fail to relax sufficiently to cause free and efficient movement.

Propelling forces.   In applying the forces that propel the body through the water, the following guides are important: (1) Almost all the forces should contribute to forward progress, and not to vertical or lateral body movement. (2) A swimmer should seek maximum water resistance against the stroking and kicking movements and minimum resistance against the counter (recovery) movements of the stroke and kick. This means that during the propelling phase, the arms, hands, and feet should present as large a surface as possible to the water, and

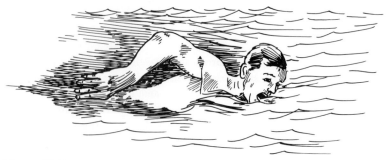

Figure 21–2.
Good body position and correct breathing techniques in the crawl stroke.

the arm and hand should *push* against the water, opposite the direction of progress. (3) The forces should be applied with speed sufficient to propel the body at an efficient rate; however, the application of forces should not be so great that they are inefficient in terms of energy cost. There is a certain pace for each swimmer which is most efficient, just as there is a certain running pace that is most efficient.

Following are analyses of the four competitive swimming strokes. Space does not permit analysis of other swimming strokes.

Front crawl stroke

It has been observed that excellent crawl-stroke swimmers get at least 70 percent of their propulsion from the arms and 30 percent or less from the legs. However, this ratio varies considerably among individuals. Occasionally, a good swimmer is observed who obtains almost all his propulsion from the arm stroke.

To reduce the resistive forces in the crawl stroke a swimmer should (1) swim with his head down (face under the water), turning the face to the side only far enough to breathe on every second stroke; (2) keep the whole body near parallel to the surface of the water, thus presenting the smallest body surface possible to the direction of movement; (3) eliminate all actions which move the body up and down or sideward; (4) wear a tight-fitting silk or nylon-type suit.

The stroke.   To benefit the most from the applied forces in the stroke, the arm and hand should push *backward* against the water's resistance. The counterforce will then be forward and equal to the applied force (Newton's third law). During the early and late phases of the stroke, it is difficult to apply the force directly opposite the direction of progress. When strong force is applied during the early phase, it tends to lift the body, whereas the late phase of the stroke tends to pull the body downward. This problem can be partly eliminated by flexing the wrist at the beginning of the stroke and hyperextending it during the late phase. This causes the palm of the hand to face the desired direction throughout the stroke. However, it still remains that the middle portion of the stroke is by far the most efficient, and the efficiency is the greatest when the arm is in the vertical position (at right angles to the body). Thus the application of force should be maximized during the middle portion of the stroke and minimized during the early and late portions. Bunn (**11**) claims that when the arm is at 45° from the horizontal, only about 70 percent of the force is effective in propelling the body forward. At 90° (vertical), 100 percent of the force is effective.

The crawl stroke starts with the arm fully extended and the hand directly in front of the shoulder. As the arm begins movement through the water, the elbow flexes slightly, and the wrist flexes enough to cause the hand to push backward instead of downward against the water. The shoulder dips deep as it moves backward with the arm. During the middle part of the stroke, medial rotation of the arm is added which speeds the movement of the hand and forearm. The hand passes directly under the midline of the body. Near completion of the stroke, the wrist hyperextends to keep the hand in a pushing position, and the elbow extends to complete the pushing action.

The muscles which contribute most to the stroke are the shoulder girdle depressors, shoulder extensors and adductors, upper-arm medial rotators, elbow extensors, and wrist flexors. During the recovery phase, the most active muscles are the shoulder girdle elevators, along with the shoulder abductors and extensors, and the elbow extensors.

The kick. The flutter kick is executed faster than the stroke. Most good swimmers execute either four or six kicks per stroke cycle. Most of the muscular force for the kick comes from the hips, but the feet actually cause the propulsion. The up-and-down drive from the hips causes the legs to follow through and finally results in a slapping (whiplike) movement of the feet. The foot action closely parallels the propelling tail action of a fish. When a fish swims, the driving force comes from movement of the fish's body, which results in slapping-type movements of the tail. The tail movements provide most of the propelling force. The fish's tail moves horizontally, but the swimmer's feet move vertically.

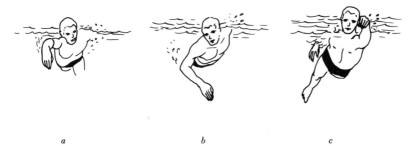

a   *b*   *c*

Figure 21–3.
Correct mechanics of the crawl stroke (front view).

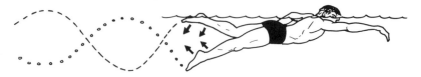

Figure 21–4.
Illustration of propelling forces from the flutter kick.

On the down kick, the knee, which has a controlled amount of tension, bends as a result of water force. This bending puts the foot in position so the top (instep) pushes backward and downward against the water, thus propelling the body forward. The ankle must be in a fully extended (plantar flexed) position during the early part of the down kick; at the completion of the down kick, the ankle is partly flexed and the knee is extended. On the up kick, the bottom (sole) of the foot provides force against the water in a backward and upward direction. The foot moves from its partially flexed position to full extension at the completion of the kick. The knee remains straight throughout the up kick.

The depth of the kicking action should be 15 to 18 inches for adult men, and proportionately less for smaller people. It has been found that increased ankle flexibility will cause more foot action and thus more propulsive force from the flutter kick.

The muscles used most extensively in the flutter kick are the hip flexors and extensors, knee extensors, and ankle flexors and extensors. In addition to the muscles causing the stroke and kick, other muscle groups are used extensively in the crawl stroke. The abdominal and lower back muscles stabilize the pelvic region, and the trunk rotator muscles rotate the trunk in time to the stroking rhythm.

Back crawl stroke

The backstroke is somewhat less powerful and less efficient than the front crawl. In the backstroke, a higher proportion of the propelling force comes from the kick (about 35 percent among good swimmers).

The principles relating to resistive forces are the same for the backstroke as those stated earlier for the front crawl. The primary differences between the two swimming methods are (1) the backstroke is performed on the back with the face above the water and the head tilted slightly upward and (2) the stroking action of the backstroke is executed more in the horizontal rather than vertical plane.

The idea of pushing with the hands opposite the direction of progress is equally important in the backstroke as in the front crawl. The main muscles

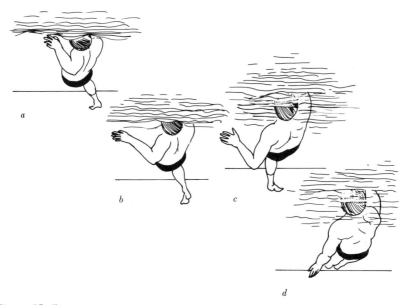

Figure 21–5.
Correct mechanics of the back crawl stroke.

involved in this stroke are the shoulder girdle depressors, shoulder adductors, flexors and medial rotators, elbow extensors, and wrist flexors.

The flutter kick on the back is the same as on the front, except in the reverse direction. The feet should ride high in the water so the toes break the surface at the completion of the up kick. But no part of the kick should be out of the water.

Breaststroke

The main guiding principle for the breaststroke, as for every other swimming style, is "maximum efficiency and minimum effort." But it has another basic rule—"symmetry of movement"—which it shares with the fourth and last stroke to be discussed, the butterfly.

Mechanically, the ideal body position is in the horizontal plane, with the body streamlined. Two factors may cause variation from this position. First, breathing necessitates that the face be clear of the water, which is likely to place the body somewhat at an angle. Second, if the body is too horizontal, the feet will break the water's surface and part of the kicking force will be destroyed.

The stroke.   The breaststroke is really only a "half-stroke," executed quickly and forcefully.

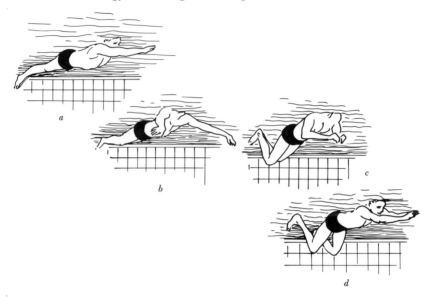

Figure 21–6.
Correct body position and mechanics of the breaststroke.

The pull starts from the glide position with the arms fully extended and the hands in front of the head. The wrists flex to a 45° angle ready to pull slightly out, down, and forcefully back. As the hands move through the water, the elbows flex slightly and are held high above the hands. The hands move through a sideward-downward arc until the upper arms reach an angle of 90° to the body. The pull is completed before the arms move past the imaginary perpendicular line extended out from the shoulders. The muscles which contribute most to the pull are wrist flexors, lower arm medial rotators, elbow flexors, upper arm medial rotators, and shoulder extensors and adductors.

The arm recovery is no more than a bringing together of the hands underneath the chin, followed by a quick smooth forward thrust of both hands as the swimmer moves into a glide position.

The kick.   The "whip kick" which is used in the breaststroke, may contribute as much as 50 percent of the total propelling force among good swimmers. In the whip kick, unlike in other kicks, the lower legs and knees play a more important part than do the hips and thighs.

Beginning from the glide position, the swimmer flexes his knees, bringing the lower legs up and over the knees. The ankles are fully flexed and the feet turned outward (Figure 21–7). While the knees are kept close together, the ankles are separated far apart. The kick is then executed by pushing the feet backward and together in a whiplike motion until the legs are fully extended. The ankles extend during the kick to cause a pushing action with the bottoms of the feet.

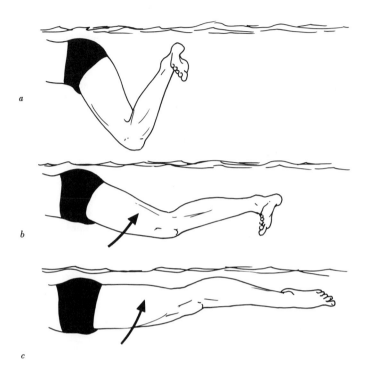

Figure 21–7.
Correct mechanics of the whip kick.

During the last half of the stroke, the legs recover from the kick (move to kicking position). As the arms recover from the stroke, the kick is executed, followed by a glide. The complete cycle is stroke-kick-glide.

The muscles used most extensively in the recovery phase of the whip kick are the knee and ankle flexors and the hip flexors and medial rotators. The knee and ankle extensors and hip adductors are the prime contributors to the power phase of the kick.

Butterfly stroke

The butterfly was derived from the orthodox breaststroke style. But the butterfly is now characterized by an overarm recovery and the dolphin kick.

The butterfly stroke is nearly the same as the front crawl stroke, except the arms and legs move simultaneously in the butterfly whereas they move alternately in the crawl stroke. The principles involved and the mechanics of the strokes and kicks are very similar.

The stroke.   Refer to pages 342 to 344 for a description of the crawl stroke. The butterfly stroke differs from that description in only two ways: (1) the arms move simultaneously and (2) the hands pass underneath the shoulders rather than under the midline of the body.

The kick.   The butterfly kick is called the *dolphin kick* because of its resemblance to that ocean mammal. The kick is difficult to master because it involves both trunk and leg movements. Also its timing with the arm pull is difficult. The driving force for the kick begins with an up-and-down movement of the hips. This initiates movements in the hip, knee, and ankle joints and results in whiplike movements of the legs and feet. The leg action is very similar to the flutter kick, but in the dolphin kick, the driving force is initiated farther up the body. The two legs move simultaneously in the same plane. Most good butterfly swimmers use two complete kicks for every complete arm cycle.

To explain the coordination of the hips and legs, one should be aware that with every downward movement of the legs, the hips tend to raise an inch or two;

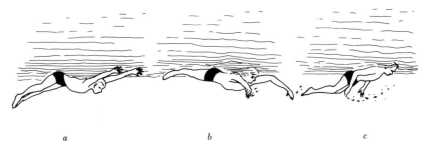

a   b   c

Figure 21–8.
Body action during the butterfly stroke.

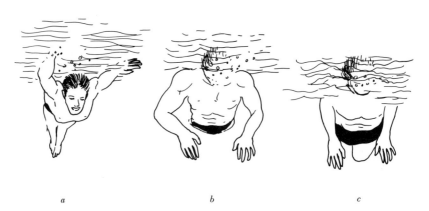

a   b   c

Figure 21–9.
Correct mechanics of the butterfly stroke.

therefore with every upward movement of the legs, the hips tend to submerge a few inches.

The muscles which contribute to the butterfly kick are the same as those that contribute to the freestyle or flutter kick (see pages 343–344).

Recommended supplementary reading

BROER, MARION R.: "Efficiency of Human Movement," 2d ed., chap. 24, W. B. Saunders Company, Philadelphia, 1966.

BUNN, JOHN W.: "Scientific Principles of Coaching," chap. 11, Prentice-Hall, Inc., Englewood Cliffs, N.J., 1955.

COOPER, JOHN M., and RUTH B. GLASSOW: "Kinesiology," 2d ed., chap. 15, The C. V. Mosby Company, St. Louis, 1968.

22

Summary of how to improve performance

*I*t is now appropriate to reintroduce the *immediate* function of the teacher, coach, and therapist: to help people increase their ability to perform. This book has aimed to prepare the reader to give people this kind of help by providing insight into the factors within and outside the body that influence performance. In summary, the present chapter identifies the components of excellent performance and discusses the contribution of each.

Three major aspects are involved in achieving excellent performance. The first aspect is psychological readiness, the extent to which the performer is psychologically ready to make his best effort at the given time. The second aspect is anatomical and physiological preparation. This includes conditioning the body and learning specific skills. The third aspect is application of natural laws and principles which influence performance. Although this text does not discuss the psychological aspect, it is very important and should not be minimized.

Anatomical and physiological components of performance

These components are two types: *general* and *specific*. The general components combined make up what is referred to as general athletic ability. The specific components are skills (neuromuscular coordinations) specific to the performance. General athletic ability includes such components as strength, endurance, agility, and flexibility. Specific skills are skills such as throwing, shooting, and jumping. If a performer has a large amount of general athletic ability (possesses general components in large amounts), we say he is a "natural athlete." But he will be unable to perform well in a particular activity until, through long hours of practice, he develops the skills specific to that performance. For example, endurance, agility, reaction time, power, and speed are all general athletic components of performance in basketball, and they are equally important in soccer, football, baseball, track, field, and various other sports. However shooting accuracy, dribbling, and rebounding are all specific skills unique to basketball, not needed in anywhere near the same amount in other sports.

A decathlon champion obviously possesses abundant general athletic ability, along with specific skills required in the decathlon events. However, he will not do well in tennis until he develops the specific skills of tennis; nor will he bowl a high score until he develops accuracy in bowling; nor will he succeed in soccer until he learns to handle the ball, play correct field positions, and execute defensive skills.

The term natural athlete does not necessarily mean "inborn." *Capacity* is inherited, but *use* greatly influences the level of general athletic ability. A gifted person may possess relatively low levels of this ability and others with less endowment may display more athletic ability due to experience in athletics.

Each kind of performance is different from any other one. In some cases different performances involve many of the same components, but in different amounts. The challenge to the teacher and coach is (1) to identify the components essential to a particular performance, (2) to determine the relative importance of the components, and (3) to design instructional and training programs which will develop the components in proportion to their importance.

Components of general athletic ability

Several components are common to good performance in a number of different activities. These components also seem to form the base on which specific skills may be developed.

Strength.   The amount of force that a person can apply with a particular part of the body is the strength of that part. This definition implies the importance of strength in athletic performance. Even though nearly all human movements are performed against some resistance, athletic movements usually involve greater resistance than normal. For instance, in putting the shot, throwing the discus, pole-vaulting, gymnastic movements, jumping, running, swimming, leaping, and other such vigorous movements, the body segments apply near-maximum force, and the amount of force that can be applied has strong influence on success of the performance. Because strength is so important to athletic performance, let us analyze how it contributes.

Strength is essentially a result of (1) the combined contractile forces of the several agonist muscles causing the movement, (2) mechanical ratios of the particular lever arrangements, and (3) ability to coordinate all the mover muscles into a unified force and to coordinate them with the antagonist and stabilizer muscles.

It is interesting to note that strength is a basic element in several other components important to performance. Thus strength takes on unusual significance. Physical *power* is the ability to project the body or an object through space (or to do work against time). Power is basic to jumping activities (projecting the body) and to throwing and putting activities (projecting an object). When expressed in a formula, power = force × velocity (or work divided by time). Increased strength causes increased ability to apply force. Therefore, if velocity remains constant, increased strength contributes to increased power. This idea is supported by several research studies.

Strength is also a basic element in *muscular endurance*. Endurance is the ability to resist fatigue and to recover quickly after fatigue. It enables a performer to persist at a given level of performance. If a weak muscle can perform a movement against a given resistance fifty times, then a stronger muscle can perform against the same resistance with greater ease; therefore, it can repeat the movement considerably more than fifty times. This means that if all else is equal, increased strength causes increased muscular endurance. This idea is well supported by research. Of course, endurance is dependent upon the efficient functioning of several different body systems, but muscular strength is one of the important elements.

Strength contributes to *agility* which is defined as the ability to change direction of the body or its parts rapidly. Agility is demonstrated in such activities as dodging shuttle runs, zigzag runs, and the squat thrust. Agility is essential to good performance in field games—such as football, soccer, and hockey—and court games—such as basketball, tennis, volleyball, and badminton. Changing the direction of the body or its parts calls for adequate muscular strength to overcome the force of momentum which tends to keep the body moving in the same direction. After the direction has been changed, strength (really power of which strength is a part) is important in regaining momentum in the new direction of movement. Without adequate strength a high level of agility is impossible.

Strength is important to *running speed*, which is basic to performance in many activities. Actually, running speed is closely related to power because running is a series of body projections made alternately from the right and left feet. In running, the body is thrust forward by the force of body levers pushing against a resistive surface. If all else remains equal, increased strength will cause increased application of force, which will improve running speed.

Thus it becomes evident that strength makes a very large contribution to many forms of athletics. The coach and athlete should give adequate attention to strengthening those muscle groups which contribute directly to the desired movements. Methods of developing desired strength are explained in Chapter 8.

Even though strength influences performance in several ways, it should not be thought of as a panacea. More strength is not always the answer to improving performance; in many cases, other components fill the need better.

Endurance (muscular and circulorespiratory).   A high level of endurance implies that the performer can persist at a given level. When endurance gives way to fatigue as a result of muscular work, several elements which are important to good performance diminish. Fatigue results in reduction of strength, neuromuscular coordination and timing, speed of movement, reaction time, accuracy, and general alertness. Increased endurance prolongs the onset of fatigue; therefore, endurance contributes to improved performance in activities where fatigue may be a restricting factor.

Power.   The ability to project the body or an object through space is dependent upon power. Obviously, the ability to project the body is important in many performances, including basketball, volleyball, football, some track and field events, gymnastics, dance, and running. The ability to project an object is equally important in such activities as track and field throwing events, baseball, softball, basketball, and football. Ability to project the body or an object can be increased by improving one or both of the factors (force and velocity) which contribute to power. The application of force is increased by increasing strength. Velocity is dependent upon the speed of muscular contractions, which can be increased as a result of speed training.

Improved coordination through a particular movement pattern will also improve power in that particular movement. Therefore, specific power can be favorably influenced by practicing specific skills. Power is specific to body segments, meaning that a person can develop a great amount of power in the legs, for instance, and remain relatively unpowerful in the arms. Power in different areas of the body is influenced by the amount and kind of training the person has.

Agility.   The ability to make a rapid change in direction of the body or its parts depends primarily on strength, reaction time, speed of movement, and specific coordinations. Agility is important in activities involving dodging and fast starting and stopping actions, as well as those requiring a series of quick movements of body segments. Agility in specific movement patterns can be increased by practicing those movements, thereby increasing coordinations contributing to the movements. Also, increased strength will increase agility in movements where momentum tends to keep the body in motion in the same direction. Other factors which determine agility, namely, speed of movement and reaction time, may be increased as a result of specific training. But these factors can be influenced only a limited amount. Like power, agility in a specific movement pattern can be favorably influenced by improving coordination in that particular movement, which is accomplished best by correctly practicing the particular movement over and over.

Running speed.   Running speed is an athletic event by itself and is also very important in performance of other athletic activities. To increase running speed, the performer must improve (1) length of stride, or (2) leg speed, or (3) length of stride and leg speed. Length of stride can be increased by *increasing power* of the muscle groups which are of prime importance in running (best possibility for improving speed) or by getting the runner to *lengthen his stride* consciously. Conscious lengthening of the stride has very limited possibilities for increasing speed, and lengthening the stride too much will have a detrimental effect.

The rate with which the legs can be moved while taking full running strides is dependent upon (1) reaction time, (2) coordination of the muscles involved, (3) speed of muscle contractions, and (4) strength (when movement is against a heavy resistance such as in projecting the body). If any of these factors is increased, then speed of leg movement will increase. But research and experience have proven that speed of movement can be increased only slightly as a result of training; nevertheless, a slight increase can have a significant effect on performance.

A sprinter may sometimes reduce his time considerably by improving parts of his race other than running speed. For instance, he may develop a better starting technique; or improve his ability to accelerate; or learn to run more efficiently, thereby becoming less tired; or improve his finishing technique.

Reaction time.   Reaction time is the time which lapses between the external stimulus and the initial response to that stimulus. It is extremely important in all performances where quick movements are required, and it has special significance in events in which individuals must defend against each other. Here contestants must respond to each other's movements. There is evidence that reaction time in specific movements will improve a limited amount as a result of extensive practice of those movements, and even a small increase may produce significant results in performance. It is difficult to say whether it is possible to improve reaction time in general by training.

Flexibility.   Flexibility is determined by the elasticity of the muscles, tendons, and ligaments. Lack of flexibility restricts full range of motion in the joints. However, range of motion may also be restricted by other factors, such as bone structure and size of tissue (muscle or other) near the joint. A certain degree of flexibility is important to performance in activities such as modern dance, gymnastics, and diving. In these performances, the body must be flexible enough to assume desired positions which demonstrate good form. The pike position, for example, requires great flexibility in the backs of the upper legs and the lower back. Specific performances which require unusual flexibility are the butterfly stroke, hurdling, high-jumping, ballet and modern dancing, and gymnastics.

Flexibility can be increased by regular stretching of the muscles, tendons, and ligaments. The best approach is to determine the tissues which need to be stretched, place them on stretch, hold the position for a few seconds, and repeat the steps several times. The muscles should be stretched until a stretch pain is felt. This procedure must be followed regularly. Bouncing is not recommended; slow stretch is both safer and more effective.

It should be remembered that too much flexibility may make a joint injury prone, because excessive flexibility reduces the stability of a joint. But in most instances, performers could profit by increased flexibility at certain joints without detrimental effects.

Specific skills

Skill is the ability to execute a combination of specific movements smoothly and efficiently. It is the effective coordination of all the different muscles involved, whether they are agonists, antagonists, neutralizers, or stabilizers. In other terms, skill may be defined as the ability to use the correct muscles at the correct time, with the exact force necessary to perform the desired movements in the proper sequence. An athletic performance consists of several specific skills, and each skill involves one or more movements of body segments. Therefore, to take a systematic and effective approach to improving performance, a person must analyze the specific skills composing the performance and then attempt to improve those skills. For example, basketball is composed of such skills as running, rebounding, jumping, dodging, dribbling, passing, and catching. Basketball performance may be improved by greater facility in one or more of these specific skills.

The problem, then, is to identify the specific skills in a performance and employ effective techniques to improve them. Essentially, skill improvement amounts to determining the correct mechanics and incorporating them into the performance. The skill must be practiced correctly over and over until the movement patterns become naturally smooth and efficient. As a result of such practice, the performer will increase his skill by judgment of speed, distance and time, smoothness and efficiency in movement, and insight into the various circumstances of the performance.

Accuracy.   Accuracy is demonstrated in such skills as shooting in basketball, throwing or passing in baseball, softball, and football, shooting in archery, or rolling a bowling ball. Regardless of how smoothly and beautifully a player shoots the basketball, unless the ball goes through the basket a high percentage of the time, the player is ineffective. The same idea applies to the archer, marksman, quarterback, pitcher, and other accuracy performers. Accuracy in specific movements can be improved considerably through practice. Such improvement calls for many hours of repetitious performance of the skill. In practicing for accuracy, it is very important for the performer to do so at typical performance speed. Throwing a baseball accurately at slow speed is different than throwing accurately at a fast speed; performing a lay-up in basketball at slow speed requires different coordinations and judgments than performing the same skill at high speed. Under competitive conditions, most skills are performed with high speed and maximum effort. Often, slowing down the performance during practice will aid in analyzing the mechanics of the skill and in improving the movement patterns; but for best results, accuracy skills should be practiced extensively at the same speed and intensity as they will be performed in competition. Accuracy is dependent upon judgment of speed, distance, and time, along with a high degree of neuromuscular coordination.

Judgment of speed, distance, and time.   Judgment of speed and distance and time is important to a football player when he throws downfield to a running receiver. The passer must be able to judge the distance to the receiver and then throw the ball at the correct angle and speed to cause it to meet the receiver. If the receiver is moving, the passer must correctly judge the receiver's speed and the speed of the ball. In shooting a basketball, the player must correctly judge his distance from the basket, then he must have the muscular coordination necessary to put the ball where he judges it should go. If the post man passes to a guard cutting in for a lay-up, the passer must correctly judge the speed of the guard. When the guard lays up the shot, he must correctly judge his speed and the rebound ability of the ball and be sure that he puts the right touch on the ball so it will rebound into the basket. Other examples could be given of activities in which judgments of speed, distance, and time must be frequently made.

Smoothness and efficiency of performance.   Smooth and efficient performances result when (1) superfluous (noncontributing) movements are reduced to a minimum, (2) tension by antagonist muscles is reduced, and (3) correct timing of all contributing muscles is accomplished. The first factor is accomplished by identifying noncontributing motions and purposely eliminating them. For instance, in swimming, excessive head movement is noncontributing and detrimental to a smooth and efficient stroke. The same can be said about extraneous head, arm, or leg movements while running. The second factor may be accomplished (1) by developing an adequate amount of flexibility in the antagonist muscles and (2) by developing the neuromuscular coordination necessary to cause these muscles (antagonists) to relax more fully during the desired movements. The third factor can be accomplished only by extensive, correct practice of the movements under gamelike conditions, which will increase the coordination and efficiency of the muscle contractions.

Application of natural laws and principles

Natural laws and principles influence all motor performances. Of course, the influence of laws varies with the nature of the performance. To approach maximum potential in any performance, the performer must identify the laws and principles which influence that performance and apply them correctly.

Leverage

The amount of force applied with any body segment and the speed of movement of that segment are partly determined by the relative lengths of the effort and resistance arms of the levers employed. Often the relative lengths may be altered purposely by changing the body position. The extent to which correct leverage is used in a performance determines good body mechanics. It is extremely important that correct mechanics be employed; otherwise, maximum performance is not possible. Therefore, it becomes necessary that students learn the correct mechanics of movement in any given performance. The details of mechanics and how they apply to performance are covered in Part 3 of this text.

Motion and force

All performances involve motion of the body and often also involve motion of an object. Force and its application are always parts of performance; therefore knowledge of how to apply the basic principles of motion and force is essential to understanding and improving performances. These principles and their applications are discussed in Chapters 12 and 13.

Balance and stability

Balance of the body in both static and dynamic positions is important to all performances. In certain kinds of performances, balance is one of the prime objectives, and the extent to which a person is able to remain in a stable position often determines his success. Therefore, the application of the principles of balance and stability becomes basic to good performance. The content of Chapter 15 provides the important information about balance and stability.

Projecting, spinning, and rebounding of objects

Many performances involve the use of implements, which must be treated in certain ways to achieve the desired results. Understanding laws and principles relating to the use of these implements and how to control them is often a key to better performance. For example, it is necessary to know the optimum angle for projecting a javelin or discus. It is important to know the influence of spin on a volleyball, baseball, or tennis ball. A good performer must have insight into how a handball, basketball, or softball will rebound. Many of these kinds of insights are developed through extensive participation, but understanding and applying the basic laws and principles of projection, spinning, and rebounding can often be a short cut to better performance. The application of these laws and principles is discussed in Chapter 14.

Warm-up in preparation for performance

It is often claimed that warm-up accomplishes the following:

1. Increases the rate and strength of muscular contraction

2. Improves the necessary coordinations in the performance
3. Helps to prevent injury
4. Brings on second wind more readily in endurance activities
5. Allows the performer to adjust to his immediate environment

In attempting to evaluate the values of warm-up, the authors reviewed eight research reports which supported the values of warm-up and seven reports which found warm-up to be of no special value. Thus the utility of warm-up still remains in question.

Most coaches and athletes want to continue with warm-up until further evidence is accumulated. The authors advocate extensive warm-up on the theory that it does contribute to better performance and prevention of injury. But it must be recognized that indiscriminate warm-up may be energy wasting and may not warm up the certain essential muscles, regardless of the total amount of warm-up. The warm-up must be specific to the activity being performed, and should be increased in intensity as the performer becomes better conditioned. The timing of the warm-up is also very important. If there is a long delay between the warm-up and the performance, the beneficial effects of the warm-up may be reduced or eliminated.

Appendix *A*
Audio-visual aids for kinesiology

The following audio-visual aids are useful for teachers of kinesiology (**59**):

Charts

Large wall charts showing the anatomy of the human body are available from several sources. Charts of the muscular and skeletal systems are of great use in kinesiology, and charts of the nervous, circulatory, and respiratory systems are also helpful. Suggested sources of the charts are:

Denoyer-Geppert Co., 5235 Ravenswood Ave., Chicago, Ill. 60640.
Anatomical Chart Company, 5732 Blackstone Ave., Chicago, Ill. 60637.
Nystron Biological Model Co., Chicago, Ill. 60600.

Models

Of greatest use are models of the muscular and skeletal systems and of specific joints and bones. Following are sources of such models:

Merck, Sharp & Dohme, West Point, Pa. 19486.
J. A. Preston Corporation, 71 Fifth Ave., New York, N.Y. 10003.
Denoyer-Geppert Company, 5235 Ravenswood Ave., Chicago, Ill. 60640.
Clay-Adams Company, 141 E. 25th St., New York, N.Y. 10010.
Nystron Biological Model Co., Chicago, Ill. 60600.

Slides

The following picture slides are very useful:

A Stereoscopic Atlas of Human Anatomy, 3-D Kodachrome slides on the human body, The C. V. Mosby Co., St. Louis, Mo.

Slides on the human body by CIBA, Box 195, Summit, N.J. 07901.
Slides on the human body by Visual Aids, Inc., Box 2411 Village Station, Los Angeles, Calif. 90024.
Slides on the human body by Logan, Inc., Box 3535 Glenstone Station, Springfield, Mo. 65804.

Loop films

Many teachers choose to make their own loop films. But the following loop films, useful in teaching kinesiology, are available for purchase:

Loop films on a variety of sports, Athletic Institute, 805 Merchandise Mart, Chicago, Ill. 60654.
Loop films of track and field events, *Track & Field News*, P.O. Box 296, Los Altos, Calif. 94022.

Movie films

The following useful films may be purchased or rented:

Muscle Status, Indiana University Motion Picture Division, Bloomington, Ind.
Muscles, Indiana University Motion Picture Division, Bloomington, Ind.
Muscles and Bones of the Body, Indiana University Motion Picture Division, Bloomington, Ind.
The Skeleton, Britannica Films, Inc., 425 N. Michigan Ave., Chicago, Ill. 60601.
The Spinal Column, Britannica Films, Inc., 425 N. Michigan Ave., Chicago, Ill. 60601.
The Nervous System, Britannica Films, Inc., 425 N. Michigan Ave., Chicago, Ill. 60601.
Simple Machines, Britannica Films, Inc., 425 N. Michigan Ave., Chicago, Ill. 60601.
Laws of Motion, Britannica Films, Inc., 425 N. Michigan Ave., Chicago, Ill. 60601.
Mechanics of Human Motion-Pitching, University of Southern California, Los Angeles, Calif.
Posture & Exercise, Indiana University Motion Picture Division, Bloomington, Ind.
The Dentists Daily Seven, University of Southern California, Los Angeles, Calif.
Champions on Film, Indiana University Motion Picture Division, Bloomington, Ind.
How to Avoid Muscle Strains, Bray Studios, Inc., 729 Seventh Ave., New York, N.Y. 10019.

Muscular System, Gaumont-British Instructional Films, Ltd., London.

Human Body—Skeleton, Coronet Productions, 65 E. South Water Street, Chicago, Ill., 60606.

Functions of the Nervous System, Knowledge Builders, Visual-Education Center Bldg., Floral Park, N.Y., 11011.

Fundamentals of the Nervous System, Britannica Films, Inc., 425 N. Michigan Ave., Chicago, Ill. 60601.

Human Body—Circulatory System, Coronet Productions, 65 E. South Water Street, Chicago, Ill., 60606.

The Blood, Britannica Films, Inc., 425 N. Michigan Ave., Chicago, Ill. 60601.

Films on the following specific skills are available from Associated Films Inc., 600 Madison Ave., New York, N.Y. 10022, or 25358 Cypress St., Hayward, Calif. 94541.

Offensive Line Play	*Hurdles*
Defensive Line Play	*Broad Jump (Long Jump)*
Backfield Fundamentals	*Shot Put*
Weight Training I	*High Jump*
Weight Training II	*Discus*
Introduction to Wrestling	*Javelin*
Sprint Crawl (Swimming)	*Triple Jump*
Offensive Drills (Basketball with Bubas)	*Pole Vault*
Sprinting with Bud Winter	*Fiberglas Vaulting*

Appendix *B*
Glossary

Abduction: The movement of any body segment away from the midline of the body.

Acceleration: Rate of increase in velocity.

Actin: A muscle protein which, along with myosin, is responsible for muscle contraction and relaxation.

Adduction: The movement of body segments toward the midline of the body.

Aerobic: Occurring in the presence of oxygen. Aerobic processes occur with oxygen present.

Afferent nervous system: Also called sensory nervous system. The bodily system that directs impulses from sensory receptors toward the spinal cord and brain.

Agility: The ability to change directions of the body or its parts rapidly. Demonstrated in such movements as dodging, zigzagging, stopping, starting, and reversing direction of movement.

Agonist muscle: A muscle which contributes to the desired movement by its concentric contraction.

Alveoli: The tiny air sacs in the lungs where external respiration takes place.

Anaerobic: Occurring in the absence of oxygen. Anaerobic processes occur with no oxygen present.

Anatomical position: A stance in which the body is at "military attention" with the palms facing forward.

Antagonist muscle: A muscle which acts in opposition to the desired movement.

Anterior: Situated before or toward the front.

Appendicular skeleton: That portion of the skeleton comprising the upper and lower extremities.

Artery: A vessel that carries blood away from the heart.

Autonomic nervous system: The bodily system that is involuntary; it cannot be consciously controlled.

363

Axial skeleton: That portion of the skeleton comprising the head, neck, and trunk.

Axis: A fixed point around which a moving object revolves.

Axon: Appendage of the neuron that conducts impulses away from the cell body.

Capillary: The smallest of the blood vessels.

Capsular ligament: A ligament which completely surrounds and encloses a joint.

Cardiac output: Volume of blood pumped through the two ventricles in one minute.

Center of gravity: The point of intersection of the three primary planes of the body. The exact center of the body. The point around which the body would rotate freely in all directions if it were free to rotate.

Central nervous system (CNS): The bodily system that includes the brain and spinal cord.

Centrifugal force: The force that tends to keep a moving object in motion along a straight line. The force that provides resistance to turning movements.

Centripital force: The force that causes a moving object to turn. The force which opposes centrifugal force.

Circumduction: Movement in a circular, cone-shaped pattern.

Concentric contraction: Shortening of a muscle due to nervous impulses.

Conditioned reflex: A reflex pattern which is learned as opposed to being inborn.

Contractile force (muscle): The amount of tension applied by a muscle or group of muscles during contraction.

Coordination: The act of various muscles working together in a smooth concerted way. Correct and precise timing of muscle contractions.

Coronary system: The body system which includes the blood vessels that service the heart muscle.

Crest (bone): A ridgelike structure upon a bone.

Deceleration: Rate of decrease in velocity.

Dendrite: The appendage of a neuron which directs impulses toward the cell body.

Diastole: The relaxation phase of each heartbeat.

Diastolic pressure: The blood pressure during the relaxation of the ventricles.

Distal: Farthest from the body midline or point of reference. The hand is at the distal end of the arm.

Dorsiflexion: The act of cocking the foot; the act of bringing the top of the foot closer to the tibia.

Dynamic contraction: Same as isotonic or phasic contraction.

Dynamic posture: The posture or position of the body while in motion.

Eccentric contraction: Controlled lengthening of a muscle. The muscle becomes longer as it contracts because the resistance is greater than the contractile force.

Ectomorph: An individual who has a slight, or slender, body build.

Efferent system: The motor nervous system which directs impulses from the brain and spinal cord to muscles, glands, and organs.

Electrogoniometer: A device used to measure and record joint action.

Electromyograph: A device used to measure and record the changes in electrical potential of muscles during contraction.

Endomorph: An individual who has a fat or heavy body build.

End plate (motor): That portion of a motor neuron which attaches to a muscle fiber.

Endurance: Ability to resist fatigue and recover quickly after fatigue.

Epicondyle (bone): A projection on or above a condyle on a bone which is used for muscle attachment.

Eversion: The act of turning the sole of the foot outward.

Extension: Movement that increases the angle at a joint, thus straightening the joint.

Extensor thrust reflex: An involuntary act caused by pressure on the bottoms of the feet, resulting in a reflex contraction of extensor muscles.

External respiration: The exchange of gases at the alveoli in the lungs.

First-class lever: A lever arrangement with the fulcrum between the effort and the resistance (*EFR*).

Flexion: Movement that decreases the angle at a joint; the act of bending the joint.

Flexibility: That property of muscles and connective tissue which allows full range of motion.

Force: The strength or energy exerted to bring about motion or a change in motion.

Fossa: A depression in a bone.

Frontal plane: An imaginary plane which dissects the body into anterior and posterior halves.

Ganglion: A collection or bundle of nerve cell bodies outside the central nervous system.

Gray matter: That tissue in the central nervous system made up of nerve cell bodies.

Hamstring muscle group: Three muscles of the posterior thigh: biceps femoris, semimembranosus, and semitendinosus.

Horizontal extension: Extension of a body segment through the transverse (horizontal) plane.

Horizontal flexion: Flexion of a body segment through the transverse (horizontal) plane.

Hyperextension: Extension of a body segment past the anatomical position.

Hypertrophy: An increase in the overall size of a tissue.

Hyperventilation: The state caused by hard breathing in which too much air pressure results in dizziness and/or unconsciousness.

Inertia: A property of matter by which it remains at rest or in uniform motion in the same straight line unless acted upon by some external force.

Inferior portion: The portion of a body that is below, or deeper than, another structure or reference point.

Insertion (of a muscle):   Muscle attachment farthest from the midline of the body; the more movable attachment.

Internal respiration: The exchange of gases between the circulatory system and the tissues throughout the body.

Internuncial neuron: A neuron in the spinal cord that serves as a connection between motor and sensory neurons.

Inversion: The act of turning the sole of the foot inward.

Isometric contraction: A contraction in which muscle tension increases, but the muscle does not shorten because it does not overcome the resistance.

Isotonic contraction: A contraction in which muscle fibers shorten as a result of stimulus.

Kinesthetic sense: A sense of awareness, without the use of the other senses, of muscle and joint positions and actions.

Lateral flexion: Flexion of the trunk or neck sidewards: sideward bend.

Lateral rotation: Rotation of a body segment outwardly away from the midline of the body.

Lever (body):   A rigid bar comprised of one or more bones which revolves about a fulcrum (joint).

Ligament: Tough connective tissue which binds bones together, forming joints.

Locomotion: Movement of the body from one point to another by its own power.

Medial rotation: Rotation of a body segment inwardly, toward the midline of the body.

Mesomorph: An individual who has a husky or muscular body build or a medium-type body build.

Metabolism: The sum total of all the chemical processes of the body.

Minute volume (heart):   The volume of blood pumped through the left ventricle in one minute.

Momentum: The property of a moving body that determines the force required to bring the body to rest. Momentum = mass × velocity.

Motor unit: A group of muscle fibers dispersed throughout a muscle and supplied by a single motor nerve fiber.

Movement time: The amount of time that it takes to accomplish the movement after the impulse to respond has been received.

Multijoint muscle: A muscle that extends over two or more joints.

Muscle boundness: A pathological condition brought on by improper training in which the joints lose some of their range of motion due to hypertrophied muscles.

Muscle bundle: A group of 20 to 100 muscle fibers, lying parallel to each other and bound together by a connective tissue.

Myosin: A muscle protein which, along with actin, is responsible for muscle contraction and relaxation.

Nerve (nerve tract) : A cablelike bundle composed of many nerve fibers.

Neuromuscular coordination: Coordination which results from nerve impulses reaching the proper muscles, with sufficient intensity, at the correct time.

Neuromyal junction: The intersection between the motor end plate of a nerve branch and the muscle fiber.

Neuron: A complete nerve cell, including the cell body and all its appendages.

Neutralizer muscle: A muscle that acts to equalize the action of another muscle.

Origin (of a muscle) : The muscle attachment closer to the midline of the body; the less movable attachment.

Overload: The process of demanding more performance from a system than is ordinarily required.

Oxygen debt: A condition which results when the demand for oxygen is greater than the supply.

Peripheral nervous system: The body system which includes all those parts of the nervous system not included in the brain and spinal cord.

Plantar flexion: Also known as ankle extension. The act of moving the top of the foot away from the tibia.

Posterior portion: Rear or back portion.

Postural muscles: Also called antigravity muscles. The muscles used to maintain posture.

Power: The product of force × velocity. The ability to apply force at a rapid rate.

Prime mover muscle: A muscle which makes a primary contribution to the desired movement.

Process (of a bone) : A prominence or projection on a bone.

Progressive resistance training: A muscle-training program in which the amount of resistance is systematically increased as the muscles gain in strength.

Pronation: The act of turning the palms of the hands downward.

Proximal: Located toward the midline of the body or nearest the point of reference.

Quadriceps muscle group: Four muscles of the anterior thigh: rectus femoris, vastus lateralis, vastus medialis, and vastus intermedius.

Range of motion: The amount of movement that can occur in a joint, expressed in degrees.

Reaction time: That time between the reception of a signal to respond and the beginning of the response.

Reflex: An immediate response to a situation in which the thought process is bypassed.

Reflex time: Time of nerve impulse travel in a reflex action.

R.M. (repetition maximum): In weight training, the maximum number of repetitions that can be accomplished against a given amount of resistance.

Rotary motion (angular): The rotation of an object about an axis with each point of the object describing an arc or a circle around the axis.

Rotation: Movement of a body segment around its own longitudinal axis.

Sagittal plane: An imaginary plane which dissects the body into right and left halves.

Second-class lever: A lever arrangement with the resistance between the fulcrum and the effort (*FRE*).

Shoulder depression: Lowering of the shoulder girdle.

Shoulder elevation: Raising of the shoulder girdle.

Shoulder protraction: Broadening of the distance between the two shoulder joints.

Shoulder retraction: Narrowing of the distance between the two shoulder joints.

6-6-6: A technique in isometric weight training consisting of near-maximum contractions for six seconds and rest for six seconds, repeated six times.

Skeletal muscle: Also called striated, motor, and voluntary muscle. A muscle which attaches to and causes movement of the skeleton.

Skill: Neuromuscular coordination.

Smooth muscle: Also called visceral and involuntary muscle. A muscle located in the internal organs, with the exception of the heart.

Stability: Firmness in position. Ability to withstand external force.

Stabilizer muscle: Any muscle that acts to stabilize or fix a body segment in order for another segment to move on it.

Static contraction: Same as tonic or isometric contraction.

Static posture: The posture or position of the body while at rest.

Static work: The condition in which no movement occurs when muscular force is applied.

Steady state: A condition where the supply of oxygen to the tissues is equal to the demand for oxygen.

Strength: The ability to apply force with a segment of the body.

Stretch reflex: An automatic reflex to contract in skeletal muscles, brought on by sudden stretching of the muscles.

Stroke volume (heart): The volume of blood pumped out of the left ventricle with each contraction.

Summation wave: A sustained muscular contraction caused by rapid firing of nerve impulses.

Superior portion: A body portion that is above, or over, another body portion or reference point.

Supination: The act of turning the palms of the hands upward.

Synapse: The intersection (junction) between two or more nerve fibers.

Systole: The contracting phase of each heart beat.

Tendon: A tough fiberous tissue that connects muscles to bones.

10-3: A technique in weight training consisting of three sets of ten repetitions each, with a rest period between each set.

Third-class lever: A lever arrangement with the effort between the fulcrum and the resistance (*FER*).

Translatory motion: Motion in which an object moves fom one point to another point, as opposed to rotary motion. It can occur in either a linear or a curvilinear path.

Transverse plane: An imaginary plane which dissects the body into upper and lower halves.

Trochanter: A large projection or prominence upon a bone.

Tuberosity: A large rounded prominence upon a bone.

Turgor: The natural pressure from fluids inside a cell.

Vasomotor tone: The tone of the muscles that line the walls of the blood vessels.

Vein: A vessel that returns blood to the heart.

Velocity: The rate at which an object travels in a given direction.

Viscosity (blood): The "thickness" of a fluid; the resistance to flow.

Vital capacity: The total amount of air that can be forced out of the lungs after a forced inhalation.

Voluntary nervous system: That part of the nervous system which is consciously controlled.

White matter: That tissue in the central nervous system made up of nerve fibers, not nerve cell bodies.

Work: A condition occurring when muscles contract. If the muscle contractions cause movement, then the work is dynamic; if no movement occurs, the work is static.

References

1. ALLEY, LOUIS E.: An Analysis of Water Resistance and Propulsion in Swimming the Crawl Stroke, *Res. Quart.*, vol. 23, p. 253, 1952.
2. ARMBRUSTER, DAVID A., SR., ROBERT H. ALLEN, and BRUCE HARLAN: "Swimming and Diving," 3d ed., The C. V. Mosby Company, St. Louis, 1958.
3. BALLARD, S. S.: "Physics Principles," The Macmillan Company, New York, 1956.
4. BARNEY, V. S., and B. L. BANGERTER: Comparison of Three Programs of Progressive Resistance Exercise, *Res. Quart.*, vol. 32, pp. 138–146, 1961.
5. BARNEY, VERMON S., CYNTHA C. HIRST, and CLAYNE JENSEN: "Conditioning Exercises," The C. V. Mosby Company, St. Louis, 1965.
6. BASMAJIAN, J. V.: New Views of Muscular Tone and Relaxation, *Canad. M.A.J.*, vol. 77, p. 203, 1957.
7. BASMAJIAN, J. V.: "Muscles Alive," The Williams and Wilkins Company, Baltimore, 1962.
8. BERGER, R. A.: Optimum Repetitions for the Development of Strength, *Res. Quart.*, vol. 33, pp. 334–338, 1962.
9. BERGER, R. A.: Comparison of Static and Dynamic Strength Increases, *Res. Quart.*, vol. 33, pp. 329–333, 1962.
10. BROER, MARION R.: "The Efficiency of Human Movement," pp. 32–60, W. B. Saunders Company, Philadelphia, 1960.
11. BUNN, JOHN W.: "Scientific Principles of Coaching," pp. 3–12, 22–92, Prentice-Hall, Inc., Englewood Cliffs, N.J., 1955.
12. CAPEN, E. K.: Study of Four Programs of Heavy Resistance Exercises for Development of Muscular Strength, *Res. Quart.*, vol. 27, pp. 132–142, 1965.
13. CLARKE, H. HARRISON: "Muscular Strength and Endurance in Man," Prentice-Hall, Inc., Englewood Cliffs, N.J., 1966.
14. CLEVELAND, HENRY G.: "The Determination of the Center of Gravity in Segments of the Human Body," Thesis, University of California, 1955.
15. COLLINS, MURRAY ROLAND: Research on Sprint Running, *Athletic J.*, vol. 32, p. 30, 1952.
16. COLLINS, MURRAY ROLAND: "The Effect of Stride Length on Efficiency in Distance Running," Thesis, University of Southern California, 1951.

17. COLLINS, PATRICIA ANN: "Body Mechanics of the Overarm and Sidearm Patterns," Thesis, University of Wisconsin, 1960.

18. COOPER, JOHN M., and RUTH B. GLASSOW: "Kinesiology," 2d ed., The C. V. Mosby Company, St. Louis, 1968.

19. COUNSILMAN, JAMES E.: Forces in Two Types of Crawl Strokes, Res. Quart., vol. 26, p. 2, 1955.

20. DELLA, DAN G.: Individual Differences in Foot Leverage in Relation to Jumping Performance, Res. Quart., vol. 21, p. 11, 1950.

21. DELORME, THOMAS L., and A. L. WATKINS: Techniques of Progressive Resistance Exercise, Arch. Phys. Med. Rehabil., vol. 29, pp. 262–273, May, 1948.

22. DEVRIES, HERBERT A.: "Physiology of Exercise for Physical Education and Athletics," William C. Brown Co., Dubuque, Iowa, 1966.

23. DOHERTY, KENNETH: "Modern Track and Field," 2d ed., Prentice-Hall, Inc., Englewood Cliffs, N.J., 1963.

24. DYSON, GEOFFREY: "The Mechanics of Athletics," Dover Publications, Inc., New York, 1967.

25. FAY, TEMPLE: The Origin of Human Movement, Am. J. Psychiat., vol. 111, p. 644, 1955.

26. GOLLNICK, P. D., and P. V. KARPOVICH: Electrogonimetric Study of Locomotion and Some Athletic Movements, Report to U.S. Army Medical and Development Command, Office of Surgeon General, Washington, D.C., 1961.

27. GROVES, WILLIAM H.: Mechanical Analysis of Diving, Res. Quart., vol. 21, p. 132, 1950.

28. GUYTON, ARTHUR C.: "Function of the Human Body," 2d ed., W. B. Saunders Company, Philadelphia, 1965.

29. HAIRABEDIAN, ARA: "The Effect of a Weight Training Program on Speed of Running," Master's Thesis, Pennsylvania State University, University Park, 1952.

30. HART, IVOR: "The Mechanical Investigations of Leonardo da Vinci," Chapman & Hall, Ltd., London, 1935.

31. HELLEBRANDT, FRANCES A.: Gravitational Influences on Postural Alignment, Physiol. Rev., vol. 22, p. 149, 1942.

32. HELLEBRANDT, FRANCES A.: Physiological Analysis of Basic Motor Skills, Am. J. Phys. Med., vol. 40, p. 14, 1961.

33. HELLEBRANDT, FRANCES A., and ELIZABETH BROGDON FRANSEEN: Physiological Study of the Vertical Stance of Man, Physiol. Rev., vol. 23, p. 220, 1943.

34. HELLEBRANDT, FRANCES A., E. T. HELLEBRANDT, and CLARENCE WHITE: Methods of Recording Movement, Am. J. Phys. Med., vol. 39, p. 5, 1960.

35. HENRY, FRANKLIN M.: Dynamic Kinesthetic Perception and Adjustment, Res. Quart., vol. 24, p. 176, 1953.

36. HETTINGER, THEODOR: "Physiology of Strength," Charles C Thomas, Publisher, Springfield, Ill., 1961.

37. HILL, A. V.: The Design of Muscles, Brit. Med. Bull., vol. 12, pp. 165–166, 1956.

38. HILL, A. V.: The Mechanics of Voluntary Muscle, Lancet, vol. 261, pp. 947–951, 1951.

39. HILL, A. V.: "Muscular Movement in Man," McGraw-Hill Book Company, New York, 1927.

40. HIRT, SUSANNE: What Is Kinesiology?, *Phys. Therap. Rev.*, vol. 35, pp. 419–426, 1955.

41. HIRT, SUSANNE E., CORRINE FRIES, and FRANCES A. HELLEBRANDT: Center of Gravity of the Human Body, *Arch. Phys. Therap.*, vol. 25, p. 280, 1944.

42. HUBBARD, A. W.: Experimental Analysis of Running and of Certain Fundamental Differences between Trained and Untrained Runners, *Res. Quart.*, vol. 10, p. 28, 1939.

43. HUXLEY, H. E.: The Contraction of Muscle, *Sci. Am.*, vol. 199, p. 67, 1958.

44. JENSEN, CLAYNE R.: Coaching the Sprints, *Athletic J.*, March, 1958.

45. JENSEN, CLAYNE R.: Controversy over Warm-up in Athletic Performance, *Athletic J.*, December, 1966.

46. JENSEN, CLAYNE R.: Facts on Weight Training for Athletics, *Coach and Athlete*, January, 1963.

47. JENSEN, CLAYNE R.: The Significance of Strength in Athletic Performance, *Coach and Athlete*, January, 1966.

48. JENSEN, CLAYNE R.: Training for Hurdles, *Athletic J.*, January 1958.

49. JOHNSON, WARREN (ed.): "Science and Medicine of Exercise and Sports," Harper & Row, Publishers, Incorporated, New York, 1960.

50. JOSEPH, J.: "Man's Posture-electromyographic Studies," Charles C Thomas, Publisher, Springfield, Ill., 1960.

51. KARPOVICH, PETER: "Physiology of Muscular Activity," 5th ed., W. B. Saunders Company, Philadelphia, 1959.

52. LOKEN, NEWTON D., and ROBERT J. WILLOUGHBY: "Complete Book of Gymnastics," Prentice-Hall, Inc., Englewood Cliffs, N.J., 1959.

53. LOWMAN, C. L.: Faulty Posture in Relation to Performance, *J. Health Phys. Educ. Recreation*, vol. 29, p. 14, 1958.

54. MAUTNER, HERMAN E.: The Relationship of Function to the Microscopic Structure of Striated Muscle (review), *Arch. Phys. Med. Rehabil.*, vol. 37, p. 268, 1956.

55. METHENY, ELEANOR: "Body Dynamics," McGraw-Hill Book Company, New York, 1952.

56. MOREHOUSE, LAURENCE E., and AUGUSTUS T. MILLER: "Physiology of Exercise," 4th ed., pp. 30–42, 50–58, The C. V. Mosby Company, St. Louis, 1963.

57. MORTON, DUDLEY J., and DUDLEY DEAN FULLER: "Human Locomotion and Body Form," The Williams & Wilkins Company, Baltimore, 1952.

58. MUYBRIDGE, E.: "The Human Figure in Motion," Dover Publications, Inc., New York, 1955.

59. NEUBERGER, TOM (ed.): "Audiovisual Aids Used in the Teaching of Kinesiology," Unpublished Document, Eastern Michigan University, Ypsilanti, Mich.

60. PALMER, CARROLL E.: Studies of the Center of Gravity in the Human Body, *Child Develop.*, vol. 15, p. 99, 1944.

61. RASCH, PHILIP J., and ROGER K. BURKE: "Kinesiology and Applied Anatomy," 3d ed., Lea & Febiger, Philadelphia, 1967.

62. STILLWELL, G. KEITH: Physiology of Skeletal Muscular Contraction (review), *Arch. Phys. Med. Rehabil.*, vol. 38, p. 682, 1957.

63. THOMPSON, CLEM W.: "Kranz Manual of Kinesiology," 5th ed., The C. V. Mosby Company, St. Louis, 1965.

64. TRICKER, R. A. R., and B. J. K. TRICKER: "The Science of Movement," American Elsevier Publishing Company of New York, 1967.

65. TUTTLE, W. W., and BYRON A. SCHOTTELIUS: "Textbook of Physiology," 15th ed., pp. 136–241, 303–308, The C. V. Mosby Company, St. Louis, 1965.

66. WELLS, KATHERINE F.: "Kinesiology," 4th ed., W. B. Saunders Company, Philadelphia, 1966.

67. WELLS, KATHERINE F.: "What We Don't Know about Posture, *J. Health Phys. Educ. Recreation*, vol. 29, p. 31, 1958.

68. WILLIAMS, MARIAN, and H. R. LISSNER: "Biomechanics of Human Motion," W. B. Saunders Company, Philadelphia, 1962.

69. ZORBAS, WILLIAM S., and PETER V. KARPOVICH: The Effect of Weight Lifting upon the Speed of Muscular Contractions, *Res. Quart.*, vol. 22, pp. 145–148, May, 1951.

Index

This book was set in Bodoni Book by Monotype Composition Company, Inc., and printed on permanent paper and bound by The Maple Press Company. The designer was Paula E. Tuerk; the drawings were done by Russell Peterson. The editors were Nat LaMar and Timothy Yohn. Sally R. Ellyson supervised the production.

DATE DUE			
MAR 2 4 1997			